Recent Advances in Anesthesiology

Recent Advances in Anesthesiology

Edited by Tiffany Johnson

hayle medical

New York

Hayle Medical,
750 Third Avenue, 9th Floor,
New York, NY 10017, USA

Visit us on the World Wide Web at:
www.haylemedical.com

ISBN: 978-1-64647-551-3

Cataloging-in-Publication Data

Recent advances in anesthesiology / edited by Tiffany Johnson.
p. cm.
Includes bibliographical references and index.
ISBN 978-1-64647-551-3
1. Anesthesiology. 2. Anesthesia. 3. Surgery. I. Johnson, Tiffany.
RD81 .R43 2023
617.96--dc23

Table of Contents

Preface

The area of medicine which specializes in the management of pain during the perioperative period is known as anesthesiology. It includes the use of various inhaled and injected medications to cause the loss of sensations in patients, for carrying out those procedures that would otherwise cause unbearable pain. Modern anesthesiology also includes providing pre-hospital emergency medicine, running intensive care units, and transportation of critically ill patients. It is also used in prehabilitation programs to ensure the successful surgery of patients. Anesthesiology procedures require knowledge of various areas including the pharmacology of inhalational anesthetics, topical anesthetics and vasopressors. It also involves electrocardiography, electroencephalography and electromyography. The topics included in this book on anesthesiology are of utmost significance and bound to provide incredible insights to readers. It strives to provide a fair idea about this discipline and to help develop a better understanding of the latest advances within this field. This book will provide comprehensive knowledge to the readers.

Significant researches are present in this book. Intensive efforts have been employed by authors to make this book an outstanding discourse. This book contains the enlightening chapters which have been written on the basis of significant researches done by the experts.

Finally, I would also like to thank all the members involved in this book for being a team and meeting all the deadlines for the submission of their respective works. I would also like to thank my friends and family for being supportive in my efforts.

Editor

1

Intraoperative management of brain-dead organ donors by anesthesiologists during an organ procurement procedure: Results from a French survey

Benoit Champigneulle[1,2], Arthur Neuschwander[1], Régis Bronchard[3], Gersende Favé[1,4], Julien Josserand[1], Benjamin Lebas[5], Olivier Bastien[3], Romain Pirracchio[1,4,6*] and in collaboration with the SFAR research network

Abstract

Background: This study aimed at describing usual anesthetic practices for brain-dead donors (BDD) during an organ procurement (OP) procedure and to assess the knowledge and self-confidence of French anesthesiologists with this practice.

Methods: An electronic and anonymous survey with closed-questions about anesthetic management of BDD was distributed to French anesthesiologists via the mailing list of the French Society of Anesthesiology and Intensive Care Medicine.

Results: Four hundred fifty-eight responses were analyzed. Respondents were mainly attending physicians with more than 10 years of clinical experience. 78% of them declared being cognizant of guidelines regarding management of BDD. Advanced hemodynamic monitoring and endocrine substitution were rarely considered by respondents (31 and 35% of respondents, respectively). 98% of the respondents used crystalloids for fluid resuscitation. During the procedure, use of neuromuscular blockers, opioids and sedative agents were considered by respectively 84, 61 and 27% of the respondents. A very high level of agreement (10 [8–10], on a ten-points Likert-style scale) was reported concerning the expected impact of intraoperative anesthetic management on the primary function of grafts.

Conclusions: Declared anesthetic practice appeared in accordance with guidelines concerning organ donor management in the ICU. Further studies are needed to evaluate the specific impact of intraoperative management during this procedure and thus the need for specific anesthetic guidelines.

Keywords: Anesthesia, Brain-dead donors, Organ procurement, Survey

Background

Brain-dead donors (BDD) currently remain the primary source of grafts for solid organ transplantation across the world [1, 2]. In this context, appropriate management of organ donors from the diagnosis of brain death to the end of the organ procurement (OP) procedure is of paramount importance to optimize the function of potential grafts. Intensive care (ICU) management of BDD is well-codified. This is an active research field [3] and many guidelines were published and regularly updated over the last years [4–7]. Conversely, intraoperative and anesthetic management of the donor during the OP procedure is far less codified [2, 8]. French guidelines mainly specify to follow the same organ resuscitation strategy initiated in the ICU and only specify that the use of neuromuscular blocking (NMB) agents and analgesics are justified [5]. Because of the lack of specific recommendations on the intraoperative and anesthetic management of OP procedure, we hypothesize that the practices are disparate.

* Correspondence: romain.pirracchio@aphp.fr
[1]Anesthesiology and Intensive Care Department, European Hospital Georges-Pompidou, Assistance Publique - Hôpitaux de Paris (AP-HP), 20 rue Leblanc, 75015 Paris, France
[4]Paris Descartes University, Sorbonne Paris Cité, Paris, France

In this context, we performed a French national survey on intraoperative management of BDD by anesthesiologists. The aims of the study were i) to describe intraoperative anesthetic practices for BDD during an OP procedure; and ii) to evaluate the knowledge of French anesthesiologists on this specific practice.

Methods

Questionnaire

We conducted a French national survey on intraoperative anesthetic management of BDD during the OP procedure. The questionnaire included 33 closed-questions and one open-ended question (see the Additional file 1). The questionnaire was anonymous and subdivided into seven sections taking into account the domains covered by the guidelines [4–7]: general and demographic data, peroperative monitoring, hemodynamic management, metabolic management, respiratory management, anesthetic drugs employment and personal feeling about the procedure. Intraoperative use of donor management goals (DMGs) was also evaluated. For questions on standard practice, a five-point Likert-style scale was provided (ranging from *never* to *always*); for questions covering provider's perception of the OP procedure, a ten-point Likert-style scale ranging from 1 (*certainly not agree*) to 10 (*absolutely agree*) was used. Before broadcasting, the questionnaire was tested and approved by the anesthesiologists of our tertiary teaching hospital (European Georges Pompidou hospital, AP-HP, Paris, France).

According to the French law, no ethic committee approval was required for this anonymous survey intended to health professionals.

Survey processing

The questionnaire was meant to target all French anesthesiologists. Expected time to complete the questionnaire was less than 10 min. An electronic form of the survey was compiled using SurveyMonkey® (https://www.surveymonkey.com). In early September 2017, French anesthesiologists were invited to answer the survey via an email, sent through the mailing-list of the French Society of Anesthesia and Intensive Care (*Société Française d'Anesthésie-Réanimation*, SFAR). The survey was available *on-line* during a 4-month period (until end of December 2017). A follow-up email was sent 2 months after the first e-mail, in November 2017.

French local organization for organ procurement

In France, OP from BDD is only performed in hospitals accredited by the French Biomedicine Agency which is the only state agency that regulates and organizes OP and transplantation in France. In 2017, 182 medical centers were accredited in France for OP from BDD. In each center, a dedicated local team (including specialized nurses) is involved from the identification of the potential BDD in the ICU to the admission of the deceased person in the mortuary room. Local OP teams are not directly involved in the medical management of the BDD in the ICU or in the OR which remains under the purview of the attending physician. National French guidelines regarding BDD management were updated in 2005 by the French society of anesthesia and intensive care medicine and the Biomedicine Agency [5]. Authorized centers are incited to develop local procedures based on guidelines.

Data analysis

Results are reported as count (%) for categorical variables and median (25th–75th percentiles) for continuous variables. For questions pertaining to practice, in order to simplify the interpretation of the results, the answers "never" and "seldom" were grouped, as well as the answers "always", "often" and "regularly". Reported responses were compared between more junior respondents (including residents and doctors with less than 10 years of clinical experience) and more senior respondents (doctors with more than 10 years of clinical experience). The Pearson chi-square test was used to compare categorial variables. Analyses were performed using Microsoft® Excel software (2017) and SPSS software version 20 (SPSS, Chicago, IL, USA). All tests were 2-sided with $p < 0.05$ considered to define statistical significance.

Results

Respondent characteristics

Four hundred and fifty-eight anesthesiologists answered the survey during the study period. General characteristics of the respondents are described in Table 1. Among the respondents, 359 (78%) declared having knowledge on ICU BDD management guidelines; less junior respondents claimed being cognizant of these recommendations than senior respondents: 72% vs. 86% ($p < 0.001$) (Additional file 1: Table S1).

Per-operative monitoring

Almost all respondents (98%) declared always using the standard intraoperative monitoring equipment required by the SFAR (i.e., electrocardiogram, blood pressure, SpO_2 and end-tidal CO_2) during the OP procedure. Detailed answers concerning other optional monitoring are presented in the Fig. 1. Invasive blood pressure and invasive temperature monitoring were reported to be frequent (97 and 89%, respectively). Blood lactate or hemoglobin monitoring during the procedure is less frequent (50 and 74%, respectively). Most of the respondents (69%) did not report the use of advanced hemodynamic monitoring in this context. When an advanced hemodynamic monitoring

Table 1 Characteristics of the respondents

	Respondents (n = 458)
Type of institution	
University hospital	267 (58%)
Non-university hospital	191 (42%)
Function of the respondent	
Resident	48 (10%)
Fellow	53 (12%)
Attending physician	335 (73%)
Professor	22 (5%)
Field of activity[a]	
Full-time anaesthesiology	188 (46%)
Full-time ICU	42 (10%)
Shared activity (both anaesthesiology and ICU)	180 (44%)
Professional experience > 10 years[a]	209 (51%)
Numbers of OP procedures occurred last year per establishment	
< 5 procedures	55 (12%)
5–10 procedures	95 (21%)
10–20 procedures	132 (29%)
> 20 procedures	176 (38%)
Numbers of BDD personally managed in the OR by respondent during last year	
None	71 (16%)
1–4	307 (67%)
≥ 5	80 (17%)
Existence of a written protocol for anaesthetic management of BDD	197 (76%)

Data are expressed as n (%)
[a]Excluding residents
ICU intensive care unit, *BDD* brain dead donor, *OP* organ procurement, *OR* operating room

is used, pulse pressure analysis seems to be the most commonly used device in this setting (63%).

Donor management during organ procurement

DMGs: 358 (78%) respondents reported to use pre-specified DMGs during the OP procedure, without significant difference according to the level of seniority (Additional file 1: Table S1). This included: targeted mean arterial pressure range of 60–70 mmHg for 305 (67%) respondents and temperature > 35 °C for 96% of the respondents.

Hemodynamic management (Additional file 1: Figure S1) presents the distribution of the answers concerning intraoperative fluid management. Briefly, 95% of the responding anesthesiologists did not used starches for fluid resuscitation and 98% of them reported using crystalloids in this context. The most frequently used crystalloids were ringer lactate (45%) and 0.9% saline (38%). A hemoglobin threshold of 7 $g.dL^{-1}$ was considered for transfusion by 298 (65%) respondents whereas 21 (5%) of them considered that blood transfusion was not indicated in this setting.

Pulmonary management: most anesthesiologists (93%) reported implementing a protective ventilation strategy in the OR and 92% of them declared realizing recruitment maneuvers during the procedure (routinely in 55% of cases). More junior respondents appeared to implement more often a protective ventilation than the senior respondents (Additional file 1: Table S1).

Endocrine substitution: during the OP procedure, hormonal resuscitation was not considered by 65% of the respondents, without significant difference between respondents (Additional file 1: Table S1). When hormonal replacement therapy was considered, hormone substitution protocol varied substantially across practitioners except for triiodothyronine that was not used by 93% of the respondents (Additional file 1: Figure S2).

Anesthetic management during organ procurement

Responses concerning anesthetic drugs utilization are reported in the Fig. 2. Use of NMB, opioids and sedative agents was considered by respectively 84, 61 and 27% of the respondents. Among anesthesiologists who declared using a sedative agent for the procedure, the most popular agents were volatile anesthetics (65%). For 76% of the respondents, administration of unfractionned heparin is only done when asked by surgeons or the OP coordinator.

Provider's perceptions

Provider's perception concerning the anesthetic management of BDD was evaluated using a numeric scale ranging from 1 to 10. The presence of an attending anesthesiologist in the OR during the procedure was deemed necessary with an agreement of 8 (7–10). The question of feeling enough prepared for OP procedure was rated with a score of 6 (5–8). Consistently, responding anesthesiologists considered that further specific recommendations on anesthetic management of BDD would be useful (score of agreement: 9 (8–10)). A very high level of agreement (10 (8–10)) was also reported concerning the expected impact of intraoperative anesthetic management on the primary function of grafts.

Discussion

Our study aimed at describing current practices and perceptions of a large panel of anesthesiologists on the intraoperative management of BDD. The few existing recommendations on the subject are essentially based on expert opinions or extrapolated from ICU guidelines for BDD management [1, 2]. Briefly, our survey suggests that anesthetic practices concerning monitoring, DMGs, fluid resuscitation and ventilatory management are in agreement with the current ICU guidelines

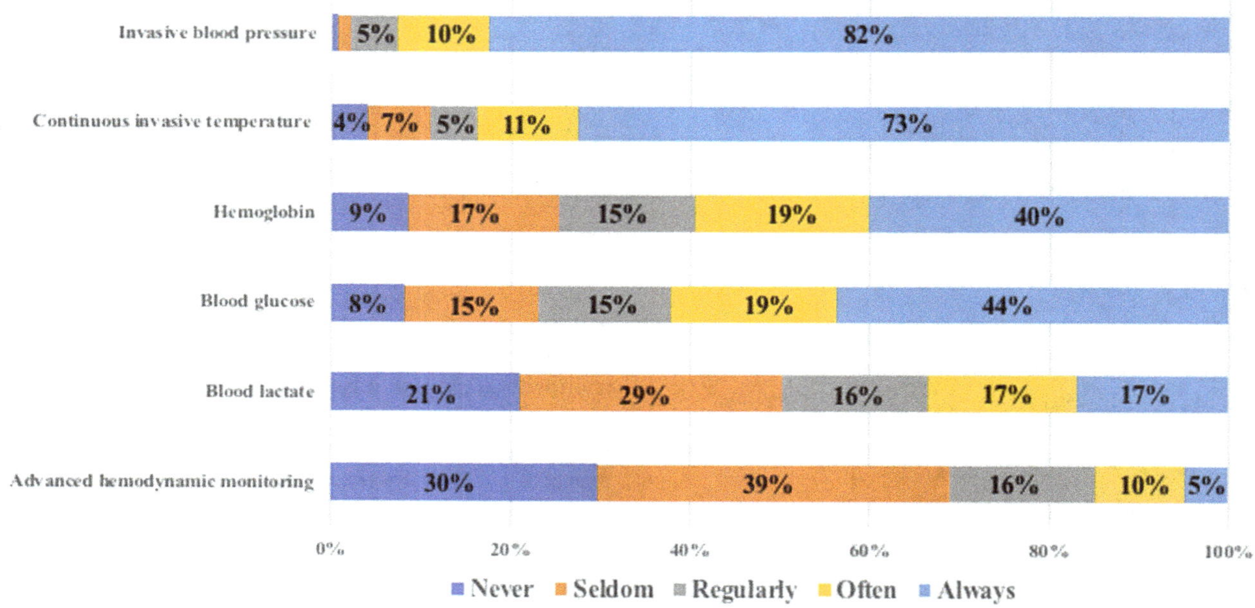

Fig. 1 Detailed answers concerning the use of complementary monitoring during the organ procurement procedure

despite significant difference between the respondents according to their level of seniority [4–7]. Particularly, more senior anesthesiologists were more likely to report knowledge of the current ICU guidelines. Conversely, more junior doctors appeared more likely to use a protective ventilation strategy, maybe because younger anesthesiologists were more trained in the era of lung-protective ventilation [9].

In the absence of specific anesthetic guidelines, maintaining the same level of care implemented in ICU is fundamental, as raised in a recent review [2]. Recent findings concerning the use of mild hypothermia (34–35 °C) to improve renal grafts recovery does not seem to be integrated into current practices [3]. The low reported use of hormone substitution may be surprising. However, this is in agreement with the French guidelines which do not

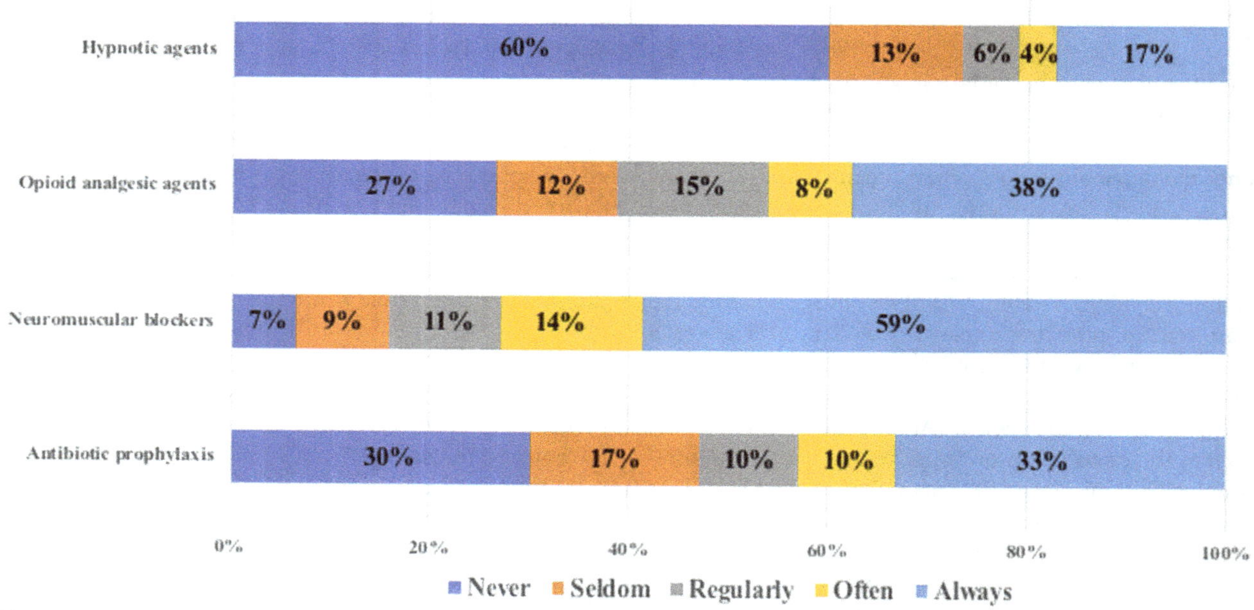

Fig. 2 Declared practices concerning anesthetic drugs utilization during the organ procurement procedure

support systematic endocrine substitution (except for vasopressin analogs in case of diabetes insipidus) [5]. This point differs with north-American guidelines [6, 7]. However, the level of evidence concerning the benefit of hormonal substitution (such as corticosteroids supplementation) remains relatively limited in this context [10]. The use of an advanced hemodynamic monitoring during the OP procedure did not seem to be a part of standard practices for a majority of the respondents in our survey. To our knowledge, there is no published data concerning the best device for hemodynamic assessment in this context. If pulse pressure variations could be use in the setting of brain death to guide fluid therapy [11], a recent randomized study failed to demonstrate any benefit (in terms of number of organs transplanted) of using a protocolized fluid therapy based on pulse-pressure variation and cardiac index [12].

The use of anesthetic drugs during the OP procedure remains a matter of debate [13]. In the context of brain death, the goal of anesthetic medications is essentially to control any possible hemodynamic and/or motor response resulting from spinal cord reflexes, thereby justifying the use of neuromuscular blocking and analgesic agents during the OP procedure [5]. Opioids alone may be insufficient to control catecholamine release induced by surgical stimulation [14]. The use of volatile anesthetic, as "vasodilator agents", may thus be justified [2, 8]. In addition, a potential beneficial effect of volatile anesthetic agents on ischemia-reperfusion injuries has been suggested and could further justify their use in this context [2, 4, 8]. However, the level of scientific evidence remains relatively limited and further investigations are needed.

Finally, the most interesting finding of our study may be the high perceived impact of intraoperative management on the primary function of the grafts. Consistently the responders reported having high expectations from the scientific societies to produce specific guidelines on anesthetic management for BDD. Further research in the area is needed to give consistency to future evidence-based guidelines.

This declarative study carries some limitations. The survey was sent to an unselected panel of French anesthesiologists, members of the French Society of Anesthesia and Intensive Care Medicine. Although this panel is supposed to be representative of the overall population of practicing anesthesiologists, we cannot rule out some degree of responder bias and thus the results may not be fully representative of the actual current practices. Furthermore, our results might not reflect the practices outside France, especially since there are some known discrepancies between current national guidelines concerning BDD management [5–7].

Conclusions

Declared anesthetic practices concerning intraoperative management of BDD during organ procurement procedures are in accordance with national French guidelines on organ donor management. Further studies are needed to investigate this specific area of donor management, to evaluate the potential impact of specific interventions (such as the use of anesthetic agents, hormone substitution or meeting intraoperative specific donor management goals...) on the graft function after transplantation and to build future high-quality anesthetic guidelines on intraoperative management of BDD.

Abbreviations

AP-HP: Assistance Publique - Hôpitaux de Paris; BDD: Brain-dead donors; DMGs: Donor management goals; ICU: Intensive Care Unit; NMB: Neuromuscular blocking; OP: Organ procurement; OR: Operating room; SFAR: French Society of Anesthesia and Intensive Care (*Société Française d'Anesthésie-Réanimation*)

Acknowledgements

Not applicable.

Authors' contributions

BC, RP, AN, GF and JJ designed the study, collected, analyzed, and interpreted the data, and wrote the manuscript. RB, BL and OB contributed to design the study and to review the manuscript. BC and RP performed the statistical analysis. BC takes the full responsibility for the integrity of the work. All authors read and approved the final version of the manuscript.

Author details

[1]Anesthesiology and Intensive Care Department, European Hospital Georges-Pompidou, Assistance Publique - Hôpitaux de Paris (AP-HP), 20 rue Leblanc, 75015 Paris, France. [2]West francilian network for organ and tissue procurement, Paris, France. [3]Agence de la Biomédecine, Direction Prélèvement Greffe Organes-Tissus, Saint-Denis La Plaine, France. [4]Paris Descartes University, Sorbonne Paris Cité, Paris France. [5]Anesthesiology and Intensive Care Department, Hautepierre Hospital, Strasbourg, France. [6]Département de biostatistiques et d'informatique médicale, INSERM U-1153, Équipe ECSTRA, Université Paris Diderot; Hôpital Saint-Louis, AP-HP, Paris, France.

References

1. Anderson TA, Bekker P, Vagefi PA. Anesthetic considerations in organ procurment surgery: a narrative review. Can J Anesth. 2015;62:529–39.
2. Souter MJ, Eidbo E, Findlay JY, Lebovitz DJ, Moguilevitch M, Neidlinger NA, et al. Organ donor management: part 1. Toward a consensus to guide anesthesia services during donation after brain death. Semin Cardiothorac Vasc Anesth. 2017;22:211–22.
3. Niemann CU, Feiner J, Swain S, Bunting S, Friedman M, Crutchfield M, et al. Therapeutic hypothermia in deceased organ donors and kidney-graft function. N Engl J Med. 2015 373:405–14.
4. McKeown DW, Bonser RS, Kellum JA. Management of the heartbeating brain-dead organ donor. Br J Anaesth. 2012;108(Suppl 1):i96–107.
5. Boulard G, Guiot P, Pottecher T, Tenaillon A. Management of subjects in a state of brain death and the preservation of organs. Ann Fr Anesth Reanim. 2005;24:836–43.
6. Kotloff RM, Blosser S, Fulda GJ, Malinoski D, Ahya VN, Angel L, et al. Management of the Potential Organ Donor in the ICU. Crit Care Med. 2015; 43:1291–325.
7. Shemie SD, Ross H, Pagliarello J, Baker AJ, Greig PD, Brand T, et al. Organ donor management in Canada: recommendations of the forum on medical management to optimize donor organ potential. CMAJ. 2006;174:S13–32.
8. Elkins LJ. Inhalational anesthesia for organ procurement: potential indications for administering inhalational anesthesia in the brain-dead organ donor. AANA J. 2010;78:293–9.

9. Kim SH, Na S, Lee WK, Choi H, Kim J. Application of intraoperative lung-protective ventilation varies in accordance with the knowledge of anaesthesiologists: a single-Centre questionnaire study and a retrospective observational study. BMC Anesthesiol. 2018;18:33.
10. Dupuis S, Amiel JA, Desgroseilliers M, Williamson DR, Thiboutot Z, Serri K, et al. Corticosteroids in the management of brain-dead potential organ donors: a systematic review. Br J Anaesth. 2014;113:346–59.
11. Cinotti R, Roquilly A, Mahé P-J, Feuillet F, Yehia A, Belliard G, et al. Pulse pressure variations to guide fluid therapy in donors: a multicentric echocardiographic observational study. J Crit Care. 2014;29:489–94.
12. Al-Khafaji A, Elder M, Lebovitz DJ, Murugan R, Souter M, Stuart S, et al. Protocolized fluid therapy in brain-dead donors: the multicenter randomized MOnIToR trial. Intensive Care Med. 2015;41:418–26.
13. Young PJ, Matta BF. Anaesthesia for organ donation in the brainstem dead--why bother? Anaesthesia. 2000;55:105–6.
14. Fitzgerald RD, Hieber C, Schweitzer E, Luo A, Oczenski W, Lackner FX. Intraoperative catecholamine release in brain-dead organ donors is not suppressed by administration of fentanyl. Eur J Anaesthesiol. 2005;20:952–6.

2

Interprofessional two-man team approach for interhospital transport of ARDS-patients under extracorporeal membrane oxygenation: A 10 years retrospective observational cohort study

Stefan Felix Ehrentraut, Barbara Schroll, Stefan Lenkeit, Heidi Ehrentraut, Christian Bode, Stefan Kreyer, Florian Kögl, Felix Lehmann, Thomas Muders, Martin Scholz, Claudia Strater, Folkert Steinhagen, Nils Ulrich Theuerkauf, Carsten Weißbrich, Christian Putensen and Jens-Christian Schewe*

Abstract

Background: Extra Corporeal Membrane Oxygenation (ECMO) has become an accepted treatment option for severely ill patients. Due to a limited availability of ECMO support therapy, patients must often be transported to a specialised centre before or after cannulation. According to the ELSO guidelines, an ECMO specialist should be present for such interventions. Here we describe the safety and efficacy of a reduced team approach involving one anaesthesiologist, experienced in specialised intensive care medicine, and a specialised critical care nurse.

Methods: This study is a 10 years retrospective, single institution analysis of all data collected between January 2007 and December 2016 from the medical records at the University Hospital Bonn, Germany.

Results: The Bonner mobile ECMO team was deployed in 170 cases for on-site evaluation for ECMO support therapy. 4 (2.4%) patients died prior to arrival or during the implementation of ECMO support. Of the remaining 166 patients, 126 were cannulated at the referring site, 40 were transported without ECMO. Of those, 21 were subsequently cannulated out our centre. 19 patients never received ECMO treatment. The primary indication for ECMO treatment was ARDS (159/166 patients). Veno-venous ECMO was initiated in 137, whilst 10 patients received veno-arterial ECMO treatment. Mean transportation time was 75 ± 36 min, and mean transport distance was 56 ± 57 km. In total, 26 complications were observed, three being directly transport-related. The overall survival was 55%.

Conclusions: Initiation of extracorporeal membrane oxygenation and subsequent transport can be safely and efficiently performed by a two-man team with good outcome.

Keywords: ECMO, Interfacility transport, ARDS, Transport safety, Transport efficiency

* Correspondence: jens-christian.schewe@ukbonn.de
Department of Anaesthesiology and Intensive Care Medicine, University Hospital Bonn, Sigmund-Freud-Str. 25, 53105 Bonn, Germany

Background

Patients affected by acute respiratory distress syndrome (ARDS) may require the use of extracorporeal membrane oxygenation (ECMO) as an emergency life-saving therapy [1]. Despite its widespread use, the availability of this ECMO is still restricted to specialised centres. Due to this limited availability, either transport of critical ill patients to the ECMO centre prior to cannulation or retrieval under ECMO support is necessary. Transport of critically ill patients holds its own risks [2, 3], but is often necessary due to rapid clinical deterioration of the patient and non-availability of other treatment options at the referring hospital. To enable a safe transport of patients, a specialised ECMO-retrieval program is crucial. Currently there are very few studies available reporting large numbers of interfacility transports on ECMO support. These have been performed at only a few programs with a great variability of team composition [4–6]. According to the Extracorporeal Life Support Organization (ELSO) General Guidelines, transport teams comprise of a cannulating physician, ECMO physician, ECMO specialist, transport nurse, and transport respiratory therapist [7]. However, there are no national standards for the exact composition of ECMO transport teams for primary transports, i.e. initiation of ECMO at the referring site and subsequent transport to the dedicated ECMO centre.

This paper aims to describe the safety and efficacy of a reduced team approach for performing primary transports of ECMO patients over a ten-year time frame.

Methods

Data from our hospital (University Hospital Bonn, tertiary German ECMO centre) were retrospectively analysed regarding ECMO indication, transport mode, duration and distance.

Type of study: retrospective cohort study. For further study details and study limitations we followed the "Strengthening The Reporting of Observational Studies in Epidemiology-STROBE" criteria [8]. The STROBE checklist for cohort studies is included in the ("Additional file 1").

Cohort of interest: All patients undergoing evaluation for ECMO initiation and primary ECMO transport by our ECMO retrieval team.

The Respiratory ECMO survival prediction (RESP) score [9] and survival after veno-arterial ECMO (SAVE) [10] score were calculated retrospectively, using all available information from our records. Where no information was available, the best option was used (e.g. no bicarbonate infusion prior to ECMO, no Nitric oxide prior to ECMO).

Data for 10 consecutive years (January 2007 – December 2016) are presented. Statistical and graphical data handling was performed using GraphPad Prism 5.0d (GraphPad Software) and Microsoft Excel for Mac 2011.

Student's paired t-test was used for statistical comparison of groups where applicable (on site pre/post initiation data: Horovitz-Index, pH, blood gas parameters, lactate; Fig. 4 a-d). All numerical data are given as mean ± standard deviation of the mean, whereas non-normal distributed data are expressed as median and interquartile range (IQR).

For comparison of observed mortality rates with the predicted mortality rates using RESP/SAVE scores, we used the Standardized Mortality Ratio (SMR) [11, 12]. The 95% confidence interval (CI) for the predicted mortality and the calculated CI in our cohort was used. A statistical significance ($p < 0.05$) is given, if the observed mortality does not fall into the 95% CI of the predicted mortality.

Disease severity – ICU scoring

24 h post admission to our hospital, standard disease severity classification systems were used to calculate each patient's *Sequential Organ Failure Assessment* (SOFA) score [13], *Simplified Acute Physiology Score (*SAPS) II [14], *and Acute Physiology And Chronic Health Evaluation* (APACHE) II score [15]. Nursing workload was assessed using the *Therapeutic Intervention Scoring System* (TISS-28) [16] and lung injury was scored using Ramsay's Lung Injury score [17].

ECMO referral standards

In compliance with the ELSO General Guidelines, veno-venous-(VV) ECMO support was indicated in all patients with conventional mechanical ventilation, as a rescue therapy to treat hypoxaemia and hypercapnia. All decisions for implantation were made following consensus between two experienced members of the ECMO team. In patients with refractory cardiogenic shock, a veno-arterial-(VA) ECMO support was established. Refractory cardiogenic shock was defined as an acute or acute on chronic heart failure with hypotension (systolic blood pressure ≤ 90 mmHg) unresponsive to fluid rescucitation requiring increasing inotropic therapy or physiologic evidence of visceral hypoperfusion. The decision regarding the mode of ECMO support and its implementation technique was left to discretion of the ECMO physician on site.

Choice of ECMO type

Depending on the underlying type of organ failure, either VV-ECMO or VA-ECMO support was implemented.

VV-ECMO support was performed by inserting either two or three cannulas, usually into both femoral veins (17–24 Ch.) and/or the right jugular vein (15–21 Ch.) after ultrasound guided percutaneous blood vessel puncture. Patients with refractory cardiogenic shock received peripheral VA-ECMO treatment through percutaneous cannulation, usually via the femoral artery/vein.

ECMO transport team

The Bonner ECMO team is comprised of 9 ECMO physicians (senior anaesthesiologist and critical care specialists) and 9 ECMO nurse specialists. All team members have long-term experience in intensive care medicine and a minimum of three years experience in the treatment of ARDS and ECMO patients, as well as the general transport of critical ill patients. This staffing allows a 24/7, 365 day availability for ECMO implantation and retrieval at external sites via an organised on call-service.

The retrieval team consists of one ECMO physician and one ECMO nurse specialist who, upon arrival at the referring hospital, re-evaluate the patient on-site and decide whether initiation of ECMO is necessary. Then, the decision regarding what type of ECMO support and what cannulation approach (VV/VA) is needed. The team performs all steps of the cannulation itself.

Following cannulation and stabilisation, a timely departure and safe transport to the University Hospital Bonn is vital.

Transport organization and logistics

To maximize patient and team safety throughout the whole high risk process of initiating ECMO therapy at an external site and the subsequent intensive care transportation of the critically ill patient, standardised checklists (Additional file 1) and operating procedures are used at all stages. Besides the fixed interdisciplinary structure of the two-man ECMO team, a regular cooperation with the Emergency Medical Service of the city of Bonn and the regional air rescue service has been established. This optimizes interactions and reduces risks concerning qualification of personnel and equipment issues. A structured debriefing structure, involving the retrieval team, is used to share important information, new insights and difficulties experienced during missions to the whole team and the involved rescue services. In combination with repetitive ECMO team trainings and team meetings, the intended crew resource management approach is reached.

External hospitals can call for support via an implemented ARDS-Hotline with around-the-clock operation. The call is received by the senior ECMO specialist on call using a standardised query protocol to collect all necessary data in consultation with the referring hospital's attending physician. Following first contact, a brief discussion between a minimum of two senior intensive care physicians from the ECMO centre takes place. In case of intention to treat with ECMO, the retrieval team is activated and the referring hospital is informed. Information about the estimated time of arrival, needful preparations in advance (e.g. Red Blood Cell (RBC) supply, informing next-of-kin/legal guardian) and potential optimizations of therapy (e.g. optimisation of ventilator settings, prone position, fluid management) is given. Availability of ultrasound and/or on site radiologist is requested. The response time for activating the ECMO -Team and the required airborne and/or ground-based transport vehicles is 30 to 90 min following a standard operating procedure, depending on the time of the day and availability of personnel on duty.

ECMO team equipment

For prompt departure and minimal time of preparation, all necessary equipment is prepacked in transport bags, sealed and stored on ICU. For safety reasons, certain equipment (e.g. cannulas, ECMO circuit) are packed in duplicate. This redundancy allows safe operation and potential re-initiation of ECMO in case of adverse events. The ECMO circuit is primed on site by the ECMO team in the referring hospital, after the final on-site decision for ECMO support is made.

During the study period, CentriMag consoles and centrifugal pumps (Levitronix, Zurich, Switzerland) were used in combination with ELS and PLS Oxygenators and tubing (Maquet Getinge Group, Rastatt, Germany) until February 2011. Since 2012, transports are carried out with the Cardiohelp System and HLS Set Advanced (Maquet Getinge Group, Rastatt, Germany). For peripheral VV or VA cannulation Fem-Flex II single-lumen cannulas (Edwards Lifescience Nordic AB, Malmö, Sweden) and Maquet HLS single-lumen cannulas were used. For ventilation during transport Oxylog 3000 or 3000plus (Drägerwerk AG&Co, Lübeck, Germany) were utilised. In the case of airborne transport Hamilton T1 (Hamilton Medical, Bonaduz, Switzerland) respirators were used. Except for a few long-term transports no blood gas analyses were assessed during the transport phase due to unavailability during transport. No heater units were used during transport, but efficient conventional measures to avoid accidental cooling were taken. Vital signs were monitored using Propaq encore (WelchAllyn Inc., Skaneateles Falls, NY, USA), Corpuls3 (GS Elektromedizinische Geräte GmbH, Kaufering, Germany) and X-Series CCT (Zoll Medical Corporation, Chelmsford, MA, USA) monitors, measuring con tinuously and standardised ECG, invasive blood pressure, $etCO_2$, SpO_2 and optional parameters as needed. For ground based transport the patient was placed on a Performance Pro XT or Power Pro XT stretcher (Stryker Corporation, Kalamazoo, MI, USA) especially modified for intensive care transportation. Until 2013 a modified equipment platform was used to mount the Levitronix, and later the Cardiohelp, console to fit different types of stretcher systems used in airborne transport. Since then the certified mobile transport carrier by Maquet is used in ground based and airborne transport.

Results

During the ten years observation period, the Bonner ECMO team was deployed 170 times. The overall number of requests from other hospitals was not consistently recorded and thus cannot be reported in sufficient detail. Three patients died prior to arrival of the mobile ECMO team (Fig. 1). 167 severely ill patients underwent ECMO evaluation on site (Fig. 1). Of these patients, 126 (75,9%) received ECMO at the referring hospital and were transported under ECMO therapy. One patient died during ECMO cannulation. 30 (18,1%) patients were transported by the ECMO team without ECMO implantation. Upon arrival at our centre, 21 patients subsequently underwent ECMO implantation. Nine (5.4%) of these transported patients were transported with the initial intention to treat with ECMO support. However, they did not receive ECMO support due to other treatment options. In addition, ten patients were transported without the intention for ECMO but in regard to upgrade of therapeutic options (Fig. 1). In those patients, decision against ECMO support therapy was either due to preexisting contraindications for ECMO support previously not reported by the referring hospital. Other reasons included non-consent for extended life support therapy by patient's living will or next of kin. Hence, transport to a tertiary university hospital environment was performed in terms of "step-up" of care.

Over the study period, we observed a constant increase in number of ECMO transports (Fig. 2a). In two years, 2009 and 2012, we observed a slightly higher number of transports.

Out of all cannulated patients, 137 (93.1%) received VV-ECMO, whilst ten patients (4%) received VA-ECMO (Fig. 2b). One patient was originally cannulated VV, however, due to rapid cardiac deterioration resulting in cardiogenic shock, subsequently switched to VA.

Transport statistics

Decisions regarding transport considering several factors like weather, time of day, distance, and availability of a dedicated transport vehicle (airborne or ground).

Whilst 24 patients were transported using a helicopter, the majority, 138 patients, were transported on ground. The remaining patients′ mode of transport was irretrievable from available records (Fig. 2c). Mean distance for airborne transport was 115 ± 105 km, with the maximum distance being 548 km. Ground distance averaged 48 ± 41, with a maximum of 251 km (Fig. 2d). On average, transport times using helicopter were 83 ± 42 min, and 75 ± 36 min for ground transport.

The mean mission time, i.e. time from alert of the ECMO centre to return with the patient, was 6.3 h. (339 min, IQR 300–480 min, Min 80 min, Max 720 min) (Fig. 2c).

Epidemiology

The mean age was 49 ± 14 (youngest 16, oldest 75) years. 94 patients were male, 73 female (Fig. 2e). Average

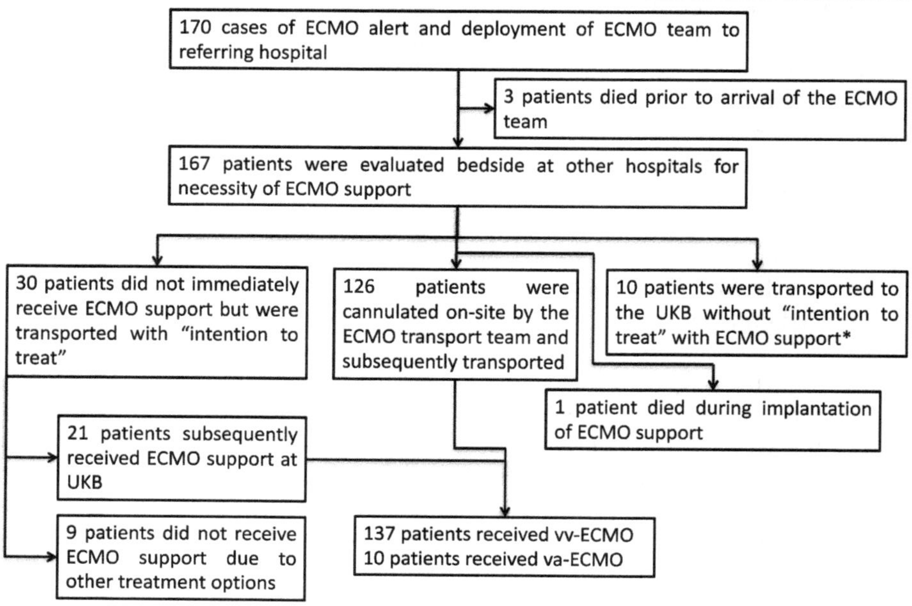

Fig. 1 Flow chart of included patients and disposition. *E.g. due to previously not reported contraindication for ECMO support by the referring hospital, and on site identified by the mobile ECMO team. Other reasons included non-consent for extended life support therapy by patient's living will or next of kin. Hence, transport was performed in terms of "step-up" of care in a tertiary university hospital environment.

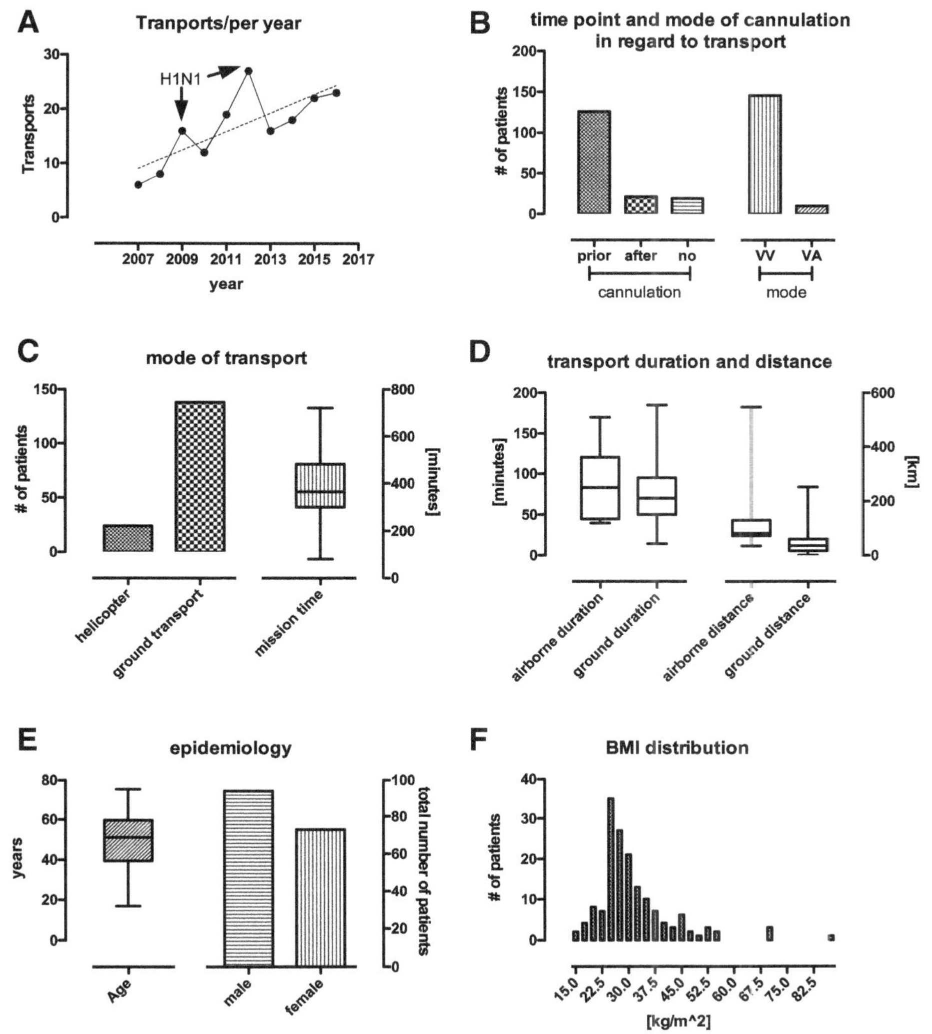

Fig. 2 **a** transports per year. Out of all peripheral ECMO requests, the ECMO team deployed in a total of 159 times. In 2009 and 2012, the observable rise in ECMO transport was traceable to the H1N1 epidemic in Germany. **b** 126 patients were cannulated at the referring site (primary transports), 30 were transported without ECMO but with intent to treat, with 21 receiving subsequent cannulation at the University Hospital Bonn. In 9 cases, subsequently no ECMO therapy was required. Out of all performed ECMO procedures, 137 were cannulated veno-venous, 10 veno-arterial. ***c:*** majority of transports ($n = 138$) were ground based, the remainder ($n = 24$) by helicopter. **d** transport duration and distance by mode of transport, airborne: Intensive care transport helicopter, ground based: ambulance, IQR: Interquartile range. Airborne duration: Median 83 min, IQR 45–120, ground based duration Median 74.8 min IQR 50–95, IHT distance Median 81.4 km IQR 72.1–129.5, ground transportation distance: Median 36 km IQR 15.7–60. **e** demographic stats: Age Median 49.3 years, IQR 39.4–59.3; 94 males, 73 females. **f** BMI distribution as histogramm, indicating the majority of patients being overweight to obese, as indicated by a BMI > 25. BMI Median 27.3, IQR 24.8–34, minimum 15.4, maximum 86.5, underlying weight for BMI calculation: Median 85.0 kg IQR 75–100, minimum 40.0, maximum 250 kg. Underlying height for BMI calculation: Median 1.74 m, IQR 1.65–1.8

height across both genders was 173 ± 10 cm. Weight ranged from 45 to 250 kg, averaging 94 ± 34 kg. The mean Body Mass Index (BMI) was 31.2 ± 10.5, indicating adipositas, as defined by a BMI > 30 (Fig. 2f). In our patient cohort, the adipose fraction of patients ranged higher compared to the general German population [18]. The total fraction of patients with a BMI > 27.5 (pre-adipose and above) was 61%.

Indication

Primary indication for ECMO referral was ARDS with different underlying aetiologies. In the majority of cases, ARDS was secondary to pneumonia with associated hypoxic and/or hypercapnic respiratory failure (Table 1). Amongst patients receiving VA-ECMO, the primary indication was refractory cardiac failure with underlying respiratory failure and ARDS (Table 2).

Table 1 Causes of ARDS: A total of 166 patients were retrospectively analysed in regard to the initial diagnoses leading to ARDS and subsequent ECMO request. In some cases a combination of causes was present (e.g. trauma and pneumonia, sepsis of other origin and pneumonia)

Primary cause ECMO indication	Total number; %of all transported patients (n = 166)
Pneumonia	59; 35,6%
Pneumonia related sepsis	15; 9%
Atypical pneumonia	3; 1,8%
Cardiac arrest	7; 4,2%
Sepsis	9; 5,4%
Influenza, other, nonspecified viral origin	11;6,6%
Trauma	3; 1,8%
H1N1 pneumonia	22; 13,2%
Decompensated COPD	9; 5,4%
unknown	1; 0,6%
Aspiration	16; 9,6%
Other (pulmonary embolism, intoxication, allergic, chemotherapy induced immunosuppression…)	19; 11,4%

Observed disease severity

The average SOFA score on admission was 12 ± 3 and SAPS II score was 40 ± 13. The mean nursing workload, estimated using TISS-28, was 30 ± 8. Mean APACHE II score was 23 ± 7 and mean Lung injury score was 3 ± 1 (Fig. 3a).

Hospital length of stay (LOS), ECMO treatment duration and days on ventilator

Mean LOS in the referring hospital was 7.8 ± 15.7 days, with 3.7 ± 4.3 days under mechanical ventilation. The duration of ECMO support was 11.5 ± 8.7 days, and overall, patients were dependent on mechanical ventilation for 26.3 ± 26.5 days. The total LOS in our hospital was 31.7 ± 29.7 days (Fig. 3b).

ECMO efficiency on site

ECMO efficiency was assessed 30–60 min post implantation. Markers of efficiency included improved patient blood gas parameters, improved pH, reduction of FiO_2 required to maintain arterial pO2 > 65 mmHg and improvement of Horowitz index. ECMO treatment significantly increased all parameters (Fig. 4a-c), when performing matched-pair analyses of pre/post-implantation data. The only parameter unaffected by ECMO implantation in our cohort were lactate levels (Fig. 4d; p = 0.12).

In-hospital survival

Survival is reported as in-hospital survival, i.e. discharge from our hospital or transfer to another hospital.

Out of 147 patients who received an ECMO support, 81 patients survived (55%). In detail, of the ten patients initially receiving VA-ECMO treatment, 3 (30%) survived. Predicted survival for VA-ECMO, determined using the SAVE-Score, was 33.5%. Of the VV-ECMO cohort, 78 (56.9%) patients survived. Predicted survival for VV-ECMO, determined using the RESP-Score, was 59.6% (Fig. 3c). Using Standardised Mortality Ratios, we compared our observed mortality with the predicted mortality calculated by the RESP/SAVE score. The SMR of the VV-cohort was 1066 (95%CI: 0,861-1271), the SMR of the VA-cohort was 1053 (95%CI 0,626-1480). No significant differences between observed and predicted mortality were found.

Table 2 Indication for VA ECMO: 1 patient received VA-cannulation due to cardiac arrest. The other 9 patients were in cardiogenic shock due to the given causes

Indication for VA-ECMO	Total number, %of all recipients (n = 10)
Cardiogenic shock following ARDS due to:	9, 90%
Pneumonia	5, 50%
Atypical pneumonia	2, 20%
Sepsis	2, 20%
Cardiac arrest	1, 10%

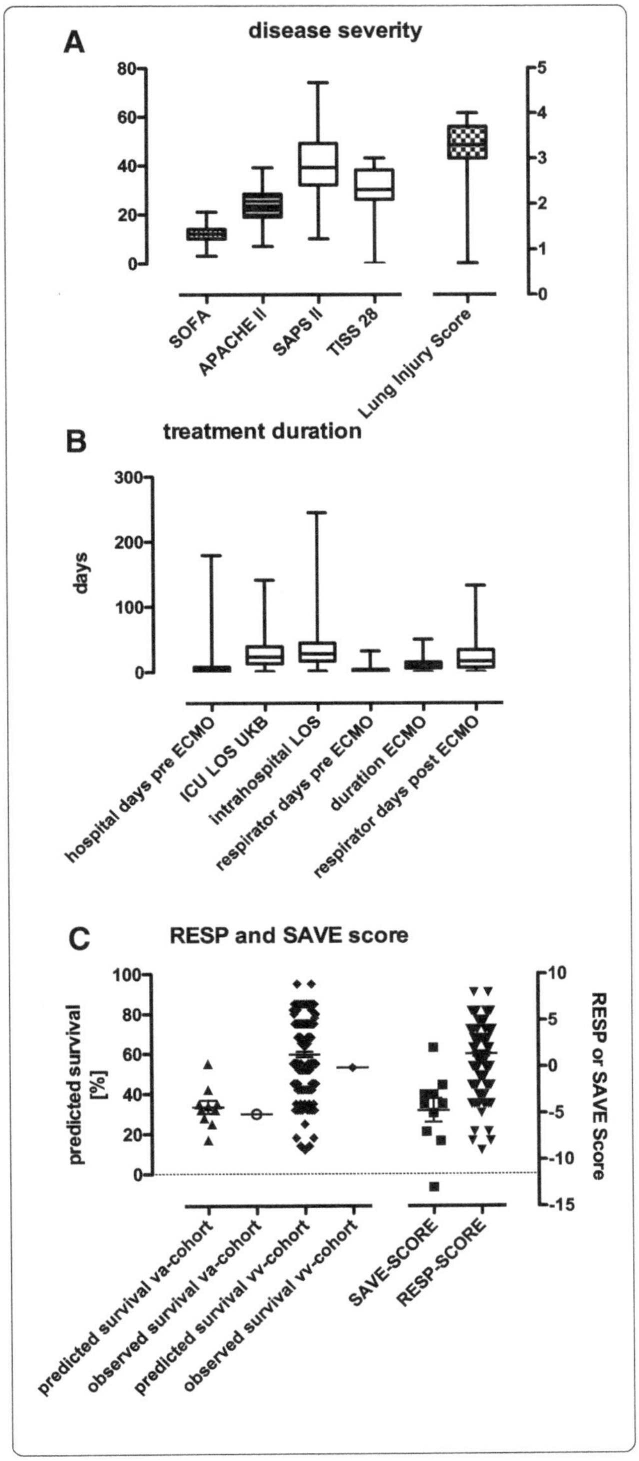

Fig. 3 a disease severity: Patients' disease severity was indicated through different well established ICU scores. SOFA was 12 ± 3, IQR 10–14; Lung Injury Score was 3 ± 0.6, IQR 3–3.7; APACHE II 23 ± 7, IQR 19–28.2: SAPS II 40 ± 13, IQR 32–49; TISS 28 30 ± 8, IQR 26–38. **b** treatment duration: total length of stay (LOS) in referring hospital: 7.8 ± 15.72 days, IQR 2–8; LOS in our hospital was 31.7 ± 29.7 days, IQR 13–39. Days with mechanical ventilation amounted to 3.7 ± 4.3 days, IQR 1–4. ECMO treatment was performed for 11.5 ± 8.7 days, IQR 6–15; overall days dependent on mechanical ventilation 26.3 ± 26.5 days, IQR 7–33.5. **c** observed and calculated mortality: SAVE score mean – 7.7 ± 4.0, IQR -7,25- -2.45. Predicted survival from score: 33.5 ± 10.1%, IQR 27.5–36.75%, observed survival in our VA-ECMO cohort: 30%. For VV-ECMO cohort, mean RESP score was 1.7 ± 3.2, IQR 0–4, predicted survival from score 59.6 ± 17.2, IQR 52–75. Observed survival in VV-ECMO cohort: 56.9%

Discharge details

Out of all surviving patients, 42 patients were transferred back to the referring hospital. 19 patients were discharged to facilities specialized in long-term rehabilitative medicine, 9 patients were transferred to a hospital closer to their residence. 7 patients were discharged from the ICU to a normal ward and consecutively fully discharged from the hospital without further rehabilitative interventions. Data for the remaining patients, were unavailable for analyses.

Observed complications

The observed complications are given in Table 3. In total 26 adverse events were observed. No observed mortality or morbidity was directly related to transport. No patient died during transport. Despite the seemingly high rate of complications, only two severe complications occurred during transport. These complications, due to hemodynamic instability and ventilator associated difficulties, were not attributable to technical difficulties during transportation, but rather due to either delayed referral and/or the generally high-risk nature of the ECMO procedure.

Discussion

Over ten years, the University Hospital Bonn ECMO retrieval team performed 166 ECMO related transports. The annual rate of ECMO transports has steadily increased over time, with two observable peaks. The first peak occurred during the German H1N1 epidemic in 2009 [19]. The second peak was in 2012, and most likely also related to seasonal influenza infections [20]. Furthermore the ECMO treatment capacity also increased in correspondence to the availability of more ECMO consoles. In recent years, the rates of transport have slightly tapered, presumably due to other ECMO centres also extending their capacities.

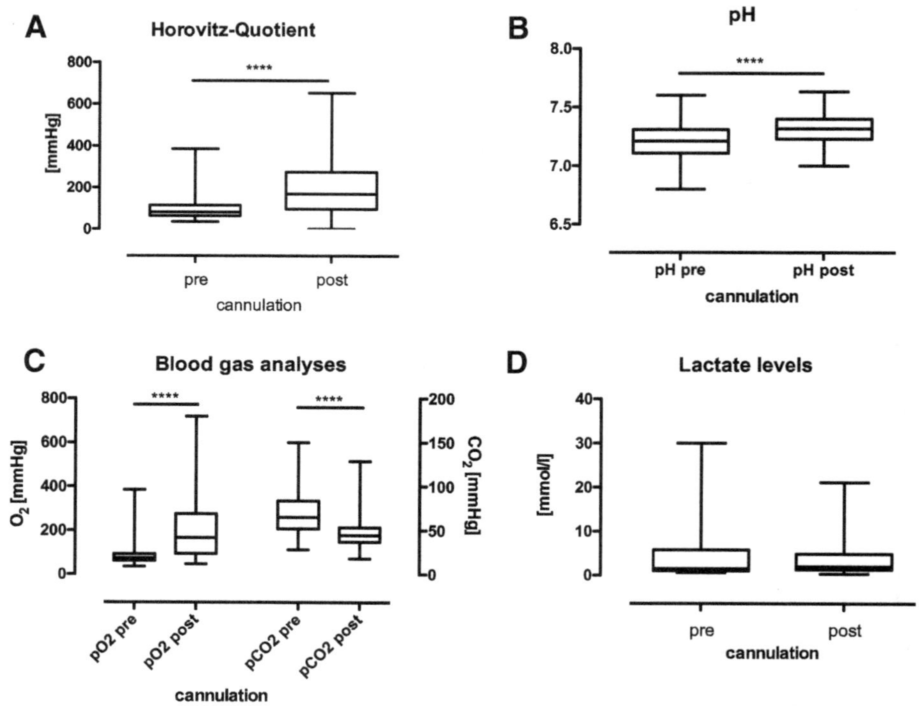

Fig. 4 Efficiency of on-site ECMO treatment: **a** Effect of ECMO on oxygenation. ECMO significantly increased Horowitz Index with 30 min post implantation. Mean Horowitz Index pre-cannulation 99.2 ± 60.6, IQR 64–114, post-cannulation 202.8 ± 133.6, IQR 95.5–273.3, $p < 0.0001$, **b** pH was significantly improved from mean 7.2 ± 0.1, IQR 7.1–7.3 pre ECMO to 7.3 ± 0.14, IQR 7.2–7.4, $p < 0.0001$. **c** Arterial blood gas analysis prior and following ECMO initiation: P_aO_2 was significantly increased from mean 86.2 ± 47.4 mmHg, IQR 61.8–93, to 206.6 ± 135.3 mmHg, IQR 94–275, $p < 0.0001$. P_aCO_2 was significantly lowered by ECMO from mean 70.2 ± 24.4 mmHg, IQR 52–83.5, to 47.98 ± 17.4 mmHg, IQR 37–53.3. **d** Lactate levels were not significantly improved by ECMO treatment. Mean arterial lactate pre ECMO initiation was 4.08 ± 5 mmol/l, IQR 1.01–5.87, and post implantation 3.9 ± 4.2 mmol/l, IQR 1.3–4.9

Survival, disease severity and ICU length of stay

The observed overall survival rate in our cohort was 55.1%, similar to previously stated survival rates reported in the ELSO Registry, and by Bryner et al. [21] with observed survival rates for respiratory failure related ARDS of 55 and 59%, respectively. Brechot colleagues also investigated survival after ECMO transport [22]. In their study, 63 of 157 (53%) transported patients survived to discharge.

Observed survival is minimally, albeit non-statistically significant, lower than the predicted survival using RESP and SAVE score. This is most likely due to a lack of data

Table 3 The most common complication observed in our cohort was necessity for several puncture attempts, followed by erroneous placement of ECMO cannulas. The observed complications are neither traceable to transport or the reduced team size. Time point of observed complication (prior to vs. during transport) is indicated in parentheses in column one

Complication	Occurrence in regard to transport	Total number, %of all patients
Cardiac arrest with ROSC	prior	4, 2.4%
Erroneous arterial cannulation	prior	1, 0,5%
Erroneous placement of cannula	prior	4, 2.4%
Arterial puncture instead of vein	prior	3, 1.8%
multiple puncture attempts	prior	7, 4.2%
Hemodynamic instability during transport	during	1, 0.5%
Bilateral pneumothorax with hemodynamic instability	during	1, 0.5%
SpO_2 loss, ventilator associated problems	during	1, 0.5%
Death during or prior to implementation	prior	4, 2.4%
Overall number of severe complications		26, 15.6%

and hence an underestimation of the underlying. Where no data was available, best possible option was used for calculation, potentially leading to confounding data.

When comparing disease severity, the patients' SOFA score 24 h post-admission/transport was comparable to data published by Strauch et al. In their retrospective analysis of SOFA scores as a mortality predictor in critically ill patients, the mean SOFA of ECMO patients was 14 and thus comparable to our observed SOFA score of 12 ± 3 (IQR 10–14). However, in their small cohort, SOFA score was not associated with outcome [23]. Brechot et al. published a mean SOFA score of 14 (IQR 10–16), also comparable to the observed scores in our cohort [22]. Mirroring this finding are data from the DACAPO study group, who reported a mean SOFA of 11 (IQR 8–13) [24].

ICU length of stay observed in our cohort was 31 ± 29 days. This is similar to ICU LOS reported by Lucchini et al., who reported a mean ICU LOS of 27 ± 28 days for all patients, and 27 ± 27 days for patients transported with ECMO [4].

Efficiency

In their description of 221 patients under ECMO Bryner et al. point out the immense strain on the involved personnel. At times, 5 staff members were deployed for one transport for a time frame of 8 to 12 h [21]. Lucchini et al. mirror this finding in their 8 year retrospective of ECMO transports [4], efficiently binding 4 members (2 intensivists, 1 ICU nurse, 1 perfusionist) for a mean mission time of 8.5 h. This amount of personnel will be difficult to maintain by ECMO centres, especially considering the continuous growing number of ECMO transports. Mean transport time for ECMO patients in the transport study performed by Strauch et al. was 9.3 h. No total mission time was reported [23]. However, they consider transport time as time from deployment of the team till return, so this is comparable to our total mission and the study by Lucchini et al. [4].

Hence, our experience with performing primary ECMO transports with a reduced team comprising only two members, may help address this problem.

The study by Brechot et al. was also performed with a two-member team (cardiovascular surgeon, perfusionist). In this regard, it is the only comparable study to our 2-member approach. They did not report a mean mission time, but rather a deployment to ECMO initiation time of 192 min. This is considerably shorter than our mean mission time of 339 min, however their transport times (35 min) and distances (15 km) are well below those reported in our study (74 min and 48 km), which might have contributed to the different times. This indicates, that a two-member approach is time efficient, thus helping reducing the personnel burden for ECMO centres.

Most recently, Heuer et al. reported a study of 75 patients transported under ECMO [25]. This study was also performed with a reduced team, consisting of three persons (2 intensivists, 1 ICU nurse). Their observed survival rate (65%) is well within the range of previously published data. However, they did not address any complication rates, mission time and, contrary to our study, deployed with a primed ECMO system. Our team deploys and primes the ECMO system on site, without any negative impact on time and safety.

Safety

We observed a total of 26 major incidents (15.6%). The majority of incidents were related to ECMO implantation or critical condition of the patient. This finding is in accordance with the observed rate of critical events in the DACAPO study, where 59 (13.6%) critical events occurred, with 42 being patient related [24]. The observed rates of ECMO implantation related complications are also in accordance with those by Brechot et al. This indicates, that out-of-centre complications are most likely secondary to the procedure itself and not the absence of a vascular surgeon in our team. Other observed complications in our cohort are lower than in the Brechot study. For example, we only experienced one patient (0.5%) with severe hemodynamic instability during transport compared to nine (5.7%) patients in the Brechot study [22]. The only other study with a two-man retrieval team, the study by Strauch et al., reports a complication rate of ~ 6,4%. According to the authors, the majority of incidents were of a technical nature [23]. Unfortunately, their study does not specify which complications were included, thus a direct comparison to our study is not possible.

Even in teams consisting of more personnel, including a cannulating surgeon, complication rates are higher than in our cohort. One of the largest of these studies, consisting of 282 primary ECMO transports, Broman et al., observed a total complication rate of 27.3%, with 22% being patient related and 5.3% being technical failure [26]. The study by Lucchini et al. reported two major complications in 42 ECMO transports (~ 4.7%). One of these complications was patient related, the other related to technical issues [4]. Due to the smaller number of patients reported in their study, comparison to our data is difficult. While offering data on complications, Bryner et al. only report total numbers for each observed type of complications. It is thus difficult to directly compare the number of observed complications. However, regarding events of a technical nature, they reported 18% "electrical complications", well above our rates. "Complications with overall aspects of patient care" and "Circuit issues" (e.g. oxygenator clotting) were observed in 4 and 9%, respectively [21].

Study limitations

Main limitation of this study is its retrospective nature and single centre experience. Due to the non-compara bility of mean survival rates, no direct comparison from our study with survival rates of other studies could be performed. Thus comparison is based on indirect standardisation and not direct comparison. Furthermore, no causality between mortality and transport can be concluded.

Conclusion

Interfacility ECMO transport by a anaesthesiology-led two-man team is feasible, safe and efficient. We did not observe increased mortality beyond the already high-risk of ECMO itself. Our reduced team approach can safely extend lifesaving therapy to patients in other institutions, whose available treatment options have been exhausted. This without increasing observed adverse events during/related to transport of the critically ill. ICU LOS and survival to hospital discharge of transported patients with ECMO is comparable to other studies with larger ECMO retrieval teams [4, 21]. We hereby show a non-inferiority of a interprofessional two-man team approach regarding primary ECMO transports.

Abbreviations

APACHE: Acute physiology and chronic health evaluation; ARDS: Acute respiratory distress syndrome; BMI: Body mass index; Ch: Charriére; COPD: Chronic obstructive pulmonary disease; ECLS: Extracorporeal life support; ECMO: Extracorporeal membrane oxygenation; ELSO: Extracorporeal Life Support Organization; EMS: Emergency medical services; ICU: Intensive care unit; IQR: Interquartile range; LOS: Length of stay; RESOP score: Respiratory ECMO survival prediction; SAPS: Simplified Acute Physiology Score; SAVE score: Survival after veno-arterial ECMO; SMR: Standard mortality ratio; SOFA score: Sequential Organ Failure Assessment; TISS: Therapeutic Intervention Scoring System; VA: Veno-arterial; VV: Veno-venous

Acknowledgements

The authors thank the specialized intensive care nurses of the Department of Anaesthesiology and Intensive Care Medicine especially the members of the ECMO transport team. Furthermore, we thank Klaus Ringelstein, Hermann Wrigge, Ulf Guenther and Marco Monnig who contributed to the initiation of the primary ECMO transport concept in Bonn.

Authors' contributions

SFE: collected, analysed and interpreted data, wrote the manuscript. BS: collected and analysed data. SL: collected, analysed and interpreted data, wrote the manuscript. HE: analysed and interpreted data, critical revision of the manuscript. SK: collected, analysed and interpreted data. CB, FK, FL, TM, MS, CS, FS, NUT, CW: collected data. CP: interpreted data, critical revision of the manuscript. JCS: conception and design; collected, analysed and interpreted data, wrote the manuscript. All authors read and approved the manuscript.

References

1. Brodie D, Bacchetta M. Extracorporeal membrane oxygenation for ARDS in adults. N Engl J Med. 2011;365:1905–14.
2. Lovell MA, Mudaliar MY, Klineberg PL. Intrahospital transport of critically ill patients: complications and difficulties. Anaesth Intensive Care. 2001;29:400–5.
3. Blakeman TC, Branson RD. Inter- and intra-hospital transport of the critically ill. Respir Care. 2013;58:1008–23.
4. Lucchini A, De Felippis C, Elli S, Gariboldi R, Vimercati S, Tundo P, et al. Mobile ECMO team for inter-hospital transportation of patients with ARDS: a retrospective case series. Heart Lung Vessel. 2014;6:262–73.
5. Zimmermann M, Bein T, Philipp A, Ittner K, Foltan M, Drescher J, et al. Interhospital transportation of patients with severe lung failure on pumpless extracorporeal lung assist. Br J Anaesth. 2006;96:63–6.
6. Foley DS, Pranikoff T, Younger JG, Swaniker F, Hemmila MR, Remenapp RA, et al. A review of 100 patients transported on extracorporeal life support. ASAIO J. 2002;48:612–9.
7. Dan Dirnberger RF. Guidelines for ECMO transport. https://www.elso.org/Portals/0/Files/ELSO%20GUIDELINES%20FOR%20ECMO%20TRANSPORT_May2015.pdf Accessed Dec 2018.
8. von Elm E, Altman DG, Egger M, Pocock SJ, Gøtzsche PC, Vandenbroucke JP, et al. The strengthening the reporting of observational studies in epidemiology (STROBE) statement: guidelines for reporting observational studies. J Clin Epidemiol. 2008;61:344–9.
9. Schmidt M, Bailey M, Sheldrake J, Hodgson C, Aubron C, Rycus PT, et al. Predicting survival after extracorporeal membrane oxygenation for severe acute respiratory failure. The respiratory extracorporeal membrane oxygenation survival prediction (RESP) score. Am J Respir Crit Care Med. 2014;189:1374–82.
10. Schmidt M, Burrell A, Roberts L, Bailey M, Sheldrake J, Rycus PT, et al. Predicting survival after ECMO for refractory cardiogenic shock: the survival after veno-arterial-ECMO (SAVE)-score. Eur Heart J. 2015;36:2246–56.
11. Everitt B, Skrondal A. Standardized mortality rate (SMR). New York: Cambridge University Press; 2010.
12. Van den Broeck J, Brestoff JR, Kaulfuss C. Statistical Estimation. In: Van den Broeck J, Brestoff JR, editors. Epidemiology: principles and practical guidelines. Dordrecht: Springer Netherlands; 2013. p. 417–38. https://doi.org/10.1007/978-94-007-5989-3_22.
13. Vincent JL, Moreno R, Takala J, Willatts S, De Mendonca A, Bruining H, et al. The SOFA (Sepsis-related organ failure assessment) score to describe organ dysfunction/failure. On behalf of the working group on Sepsis-related problems of the European Society of Intensive Care Medicine. Intensive Care Med. 1996;22:707–10.
14. Le Gall JR, Lemeshow S, Saulnier F. A new simplified acute physiology score (SAPS II) based on a European/north American multicenter study. JAMA. 1993;270:2957–63.
15. Knaus WA, Zimmerman JE, Wagner DP, Draper EA, Lawrence DE. APACHE-acute physiology and chronic health evaluation: a physiologically based classification system. Crit Care Med. 1981;9:591–7.
16. Miranda DR, de Rijk A, Schaufeli W. Simplified therapeutic intervention scoring system: the TISS-28 items--results from a multicenter study. Crit Care Med. 1996;24:64–73.
17. Murray JF, Matthay MA, Luce JM, Flick MR. An expanded definition of the adult respiratory distress syndrome. Am Rev Respir Dis. 1988;138:720–3.
18. Robert-Koch-Institut. Gesundheit in Deutschland. Gesundheitsberichterstattung des Bundes. Gemeinsam getragen von RKI und Destatis. Berlin: Robert Koch-Institut Nordufer 20 13353 Berlin; 2015.
19. Buda S, Köpke K, Luchtenberg M, Schweiger B, Biere B, Duwe S, et al. Bericht zur Epidemiologie der Influenza in Deutschland Saison 2009/10. Berlin: Robert Koch-Institute; 2010.
20. Buda S, Köpke K, Prahm K, Schweiger B, Wedde M, Duve S, et al. Bericht zur Epidemiologie der Influenza in Deutschland Saison 2012/13. Berlin: Robert Koch Institute; 2012.
21. Bryner B, Cooley E, Copenhaver W, Brierley K, Teman N, Landis D, et al. Two decades' experience with interfacility transport on extracorporeal membrane oxygenation. Ann Thorac Surg. 2014;98:1363–70.
22. Brechot N, Mastroianni C, Schmidt M, Santi F, Lebreton G, Hoareau AM, et al. Retrieval of severe acute respiratory failure patients on extracorporeal membrane oxygenation: any impact on their outcomes? J Thorac Cardiovasc Surg. 2017;155:1621–29.

23. Strauch U, Bergmans DC, Winkens B, Roekaerts PM. Short-term outcomes and mortality after interhospital intensive care transportation: an observational prospective cohort study of 368 consecutive transports with a mobile intensive care unit. BMJ Open. 2015;5:e006801.
24. Blecha S, Dodoo-Schittko F, Brandstetter S, Brandl M, Dittmar M, Graf BM, et al. Quality of inter-hospital transportation in 431 transport survivor patients suffering from acute respiratory distress syndrome referred to specialist centers. Ann Intensive Care. 2018;8:5.
25. Heuer JF, Mirschel M, Bleckmann A, Quintel M, Moerer O. Interhospital transport of ARDS patients on extracorporeal membrane oxygenation. J Artif Organs. 2018. https://doi.org/10.1007/s10047-018-1065-y.
26. Broman LM, Holzgraefe B, Palmer K, Frenckner B. The Stockholm experience: interhospital transports on extracorporeal membrane oxygenation. Crit Care. 2015;19:278.

3

The influences of anesthesia methods on some complications after orthopedic surgery

Yuqing Zeng[1,2], Junming Wan[2], Haiyong Ren[2], Jianwei Lu[2], Fuhua Zhong[2] and Shu Deng[3*]

Abstract

Background: Although several anesthesia procedures have been explored for orthopedic surgery, the complications of anesthesia remain not well resolved. This study aimed to explore the influence of different anesthesia methods on the complications after orthopedic surgery.

Methods: According to the searching strategy, anesthesia associated studies in orthopedic surgery were screened from Pubmed, Embase, and the Cochrane Library up to Mar. 10th, 2018. Then, complications and demographic data were extracted and quality of studies was assessed using Cochrane Collaboration recommendations. ADDIS software was used to perform the network meta-analysis. Pooled effect size was calculated using random effective model or consistency model, and presented with odds ratio (OR) and 95% confidence interval (CI).

Results: According to the selective criteria, a total of 23 studies with 2393 patients were enrolled in this study. Quality assessment revealed all studies had an ordinary quality. Network meta-analyses revealed that nerve block analgesia (NBA) presented a lower effect on the occurrence of post-operative nausea or vomiting (PONV; OR = 0.17, 95% CI: 0.06–0.39) and urine retention (OR = 0.07, 95% CI: 0.01–0.37) compared with epidural anesthesia (EA). Interscalene block (ISB) and local infiltration analgesia (LIA) could significantly reduce the occurrence of back pain compared with EA (OR = 0.00, 95% CI = 0.00–0.30; OR = 0.00, 95% CI = 0.00–0.25).

Conclusion: NBA presented an effective role in reliving the occurrence of PONV and urine retention, and ISB and LIA relieved the back pain compared with EA after orthopedic surgery.

Keywords: Orthopedic surgery, Nerve block analgesia, Local infiltration analgesia, Interscalene block, Complication

Background

Since it emerged in the eighteenth century, the discipline of orthopedic surgery has been remarkably developed [1]. Till now, several orthopedic surgeries have been explored, including total knee replacement, hip fracture, and total hip replacement [2]. However, there are still some deficiencies to limit the application of orthopedic surgery in clinic, such as pain control, prevention of post-operative nausea or vomiting (PONV), rapid recovery, cognitive impairment, and surgical site infection [3–5]. Specifically, anesthesia is a common procedure during orthopedic surgery, which could affect the temperature regulation, infection, bleeding, oxygen consumption, and other complications to influence the outcome of orthopedic surgery [6]. Therefore, it is important to innovate appropriate anesthesia manner to improve the outcomes and prognosis of orthopedic surgery.

With the development of few decades, although several anesthesia manners have been explored for orthopedic surgery, the complications of anesthesia are still not well resolved. A previous study has revealed that patients managed with general anesthesia perform a low risk of complications compared with patients undergoing spinal anesthesia during the total knee arthroplasty [7]. However, compared with the general anesthesia, regional anesthesia presents a better outcome than general anesthesia in total hip arthroplasty, including reductions

* Correspondence: ShushuDeng55@outlook.com
[3]Department of Hematology, The First Affliated Hospital of Zhejiang Chinese Medical University, 54 Youdian Road, Hangzhou, Zhejiang Province, People's Republic of China

of deep surgical site infection, length of hospital stay, and pulmonary complication [8]. Moreover, Stundner et al. have revealed that neuraxial anesthesia reduces the occurrence rates of blood transfusions and morbidity in the perioperative period of compared with general anesthesia for simultaneous bilateral total knee arthroplasty [9]. In addition, Ewan et al. have documented that general anesthesia increases the risk of post-operative cognitive dysfunction compared with other anesthesia methods [10]. Considering of these evidences, there is still no clear consensus in anesthesia during orthopedic surgery.

In the current study, a network meta-analysis was performed to comprehensively estimate the effects of different anesthesia manners, such as general anesthesia on the outcomes of orthopedic surgery. According to this analysis, we hope to provide some new insights for improving the outcomes of orthopedic surgery.

Methods

Data sourcing

According to the searching strategy, studies focused on the associations between anesthesia methods and adverse effects after orthopedic surgery published in English were downloaded from the Pubmed (http://www.ncbi.nlm.nih.gov/pubmed), Embase (http://www.embase.com), and the Cochrane Library (http://www.cochranelibrary.com) databases. The searching date was ranged from its recording to Mar. 10th, 2018. The searching strategy was designed as follows: "general anesthesia" (OR "general anaesthesia" OR "local anesthesia" OR "topical anesthesia" OR "local anaesthesia" OR "toponarcosis" OR "medullary anesthesia" OR "rachianalgesia" OR "rachianesthesia" OR "medullary narcosis" OR "spinal anesthesia" OR "rhachiaesthesia" OR "rhachianalgesia" OR "lumbar anesthesia" OR "epidural anesthesia" OR "epidural block" OR "epidural anaesthesia" OR "caudal anaesthesia" OR "caudal anesthesia" OR "caudalanaesthesia" OR "infiltration analgesia" OR "intrathecal analgesia") AND "orthopedics" (OR "orthopedic" OR "osteology") AND "Rando".

Inclusive and exclusive criteria

In the present study, studies were included if they met the following terms: (1) published in English; (2) reported on the influences of different anesthesia methods on the effective of patients (P) undergoing orthopedic surgery; (3) patients in different groups receiving different anesthesia methods (Intervention, I; and Control, C); (4) study outcome variables including PONV, urine retention, back pain, sore throat, and headache, and so on (Outcomes, O); and (5) randomized controlled trial (RCT; S). Studies were excluded if they were met the following criteria: (1) incomplete data which could not be used for statistical analysis; (2) reviews, letters and comments; (3) for duplicate publication or data used for several studies, only the study with complete data was included, and others were excluded.

Data extraction and quality assessment

Data was independently extracted from the included studies by two censors in this study, respectively. The extracted information included the first author, published year, study year, study area, anesthesia method, sample size in different groups, length of operation, and the demographic characteristics of included patients, including age, gender, height, weight and so on. Quality of the enrolled studies were assessed using the Cochrane Collaboration recommendations recommended by the Cochrane system [11]. During the data extraction and quality assessment, divergences were solved by discussing with the third censors.

Statistical analyses

ADDIS is a non-programming software based on Bayesian framework, and can be used for data evaluation using the Markov chain Monte Carlo theory [12, 13]. All data in the current study was analyzed using the ADDIS software (version 1.16.5), and presented with odd ratio (OR) and 95% confidence interval (CI). For $P < 0.05$ in node-splitting analysis, the random effects model was used to calculate pooled effect size; otherwise, the consistency model were used to calculate the pooled effect size. Convergence degree of model was estimated using Brooks-Gelman-Rubin method, and presented with the potential scale reduction factor (PSRF). The more PSRF approximate to 1, the better convergence was obtained [14].

Results

Characteristics of enrolled studies

According to the searching strategy, a total of 3196 studies were recruited in this study. After removing the repetitions, 1945 studies were obtained. Following this, 1779 papers among 1945 were rejected after scanning title and abstract. Subsequently, 143 studies among remains were removed after reviewing the full text. Finally, 23 studies were obtained [15–37] and the process of study enrollment was presented in Fig. 1A.

Characteristics of the enrolled studies were summarized in Table 1. For these enrolled studies, the published years of them were ranged from 1978 to 2017, and the research areas were concentrated on Germany, Japan, America, China, French, and Turkey. A total of 2393 patients were enrolled in this study, including 753 in general anesthesia (GA) group, 215 in epidural anesthesia (EA) group, 473 in local infiltration analgesia (LIA) group, 238 in nerve block analgesia (NBA) group,

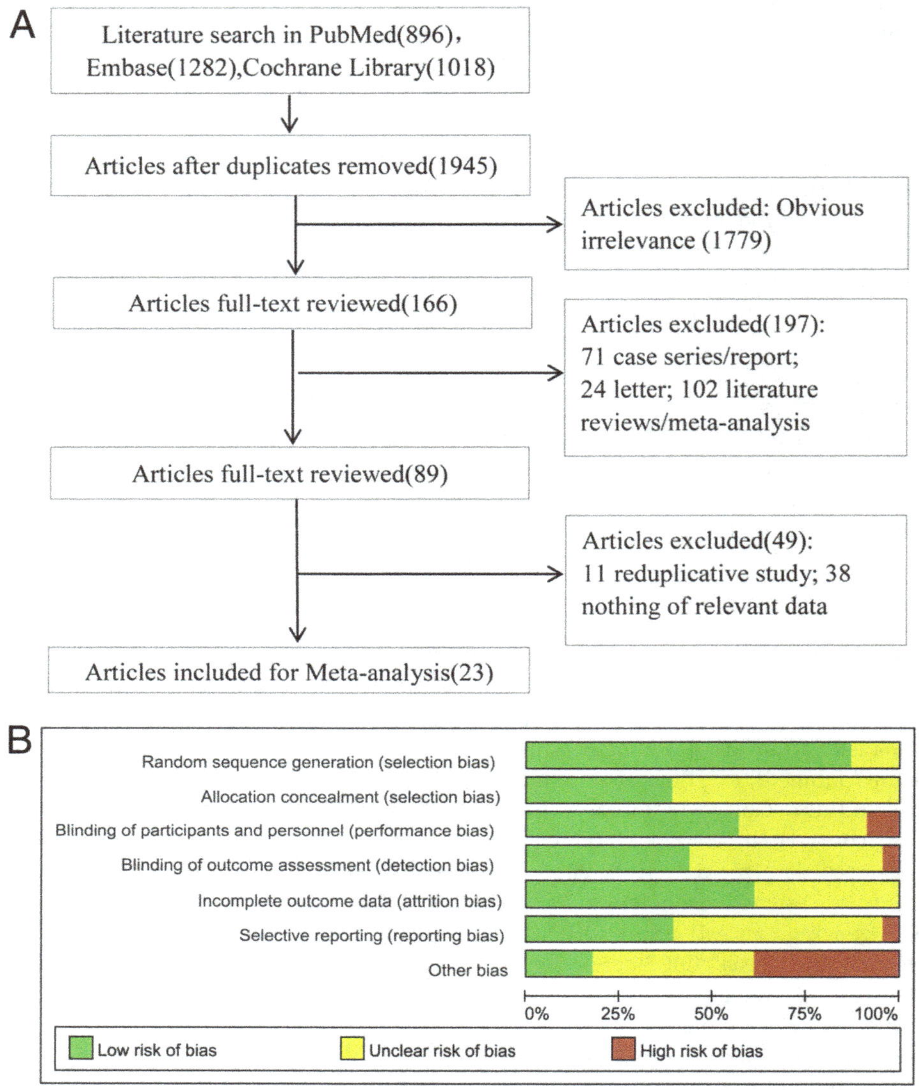

Fig. 1 Study enrollment and quality assessment. **a**, Flow chart of study enrollment; **b**, Quality assessment of enrolled studies

630 in spinal anesthesia (SA) group, 65 in interscalene block (ISB) group, and 81 in GA + ISB group. Moreover, the number of male patients was slightly higher than female patients, but there was no significantly difference for gender ratio in each study. In addition, there were no significantly difference identified in the age, height, weight, and length of operation among groups. Quality assessment indicated that the enrolled studies presented an ordinary quality (Fig. 1B). Despite the random sequence generation (selection bias), most of studies didn't report more information on other quality assessment terms.

Network meta-analyses for adverse effects after orthopedic surgery

According to the extracted data, parameters of ADDIS were set as follows: Number of chains: 4, Tuning iterations: 20000, Simulation iterations: 50000, Thinning interval: 10, Inference samples: 10000, Variance scaling factor: 2.5, and the network meta-analyses for PONV, urine retention, sore throat, back pain and headache were analyzed.

Network analysis for PONV

For PONV, the PSRF value was ranged from 1.00 to 1.01, indicating model had a good convergence. The node-splitting analysis presented that *P* values of all comparisons were more than 0.05 (Table 2A), and the consistency model was used to calculate the pooled effect sizes. The result presented that NBA had lowest influence on PONV after orthopedic surgery, and GA presented the worst effect on PONV after orthopedic surgery (Fig. 2A). Compared with NBA group, SA (OR

Table 1 Characteristics of enrolled studies

Author	Public Year	Location	Study Yeat	Group	N	Age (years)*	Male/ Female	Weight(kg)*	Height (cm)*	Length of operation (min)*
Arcioni R	2007	Italy	2004.9–2004.12	EA	25	59.1 ± 19.4	12/13	68.0 ± 8.7	166.2 ± 8.4	NA
				SA	23	60.2 ± 21.2	9/14	68.3 ± 10.4	164.7 ± 7.9	NA
Kuchalik J	2013	Sweden	NA	SA	39	66(51–84)	23/16	84 ± 23	170 ± 10	106 ± 17
				LIA	39	67(50–85)	21/18	86 ± 20	173 ± 8	112 ± 28
Dadure C	2006	France	2001.7–2002.12	EA	27	1–12	NA	7–56	72–160	65–190
				NBA	25	1–11	NA	10–52	80–151	45–180
Dunn WR	2006	USA	NA	LIA	18	Mean:51	11/7	Mean:75.0	Mean:170.3	Mean:27.4
				SA	14	Mean:55	5/9	Mean:74.2	Mean:169.6	Mean:30.9
Hadzic A	2005	USA	2000.4–2002.3	ISB	25	49 ± 13	17/8	85 ± 20	173 ± 10	127 ± 35
				GA	25	49 ± 12	13/12	86 ± 21	172 ± 10	147 ± 49
Hadzic A	2004	USA	NA	NBA	25	45 ± 15	12/13	81 ± 18	173 ± 10	72(50–165)
				GA	25	40 ± 16	11/14	77 ± 15	170 ± 10	70(30–330)
Janssen H	2014	Germany	NA	GA	42	51 ± 10	19/23	80 ± 14	170 ± 7	56.0 ± 12.4
				GA + ISB	41	53 ± 9	18/23	81 ± 16	170 ± 8	46.0 ± 15.3
Karaarslan S	2015	Turkey	NA	SA	30	43 ± 13	13/17	75 ± 13	170 ± 7	79 ± 22
				NBA	30	43 ± 10	19/11	77 ± 16	169 ± 9	85 ± 23
Krobbuaban B	2005	Thailand	NA	SA	86	41 ± 20	45/41	58 ± 13	161 ± 8	86 ± 52
				GA	85	38 ± 17	47/38	56 ± 8	168 ± 7	71 ± 15
Lehmann LJ	2014	Germany	2011.7–2012.5	GA	40	54.1 ± 11.7	22/18	83.3 ± 16.6	172.6 ± 10.7	NA
				ISB	40	49.3 ± 13.6	27/13	88.2 ± 19.2	172.2 ± 9.9	NA
				GA + ISB	40	53.8 ± 15.2	18/22	81.5 ± 16.3	169 ± 9.8	NA
Nagafuchi M	2015	Japan	2012.10–2013.7	NBA	17	72 ± 10	2/15	55 ± 8.2	NA	71 ± 15
				LIA	16	73 ± 5.9	3/13	62 ± 12.5	NA	81 ± 20
Seeberger MD	1994	Switzerland	NA	SA	96	33.7 ± 12.3	73/23	73.7 ± 12.6	174.2 ± 5.3	62 ± 35
				EA	96	32.0 ± 9.0	67/29	72.7 ± 11.0	174.7 ± 5.4	68 ± 46
Spangehl MJ	2015	NA	NA	NBA	79	67.8 ± 7.9	41/37	NA	NA	NA
				LIA	81	67.7 ± 7.2	48/43	NA	NA	NA
Standl T	1996	Germany	NA	SA	221	41.3 ± 17.8	112/109	70.4 ± 11	170.5 ± 8	120 ± 19
				GA	212	43.2 ± 17.3	106/106	70.9 ± 9	172.1 ± 6	116 ± 5
Gi E	2014	Japan	NA	LIA	25	77 ± 7	24/1	61 ± 13	149 ± 7	174 ± 23
				NBA	24	78 ± 5	21/3	64 ± 13	151 ± 7	173 ± 27
Bigler D	1985	NA	NA	GA	20	77.6 ± 2.3	5/15	NA	NA	59 ± 10
				SA	20	80.1 ± 1.6	2/18	NA	NA	67 ± 8
Hole A	1980	Norway	NA	GA	31	71.7(61–82)	11/20	NA	NA	207 ± 6
				EA	29	69.9(56–84)	10/19	NA	NA	190 ± 6
Kudoh A	2004	Japan	NA	SA	75	75.9 ± 4.0	69/6	60.4 ± 8.7	151.3 ± 7.3	106.7 ± 31.5
				GA	75	75.1 ± 4.2	66/9	59.2 ± 5.9	149.3 ± 5.4	104.2 ± 11.8
McLaren AD	1978	UK	NA	GA	29	76 ± 9.7	NA	NA	NA	NA
				SA	26	75.6 ± 10.3	NA	NA	NA	NA
Tanikawa H	2014	Japan	NA	LIA	23	71(69–76)	19/4	55.0(53.5–66.0)	151(148–152)	82.4 ± 26.0
				NBA	23	72(67.5–76.5)	20/3	54.5(48.0–66.5)	150(143.5–155.5)	75.0 ± 27.3

Table 1 Characteristics of enrolled studies *(Continued)*

Author	Public Year	Location	Study Yeat	Group	N	Age (years)*	Male/ Female	Weight(kg)*	Height (cm)*	Length of operation (min)*
Trker G	2003	Turkey	NA	EA	15	62.2 ± 6.6	9/6	72.2 ± 7.5	166.6 ± 3	129.2 ± 26.4
				NBA	15	62.3 ± 7.2	8/7	73.7 ± 6.3	167.4 ± 4.4	131.3 ± 18.7
Wang H	2017	China	2008.1–2015.12	GA	169	52.9 ± 9.7	89/80	NA	NA	52.5 ± 9.3
				LIA	187	51.4 ± 9.1	93/94	NA	NA	48.1 ± 9.9
Yukawa Y	2005	Japan	NA	LIA	22	58.9 ± 14.5	15/7	60.3 ± 9.5	159.2 ± 7.9	160.7 ± 27.0
				EA	23	59.1 ± 15.2	10/13	59.0 ± 9.7	160.1 ± 8.7	157.5 ± 29.5

Abbreviations: PONV: post-operative nausea or vomiting; GA: general anesthesia; LIA: local infiltration analgesia; ISB: interscalene block; EA: epidural anesthesia; NBA: nerve block analgesia; SA: spinal anesthesia; min: minutes; *: mean ± standard deviation/median(min-max)

= 0.31, 95%CI: 0.10, 0.86), EA (OR = 0.17, 95%CI: 0.06–0.39), GA (OR = 0.07, 95%CI: 0.02–0.18), and GA + IBS (OR = 0.19, 95%CI: 0.04–0.81) presented significantly worse effect on PONV after orthopedic surgery (Table 3A).

Network analysis for urine retention

The PSRF for urine retention was ranged from 1.00 to 1.02 indicating a good convergence for PSRF. Node-splitting analysis presented that $P > 0.05$, thus, the consistency model was used to calculate the pooled effect size of urine retention (Table 2B). The network analysis presented that the NBA group presented the lowest incidence of urine retention, and its incidence was significantly lower than that in the EA group (OR = 0.07, 95%CI: 0.01–0.37, Table 3B and Fig. 2B).

Analysis for sore throat

For sore throat, all PSRF values were 1.01, indicating a good convergence. Because no closed ring formed, consistency model was utilized to calculate the pooled side effect of sore throat. The analytical results presented that both the SA and NBA groups had lower incidences of sore throat, but no significant differences were identified compared with other groups (Fig. 3, Table 4).

Analysis for back pain

For back pain, all PSRF values were 1.01, indicating a good convergence. Because no closed ring formed, consistency model was utilized to calculate the pooled side effect of back pain. Compared with the EA group, both ISB (OR = 0.00, 95%CI: 0.00–0.30) and LIA (OR = 0.00, 95%CI: 0.00–0.25) groups presented lower

Table 2 Node-splitting analysis for PONV and urine retention

Name	Direct Effect	Indirect Effect	Overall	*P*-Value
A: PONV				
EA, GA	1.02 (−0.47, 2.42)	0.88 (−0.31, 2.09)	0.91 (0.02, 1.88)	0.89
EA, SA	0.25 (−1.15, 1.85)	−1.24 (−2.46, −0.20)	−0.68 (−1.58, 0.25)	0.10
EA, LIA	−2.46 (−4.33, − 0.74)	−1.38 (−2.44, − 0.38)	−1.74 (−2.67, − 0.89)	0.29
EA, NBA	−2.03 (−4.03, − 0.76)	−1.46 (− 2.79, − 0.21)	−1.80 (− 2.82, − 0.93)	0.47
GA, LIA	− 2.43 (− 4.62, − 0.74)	−2.77 (−3.90, − 1.76)	−2.64 (−3.70, − 1.75)	0.78
GA, NBA	−1.80 (− 4.09, − 0.11)	− 2.95 (− 4.22, − 1.99)	− 2.71 (−3.88, − 1.74)	0.41
GA, SA	−1.78 (− 2.62, − 0.96)	−0.91 (− 2.41, 0.54)	−1.57 (− 2.27, − 0.88)	0.30
GA + ISB, ISB	− 1.03 (− 3.23, 0.72)	−1.62 (− 3.68, 0.32)	−1.23 (− 2.76, 0.23)	0.65
LIA, SA	0.83 (− 0.50, 2.13)	1.29 (0.13, 2.66)	1.08 (0.20, 2.04)	0.62
LIA, NBA	− 0.08 (− 0.90, 0.65)	0.04 (−1.68, 1.49)	−0.07 (− 0.81, 0.63)	0.89
B: Urine retention				
EA, GA	−0.47 (− 2.91, 1.86)	−1.37 (− 4.68, 1.53)	−0.68 (− 2.52, 0.87)	0.60
EA, NBA	−2.93 (−5.49, − 0.99)	− 1.35 (−5.92, 2.38)	−2.59 (− 4.56, − 1.00)	0.45
EA, SA	−0.66 (− 4.75, 2.23)	−0.67 (− 3.34, 1.44)	−0.76 (− 2.71, 0.86)	0.96
GA, SA	0.20 (− 1.68, 2.06)	− 0.94 (− 4.47, 2.55)	−0.08 (− 1.60, 1.43)	0.55
NBA, SA	0.81 (− 2.34, 4.35)	2.50 (− 0.56, 5.47)	1.84 (− 0.26, 3.93)	0.48

Abbreviations: PONV: post-operative nausea or vomiting; GA: general anesthesia; LIA: local infiltration analgesia; ISB: interscalene block; EA: epidural anesthesia; NBA: nerve block analgesia; SA: spinal anesthesia. Data was presented with odds ratio and 95% confidence interval

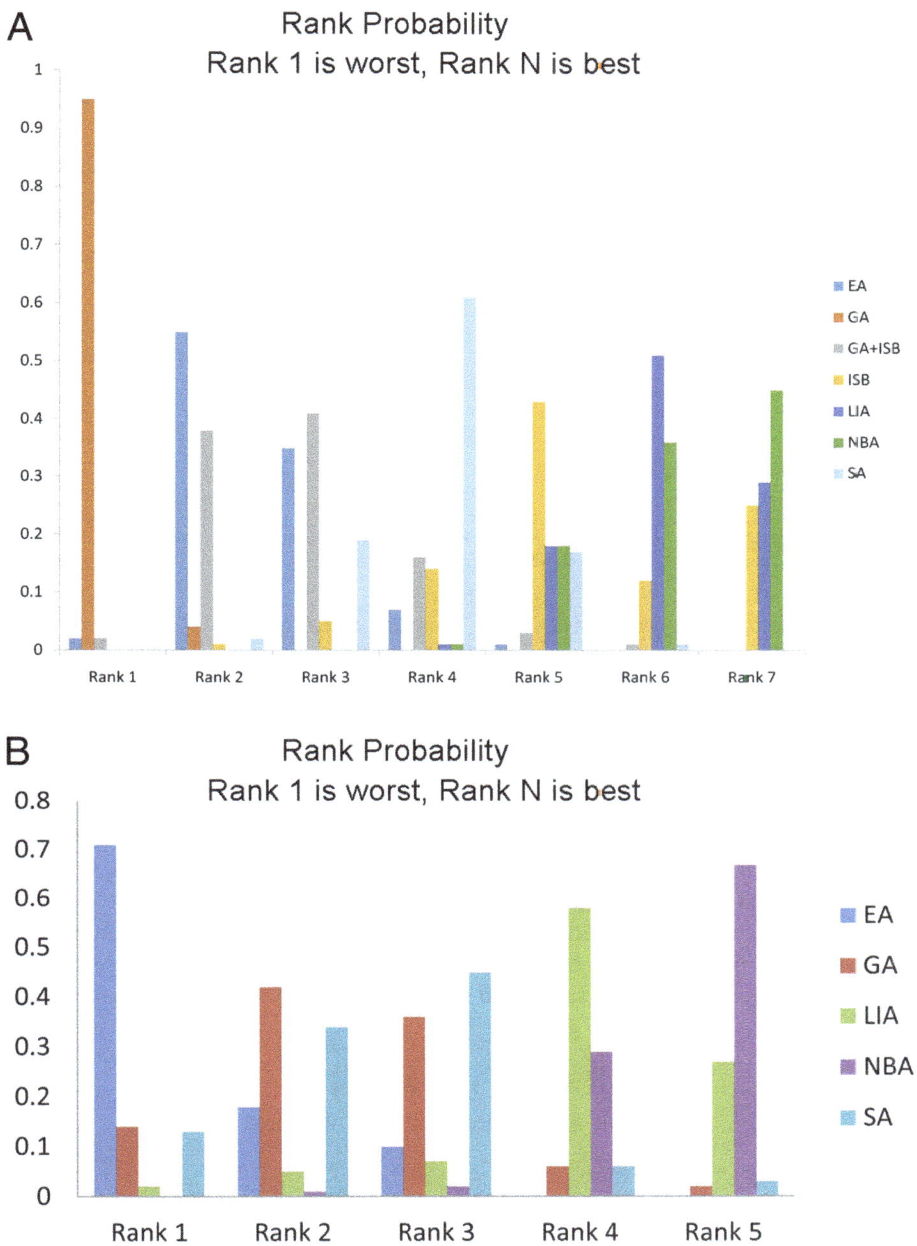

Fig. 2 Network meta-analyses for PONV and urine retention. **a**, Network meta-analyses for PONV; **b**, Network meta-analyses for urine retention. PONV: post-operative nausea or vomiting; GA: general anesthesia; LIA: local infiltration analgesia; ISB: interscalene block; EA: epidural anesthesia; NBA: nerve block analgesia; SA: spinal anesthesia

incidences of back pain; however, no other significant difference was identified in comparison between other groups (Fig. 4A, Table 5A).

Analysis for headache

For back pain, all PSRF values were 1.01, indicating a good convergence. Because no closed ring formed, consistency model was utilized to calculate the pooled side effect of back pain. The network analysis presented that LIA group had the lowest incidence of headache, but no significant difference was revealed compared with other groups (Fig. 4B, Table 5B).

Discussion

According to the selective criteria, a total of 23 studies with 2393 patients were enrolled in this study. With the network meta-analysis, patients undergoing NBA presented lower occurrence rates of PONV and urine

Table 3 Network meta-analyses for PONV and urine retention

A: PONV

EA	2.48 (1.02, 6.55)	0.85 (0.23, 3.54)	0.26 (0.05, 1.17)	0.18 (0.07, 0.41)	0.17 (0.06, 0.39)	0.51 (0.21, 1.29)
0.40 (0.15, 0.98)	GA	0.34 (0.13, 0.97)	0.10 (0.03, 0.36)	0.07 (0.02, 0.17)	0.07 (0.02, 0.18)	0.21 (0.10, 0.42)
1.17 (0.28, 4.42)	2.91 (1.03, 7.79)	GA + ISB	0.29 (0.06, 1.25)	0.20 (0.05, 0.76)	0.19 (0.04, 0.81)	0.59 (0.17, 1.94)
3.81 (0.86, 18.19)	9.67 (2.78, 36.55)	3.42 (0.80, 15.77)	ISB	0.68 (0.14, 3.40)	0.63 (0.11, 3.34)	2.02 (0.48, 8.87)
5.71 (2.44, 14.43)	13.98 (5.74, 40.29)	4.91 (1.32, 21.15)	1.48 (0.29, 7.31)	LIA	0.93 (0.44, 1.87)	2.95 (1.22, 7.69)
6.02 (2.53, 16.79)	15.08 (5.69, 48.64)	5.24 (1.24, 25.69)	1.58 (0.30, 8.71)	1.07 (0.53, 2.26)	NBA	3.22 (1.16, 9.67)
1.97 (0.78, 4.85)	4.82 (2.40, 9.66)	1.69 (0.52, 5.87)	0.49 (0.11, 2.08)	0.34 (0.13, 0.82)	0.31 (0.10, 0.86)	SA

B: Urine retention

EA	0.51 (0.08, 2.38)	0.10 (0.01, 1.18)	0.07 (0.01, 0.37)	0.47 (0.07, 2.37)
1.98 (0.42, 12.43)	GA	0.21 (0.01, 3.65)	0.15 (0.02, 1.36)	0.92 (0.20, 4.18)
9.84 (0.84, 151.97)	4.87 (0.27, 82.03)	LIA	0.71 (0.11, 5.12)	4.34 (0.25, 77.47)
13.36 (2.73, 95.12)	6.83 (0.74, 57.95)	1.41 (0.20, 9.26)	NBA	6.27 (0.77, 51.01)
2.14 (0.42, 15.04)	1.09 (0.24, 4.94)	0.23 (0.01, 3.95)	0.16 (0.02, 1.29)	SA

PONV: post-operative nausea or vomiting; GA: general anesthesia; LIA: local infiltration analgesia; ISB: interscalene block; EA: epidural anesthesia; NBA: nerve block analgesia; SA: spinal anesthesia. Data was presented with odds ratio and 95% confidence interval

retention compared with patients managed with SA, EA, GA, and GA + ISB during the perioperative period of orthopedic surgery. Meanwhile, patients managed with ISB and LIA were presented a significant lower occurrence rate of back pain compared with patients undergoing EA. However, there was no significant difference identified in the occurrence of headache among these groups.

NBA is a common anesthesia method utilized in orthopedic surgery, such as total knee arthroplasty [38], shoulder arthroscopy [39], and hip fracture [40]. It has been revealed that nerve blocks may present some benefits in lower risk of PONV, enhanced pain relief and earlier discharge [41, 42]. Park et al. have demonstrated that interscalene brachial plexus block could significantly reduce the nausea and vomiting, while suprascapular nerve anesthesia and intra-articular local anesthesia can't reduce the nausea and vomiting compared with the non-pain controlled group [43]. Hadzic et al. have identified that NBA can reduce the PONV compared with the general anesthesia for patients undergoing outpatients rotator cuff surgery [44]. During podiatric surgery in children, patients managed with EA present a higher risks for adverse events, including PONV and urine retention [18]. However, a previous meta-analysis has summarized that patients managed with NBA present a

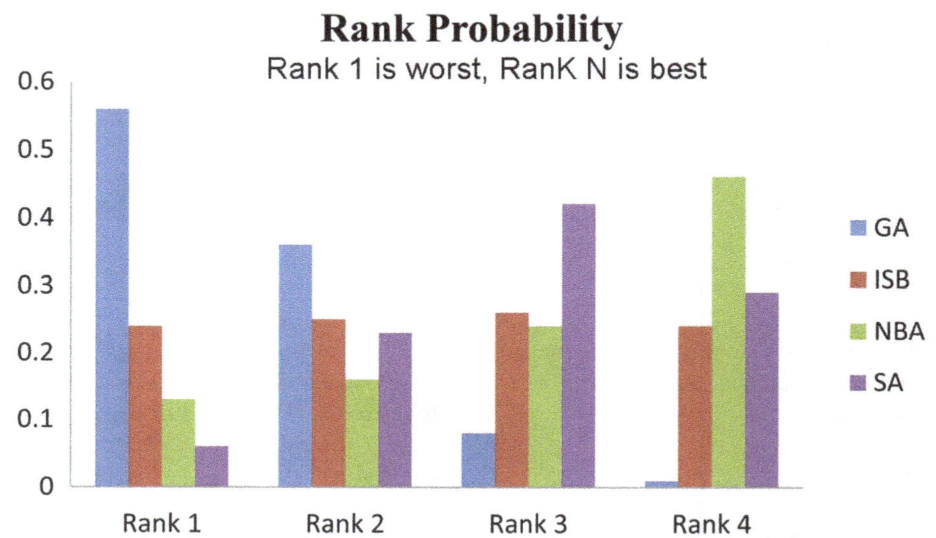

Fig. 3 Network meta-analyses for sore throat. GA: general anesthesia; LIA: local infiltration analgesia; ISB: interscalene block; NBA: nerve block analgesia; SA: spinal anesthesia

Table 4 Network meta-analysis for sore throat

GA	0.18 (0.00, 107.05)	0.05 (0.00, 36.33)	0.09 (0.00, 4.78)
5.43 (0.01, 3647.30)	ISB	0.25 (0.00, 2894.67)	0.48 (0.00, 868.90)
20.89 (0.03, 21,288.40)	3.93 (0.00, 56,736.22)	NBA	1.74 (0.00, 5921.00)
11.51 (0.21, 588.42)	2.09 (0.00, 4009.84)	0.57 (0.00, 1205.54)	SA

GA: general anesthesia; ISB: interscalene block; NBA: nerve block analgesia; SA: spinal anesthesia. Data was presented with odds ratio and 95% confidence interval

lower incidence of urine retention than patients undergoing EA, but there is no difference in the incidence of PONV [45]. With an updated meta-analysis, NBA was identified to put a significant lower effects on the occurrence rates of PONV, urine retention, and sore throat compared with patients managed with SA, EA, GA, and GA + ISB during the perioperative period of orthopedic surgery in the current study. All of these findings indicated that NBA might perform a better outcome on the prognosis of patients undergoing orthopedic surgery.

ISB is one of the most reliable and commonly anesthetic method applied for the upper extremity with less opioid consumption and opioid-associated adverse effect [46]. Meanwhile, LIA is a safety and effective method for pain control during the perioperative periods of knee and hip surgery [47]. In this study, patients managed with ISB and LIA presented a significant lower occurrence rate of back pain compared with patients undergoing EA, indicating that ISB and LIA might play a better outcome for relieving back pain during orthopedic surgery. Adersen et al. have revealed that LIA

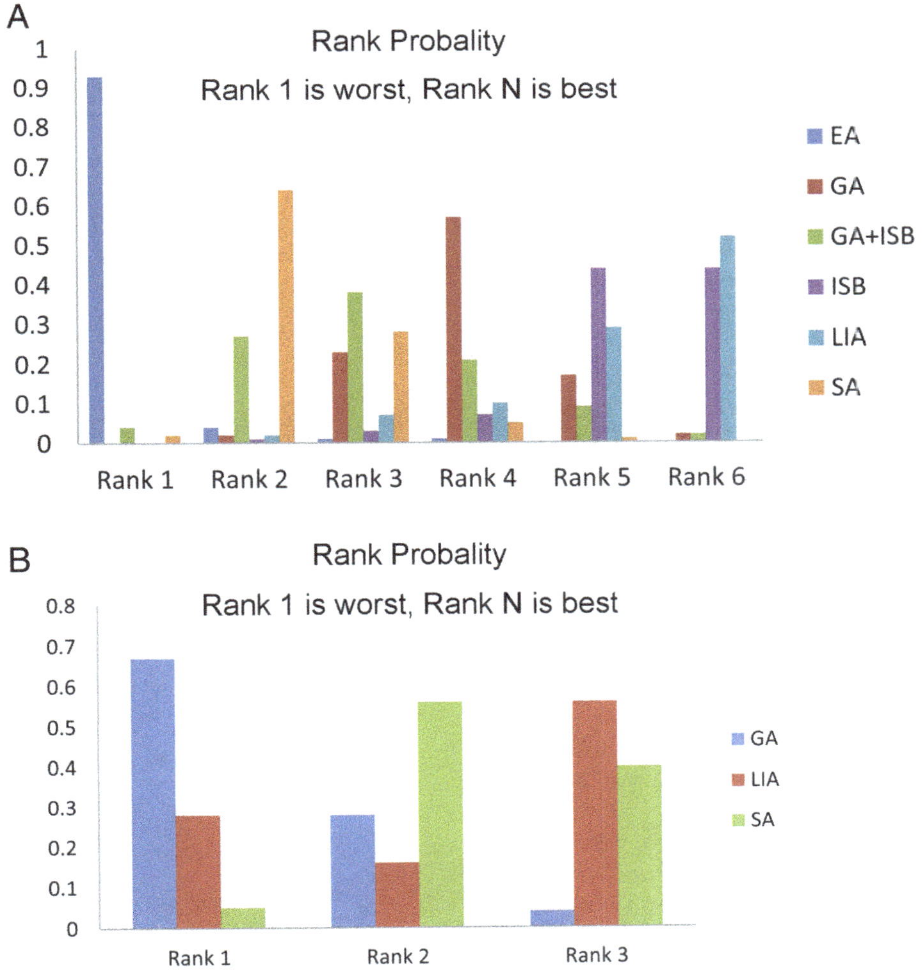

Fig. 4 Network meta-analyses for back pain and headache. **a**, Network meta-analyses for back pain; **b**, Network meta-analyses for headacheGA: general anesthesia; LIA: local infiltration analgesia; ISB: interscalene block; EA: epidural anesthesia; SA: spinal anesthesia.

Table 5 Network meta-analyses for back pain and headache

A: Back pain					
EA	0.02 (0.00, 0.57)	0.04 (0.00, 2.38)	0.00 (0.00, 0.30)	0.00 (0.00, 0.25)	0.06 (0.00, 1.38)
51.32(1.75,3339.72)	GA	1.79 (0.14, 23.31)	0.20 (0.01, 3.35)	0.18 (0.00, 5.98)	2.98 (0.75, 20.40)
27.51(0.42,4086.82)	0.56 (0.04, 7.20)	GA + ISB	0.12 (0.01, 1.81)	0.10 (0.00, 8.09)	1.69 (0.10, 43.87)
267.22(3.36,44,447.31)	4.89 (0.30, 104.69)	8.53 (0.55, 176.80)	ISB	0.82 (0.01, 96.19)	15.26 (0.73, 591.84)
306.91(3.94,62,665.12)	5.69 (0.17, 374.21)	10.33(0.12,1263.02)	1.22 (0.01, 173.76)	LIA	17.27 (0.82, 906.94)
15.74 (0.72, 650.35)	0.34 (0.05, 1.33)	0.59 (0.02, 9.74)	0.07 (0.00, 1.37)	0.06 (0.00, 1.22)	SA
B: Headache					
GA	0.32 (0.00, 25.48)		0.42 (0.10, 1.60)		
3.17 (0.04, 217.06)	LIA		1.39 (0.02, 63.62)		
2.40 (0.63, 10.17)	0.72 (0.02, 55.14)		SA		

GA: general anesthesia; LIA: local infiltration analgesia; ISB: interscalene block; EA: epidural anesthesia; SA: spinal anesthesia. Data was presented with odds ratio and 95% confidence interval

presents a superior outcome with less adverse effect, including pain control, than EA during total knee arthroplasty [48]. Another study has also demonstrated that LIA performs a better outcome in pain controlling during total knee arthroplasty [49]. These findings demonstrated LIA and ISB might perform effective roles in relieving pains, such as back pain, during the perioperative period of orthopedic surgery. Despite of these, LIA was also identified to play critical role in relieving headache during the perioperative period of orthopedic surgery, but no statistically difference was identified compared with other group. Therefore, further investigation with large sample size might be required.

Although this study was the first to compare the effects of different anesthesia methods on the complications of orthopedic surgery, but there were still some limitations in this study. First, due to the incomplete data in studies, correction of concomitant variables was not performed, which might affect the results identified in this study. Meanwhile, the subgroup analysis was also not conducted. Second, limited by the property of ADDIS, the calculation of pooled effect size might be influenced. Third, some complications, such as headache and back pain, were not reported in several anesthesia methods; thus, there might be some bias contained in this study.

Conclusions

In conclusion, according to the network analysis, NBA was a superior anesthesia method in reliving the occurrence of PONV, urine retention, and sore throat compared with patients managed with SA, EA, GA, and GA + ISB during the perioperative period of orthopedic surgery. ISB and LIA were two effective anesthesia methods in lowering the occurrence rate of back pain during the perioperative period of orthopedic surgery. Therefore, it is important to surgeons to select appropriate anesthesia methods during the perioperative period of orthopedic surgery according to the physical fitness of patients and the effects of anesthesia methods on the occurrence of complications.

Abbreviations

CI: confidence interval; EA: epidural anesthesia; ISB: interscalene block; LIA: local infiltration analgesia; NBA: nerve block analgesia; OR: odd ratio; PSRF: potential scale reduction factor; SA: spinal anesthesia

Acknowledgements

Not applicable.

Authors' contributions

YZ, JW and SD conceived the research. HR and JL acquired the data. YZ and FZ performed the statistics analysis. YZ and JW drafted the manuscript. SD revised the manuscript. All authors have read and approved the manuscript.

Author details

[1]The First Clinical Medical College, Guangzhou University of Chinese Medicine, 16 Jichang Road, Baiyun District, Guangzhou 510405, Guangdong Province, People's Republic of China. [2]Department of Orthopaedics, Tongde Hospital of Zhejiang Province, Hangzhou, Zhejiang Province, People's Republic of China. [3]Department of Hematology, The First Affliated Hospital of Zhejiang Chinese Medical University, 54 Youdian Road, Hangzhou, Zhejiang Province, People's Republic of China.

References

1. Waheeb A, Zywiel MG, Palaganas M, Venkataramanan V, Davis AM. The influence of patient factors on patient-reported outcomes of orthopedic surgery involving implantable devices: a systematic review. Seminars in Arthritis & Rheumatism. 2015;44:461–71.
2. Huang F, Wu D, Ma G, Yin Z, Wang Q. The use of tranexamic acid to reduce blood loss and transfusion in major orthopedic surgery: a meta-analysis. Transfusion & Apheresis Science. 2014;186:318–27.
3. Andrade N, Schmiedt CW, Cornell K, Radlinsky MG, Heidingsfelder L, Clarke K, et al. Survey of intraoperative bacterial contamination in dogs undergoing elective orthopedic surgery. Veterinary Surgery Vs. 2016;45:214–22.
4. Veljkovic A, Dwyer T, Lau JT, Abbas KZ, Salat P, Brull R. Neurological complications related to elective orthopedic surgery: part 3: common foot and ankle procedures. Regional Anesthesia & Pain Medicine. 2015;40:455.
5. Hu N, Guo D, Wang H, Xie K, Wang C, Li Y, et al. Involvement of the blood-brain barrier opening in cognitive decline in aged rats following orthopedic surgery and high concentration of sevoflurane inhalation. Brain Res. 2014; 1551:13–24.

6. Safavi M, Honarmand A, Negahban M. Attari M. Prophylactic effects of intrathecal Meperidine and intravenous Ondansetron on shivering in patients undergoing lower extremity orthopedic surgery under spinal anesthesia. 2014;3:94–9.
7. Pugely AJ, Martin CT, Gao Y, Mendozalattes S, Callaghan JJ. Differences in short-term complications between spinal and general anesthesia for primary Total knee arthroplasty. Jbjs. 2013;95:193–9.
8. Helwani MA, Avidan MS, Abdallah AB, Kaiser DJ, Clohisy JC, Hall BL, et al. Effects of regional versus general anesthesia on outcomes after Total hip arthroplasty. J Bone Joint Surg (Am Vol). 2015;97:186–93.
9. Stundner O, Chiu YL, Sun X, Mazumdar M, Fleischut P, Poultsides L, et al. Comparative perioperative outcomes associated with neuraxial versus general anesthesia for simultaneous bilateral total knee arthroplasty. Regional Anesthesia & Pain Medicine. 2012;37:638.
10. Mason SE, Noel-Storr A, Ritchie CW. The impact of general and regional anesthesia on the incidence of post-operative cognitive dysfunction and post-operative delirium: a systematic review with meta-analysis: Centre for Reviews and Dissemination (UK); 2010. 67–79 p.
11. Higgins JE. Cochrane Handbook for Systematic Reviews of Interventions. http://wwwcochrane-handbookorg. 2008; 5: S38.
12. Hillege H, Brock BD, Valkenhoef GV, Zhao J. ADDIS: an automated way to do network meta-analysis. Research Report. 2016.
13. Van Valkenhoef G, Tervonen T, Zwinkels T, De Brock B, Hillege H. ADDIS: a decision support system for evidence-based medicine. Decis Support Syst. 2013;55:459–75.
14. Brooks SP, Gelman A. General methods for monitoring convergence of iterative simulations. Journal of Computational & Graphical Statistics. 1998;7:434–55.
15. Hole A, Terjesen T, Breivik H. Epidural versus general anaesthesia for total hip arthroplasty in elderly patients. Acta Anaesthesiol Scand. 1980;24:279–87.
16. Arcioni R, Palmisani S, Tigano S, Santorsola C, Sauli V, Romanò S, et al. Combined intrathecal and epidural magnesium sulfate supplementation of spinal anesthesia to reduce post-operative analgesic requirements: a prospective, randomized, double-blind, controlled trial in patients undergoing major orthopedic surgery. Acta Anaesthesiol Scand. 2007;51: 482–9.
17. Bigler D, Adelhøj B, Petring OU, Pederson NO, Busch P, Kalhke P. Mental function and morbidity after acute hip surgery during spinal and general anaesthesia. Anaesthesia. 1985;40:672–6.
18. Dadure C, Bringuier S, Nicolas F, Bromilow L, Raux O, Rochette A, et al. Continuous epidural block versus continuous popliteal nerve block for postoperative pain relief after major podiatric surgery in children: a prospective, comparative randomized study. Anesth Analg. 2006;102:744.
19. Dunn WR, Cordasco FA, Flynn E, Jules K, Gordon M, Liguori G. A prospective randomized comparison of spinal versus local anesthesia with Propofol infusion for knee arthroscopy. Arthroscopy the Journal of Arthroscopic & Related Surgery. 2006;22:479–83.
20. Gi E, Yamauchi M, Yamakage M, Kikuchi C, Shimizu H, Okada Y, et al. Effects of local infiltration analgesia for posterior knee pain after total knee arthroplasty: comparison with sciatic nerve block. J Anesth. 2014;28:696–701.
21. Hadzic A, Arliss J, Kerimoglu B, Karaca PE, Yufa M, Claudio RE, et al. A comparison of infraclavicular nerve block versus general anesthesia for hand and wrist day-case surgeries. Anesthesiology. 2004;101:127–32.
22. Hadzic A, Williams BA, Karaca PE, Hobeika P, Unis G, Dermksian J, et al. For outpatient rotator cuff surgery, nerve block anesthesia provides superior same-day recovery over general anesthesia. Anesthesiology. 2005;102:1001–7.
23. Janssen H, Stosch RV, Pöschl R, Büttner B, Bauer M, Hinz JM, et al. Blood pressure response to combined general anaesthesia/interscalene brachial plexus block for outpatient shoulder arthroscopy. BMC Anesthesiol. 2014;14:50.
24. Karaarslan S, Tekgül ZT. E Ş, Turan M, Karaman Y, Kaya A, et al. Comparison Between Ultrasonography-Guided Popliteal Sciatic Nerve Block and Spinal Anesthesia for Hallux Valgus Repair. 2015;37.
25. Krobbuaban B, Kumkeaw S, Pakdeesirivong N, Diregpoke S. Comparison of postanesthetic complaints after general and spinal anesthesia in patients undergoing lower limb surgery. Journal of the medical Association of Thailand =. Chotmaihet thangphaet. 2005;88:909.
26. Kuchálik J, Granath B, Ljunggren A, Magnuson A, Lundin A, Gupta A. Postoperative pain relief after total hip arthroplasty: a randomized, double-blind comparison between intrathecal morphine and local infiltration analgesia. Br J Anaesth. 2013;111:793–9.
27. Kudoh A, Takase H, Takazawa T. A comparison of anesthetic quality in propofol-spinal anesthesia and propofol-fentanyl anesthesia for total knee arthroplasty in elderly patients. J Clin Anesth. 2004;16:405.
28. Lehmann LJ, Loosen G, Weiss C, Schmittner MD. Interscalene plexus block versus general anaesthesia for shoulder surgery: a randomized controlled study. European Journal of Orthopaedic Surgery & Traumatology. 2015;25:255.
29. Mclaren AD, Stockwell MC, Reid VT. Anaesthetic techniques for surgical correction of fractured neck of femur. A comparative study of spinal and general anaesthesia in the elderly. Anaesthesia. 1978;33:10–4.
30. Nagafuchi M, Sato T, Sakuma T, Uematsu A, Hayashi H. Tanikawa H, et al. Femoral nerve block-sciatic nerve block vs femoral nerve block-local infiltration analgesia for total knee arthroplasty: a randomized controlled trial Bmc Anesthesiology. 2015;15:182.
31. Seeberger MD, Lang ML, Drewe J, Schneider M, Hauser E, Hruby J. Comparison of spinal and epidural anesthesia for patients younger than 50 years of age. Anesth Analg. 1994;78:667–73.
32. Standl T, Eckert S, Schulteam EJ. Postoperative complaints after spinal and thiopentone-isoflurane anaesthesia in patients undergoing orthopaedic surgery. Spinal versus general anaesthesia. Acta Anaesthesiol Scand. 1996;40:222–6.
33. Tanikawa H, Sato T, Nagafuchi M, Takeda K, Oshida J, Okuma K. Comparison of local infiltration of analgesia and sciatic nerve block in addition to femoral nerve block for total knee arthroplasty. J Arthroplasty. 2014;29:2462–7.
34. Türker G, Uçkunkaya N, Yavaşcaoğlu B, Yilmazlar A, Ozçelik S. Comparison of the catheter-technique psoas compartment block and the epidural block for analgesia in partial hip replacement surgery. Acta Anaesthesiol Scand. 2010;47:30–6.
35. Wang H, Ma L, Yang D, Wang T, Wang Q, Zhang L, et al. Cervical plexus anesthesia versus general anesthesia for anterior cervical discectomy and fusion surgery: a randomized clinical trial. Medicine. 2017;96:e6119.
36. Yukawa Y, Kato F, Ito K, Terashima T, Horie Y. A prospective randomized study of preemptive analgesia for postoperative pain in the patients undergoing posterior lumbar interbody fusion: continuous subcutaneous morphine, continuous epidural morphine and diclofenac sodium. Spine. 2005;30:2357.
37. Spangehl MJ, Clarke HD, Hentz JG, Misra L, Blocher JL, Seamans DP. The Chitranjan Ranawat Award: Periarticular Injections and Femoral & Sciatic Blocks Provide Similar Pain Relief After TKA: A Randomized Clinical Trial. Clinical Orthopaedics and Related Research®. 2015; 473: 45–53.
38. Ng FY, Chiu KY, Yan CH, Ng KF. Continuous femoral nerve block versus patient-controlled analgesia following total knee arthroplasty. J Orthop Surg. 2012;20:23.
39. Chang KV, Hung CY, Wu WT, Han DS, Yang RS, Lin CP. Comparison of the effectiveness of suprascapular nerve block with physical therapy, placebo, and intra-articular injection in Management of Chronic Shoulder Pain- a meta-analysis of randomized controlled trials. Archives of Physical Medicine & Rehabilitation. 2015;97:1366–80.
40. Beaudoin FL, Haran JP, Liebmann O. A comparison of ultrasound-guided three-in-one femoral nerve block versus parenteral opioids alone for analgesia in emergency department patients with hip fractures: a randomized controlled trial. Acad Emerg Med. 2013;20:584–91.
41. Junger A, Klasen J, Benson M, Sciuk G, Hartmann B, Sticher J, et al. Factors determining length of stay of surgical day-case patients. Eur J Anaesthesiol. 2001;18:314–21.
42. Chung F, Ritchie E, Su J. Postoperative pain in ambulatory surgery. Anesth Analg. 1997;85:808–16.
43. Park SK, Choi YS, Choi SW, Song SW. A comparison of three methods for postoperative pain control in patients undergoing arthroscopic shoulder surgery. Korean J Pain. 2015;28:45–51.
44. Hadzic MDPDA, Arliss MDJ, Kerimoglu MDB, Karaca MD Pelin E, Yufa MDM, Claudio BS,Richard E, et al. A comparison of Infraclavicular nerve block versus general anesthesia for hand and wrist day-case surgeries. Anesthesiology. 2004; 101: 127–132.
45. Fowler SJ, Symons J, Sabato S, Myles PS. Epidural analgesia compared with peripheral nerve blockade after major knee surgery: a systematic review and meta-analysis of randomized trials. Br J Anaesth. 2008;100:154–64.
46. McNaught A, Shastri U, Carmichael N, Awad IT, Columb M, Cheung J, et al. Ultrasound reduces the minimum effective local anaesthetic volume compared with peripheral nerve stimulation for interscalene block. British Journal of Anaesthesia. 106: 124–130.

47. Kerr DR, Kohan L. Local infiltration analgesia: a technique for the control of acute postoperative pain following knee and hip surgery: a case study of 325 patients. Acta Orthop. 2008;79:174–83.
48. Andersen KV, Bak M, Christensen BV, Harazuk J, Pedersen NA, Søballe K. A randomized, controlled trial comparing local infiltration analgesia with epidural infusion for total knee arthroplasty. Acta Orthop. 2010;81:606–10.
49. Spreng UJ, Dahl V, Hjall A, Fagerland MW, Ræder J. High-volume local infiltration analgesia combined with intravenous or local ketorolac +morphine compared with epidural analgesia after total knee arthroplasty. Br J Anaesth. 2010;105:675–82.

4

Ice versus lidocaine 5% gel for topical anaesthesia of oral mucosa

Nishma Hindocha[1], Filip Manhem[2], Emmanuel Bäckryd[3] and Mats Bågesund[4*]

Abstract

Background: Topical anaesthesia is important to optimize pain control during dental injection. Our aim was to describe a new simple method for topical anaesthesia of oral mucosa and to compare the effectiveness of ice and lidocaine 5% gel for topical anaesthesia of oral mucosa.

Methods: A total of 40 patients aged 10.7–19.5 years were included. The side and method of application were both randomized. Heart rate was recorded, and discomfort and pain were evaluated with a visual analogue scale (VAS). A paired t-test was used to compare mean values, a chi^2 test was used to compare proportions, and a Pearson correlation test was used to examine correlations between variables.

Results: When ice was used, buccal injection VAS pain was rated lower ($p = 0.044$), and VAS discomfort was rated higher ($p = 0.001$), in comparison to when lidocaine 5% gel was used. There was no significant difference in relative heart rate change between ice and lidocaine 5% gel at either needle stick or injection. Lidocaine 5% gel produced a relative heart rate reduction after palatal injection (0.99 ± 0.06) while buccal injection produced an increased relative heart rate (1.02 ± 0.08) ($p = 0.010$). Unpleasant taste was more frequently reported when lidocaine 5% gel was used ($p = 0.025$). An application time of 1 min was sufficient for both ice and lidocaine 5% gel to achieve pain reduction from needle stick in buccal mucosa.

Conclusion: The cheap and readily available described method using ice for topical anaesthesia of oral mucosa before dental injection is an effective alternative to lidocaine 5% gel.

Keywords: Administration, Topical, Anaesthesia, Ice, Lidocaine

Background

Despite the continuous development of new dental injection techniques, the injection of local anaesthesia still causes discomfort and pain for many patients and has been described as a major reason for dental anxiety [1–3]. Topical anaesthesia should therefore be used to eliminate or minimize the pain caused by the needle.

Topical anaesthetic gels are common in dentistry [4], but studies have shown varying results on their effects. Topical anaesthesia does not guarantee completely pain-free injections, and the efficacy is dependent on several factors such as time (injection speed) and gauge size of the needle [5]. Some authors have stated that lidocaine 5% gel only relieves pain caused by the needle insertion, but not the pain caused by the actual injection, unless a 10-min period has passed since administration of topical anaesthesia [6]. There are even studies questioning whether topical anaesthesia has any effect on pain during either needle insertion or injection [7].

The methods used today for topical anaesthesia before dental injections mainly include different types of gel (e.g. lidocaine, prilocaine or benzocaine). Unfortunately, these gels have a tendency to spread in the mouth due

* Correspondence: mats.bagesund@regionostergotland.se
[4]Centre for Orthodontics and Paediatric Dentistry, Norrköping, Public Dental Service Östergötland, Region Östergötland, and Department of Biomedical and Clinical Sciences, Linköping University, Linköping, Sweden

to lack of bioadhesion, which may result in a reduced anaesthetic effect [8], unpleasant taste, and/or discomfort for the patient [9]. Furthermore, there is a risk of allergic reactions to several components in the different gels available for topical anaesthesia [10]. These factors are important reasons for developing and evaluating other substances and techniques for topical anaesthesia.

Ice was introduced during the nineteenth century as a safe method of local anaesthesia [11], and the use of cooling for reduction of injection pain in the skin is well documented. However, published studies evaluating ice as topical anaesthesia in dentistry are very rare [12]. One study from 1989 described how ice on the palate before and during local infiltration anaesthesia could relieve discomfort, but did not compare ice with other agents for topical anaesthesia [13]. Another study found that cooling increased the efficacy of conventional topical anaesthesia, but did not evaluate ice as the only topical anaesthetic agent [14]. Thus, ice as topical anaesthesia of the oral mucosa is not an established method in dentistry today [12].

Several explanations for the anaesthetic effect of cooling have been proposed [15]. Topical cold application would for instance stimulate myelinated A fibers, thereby activating inhibitory pain pathways [16], perhaps as part of the gate control system at the spinal cord level [15]. Furthermore, cooling causes cold-induced neuropraxia by decreasing the activation threshold of tissue nociceptors and the conduction velocity of nerve signals conveying pain [17, 18].

The aim of this study was to describe a new simple method for topical anaesthesia of oral mucosa and to compare the anaesthetic effect and subjective experience of two topical anaesthetic agents, lidocaine 5% gel and ice, applied on the oral mucosa prior to needle stick and injection of local anaesthesia.

Methods

The study was approved by the Regional Ethical Review Board in Linköping (ref: 2013/315–31 – December 11th, 2013) and the Swedish Medical Products Agency (EudraCT no: 2013–005305-31 - date of registration of TRN: February 10th, 2014) before the start of the clinical investigations, and the process was monitored by Forum Östergötland, Linköping, Sweden. Our study adheres to the CONSORT guidelines (http://www.consort-statement.org/) for reporting clinical trials.

The clinical part of the study (data collection) was performed by two general dentists at a public dental clinic from August 2014 to August 2017.

Inclusion criteria

Healthy patients (ASA 1; see [19]), who were aged under 20 years, did not express any dental fear, and were planned for orthodontic treatment including extractions of two contralateral maxillary premolars without pathology, were invited to participate in the study. Participants as well as their legal guardians (for those aged under 18) had to be positive to participate in the study.

Exclusion criteria

Patients were excluded if they had any medical conditions considered to affect patient safety or the quality of the study, or if they had any known hypersensitivity to local anaesthetics of amide type or any of the other contents in the substance used. If the study protocol was not followed in a way that made it impossible to compare the anaesthetic effect and subjective experience of the two topical anaesthetic agents according to the aim of the study, the patient was excluded from the study. Patients without written consent signed by themselves and by both parents/guardians were excluded. If a patient or parent/guardian denied further participation the patient was immediately excluded from the study without any further questions.

Information and consent

The orthodontist referred the patients, who were positive to participate, to the principal investigator (PI). All patients, who were suitable according to the inclusion and exclusion criteria, received a phone call from the PI, who informed them further about the study and asked if they were willing to participate in the study. Patients and guardians were informed that they had the right to discontinue their participation in the study at any time and for any reason without having to motivate their decision, and that not participating, or leaving the study, would not influence the remaining or planned treatment. They also received verbal and written information about the study and were encouraged to ask questions about it. If they decided to participate in the trial, they had to bring a consent form to the first treatment session, signed by both the patient and, when applicable, by the legal guardians.

First appointment

At the first visit, the PI verified that the patient and the legal guardians (when applicable) had received and understood the information given and that they had given their consent to participate in the study. A set of envelopes numbered consecutively by a statistician according to inclusion in the study was used to conduct the randomisation in blocks of four. Before starting the procedure, an envelope was opened to see which side of the maxilla (right or left) and which topical anaesthesia (lidocaine 5% gel or ice) to use at the first and second appointment, respectively.

The procedure for each treatment session is presented in Fig. 1. A pulse oximeter (Contec PM60A, Contec Medical Systems, Qinhuangdao, China) was applied to the patient's left index finger.

Technique for application of topical anaesthetics

The oral mucosa was dried with a cotton roll before application of the topical anaesthesia. Application of 0.2 mL lidocaine 5% gel (Apoteket, Stockholm, Sweden) was performed with a cotton roll on the oral mucosa (Fig. 2). Ice was prepared by filling a 2.5 ml plastic syringe (BD Plastipak, 2 ml, Ref 300,185, Becton Dickinson, San Agustín del Guadalix, Madrid, Spain) with tap water and freezing it in a freezer at the clinic. The ice temperature was between – 4 °C and 0 °C to avoid any risk of frostbite. Before administration, the tip of the plastic syringe was cut off with a scalpel (Figs. 3 and 4), allowing the ice to be pressed out on the mucosa while it melted (Figs. 5 and 6). The patient answered the questionnaire (Table 1) after each sequence of the study (Fig. 1).

Buccal evaluation

The effect of the topical anaesthesia on the buccal site was evaluated with a 1 mm deep needle stick (with a 30-gauge ½ inch short needle) apically of the tooth, without bone contact, for 1 s at 1, 2.5, and 5 min, counted from when the topical anaesthesia was first applied to the mucosa. Injection of 1.5 ml Xylocain Dental Adrenalin 20 mg/ml lidocaine + 12.5 micrograms/ml adrenaline (AstraZeneca, Södertälje, Sweden) was performed with the same 30-gauge ½ inch short hypodermic needle applied to The Wand (Milestone Scientific, Livingston, NJ, USA), 5 min after application of topical anaesthesia. The injection was performed with the lowest possible injection speed for The Wand. Pain was graded by the patient on a 100 mm visual analogue scale (VAS) after each stick and after each injection (Table 1). Discomfort was also graded on a VAS scale after injection. The patients reported if there was any irritation in the mucosa, and graded the taste of the topical anaesthesia on a five-point Likert scale (Table 1).

Palatal evaluation

Topical anaesthesia was not applied to the palatal mucosa until after the injection and evaluation of the buccal side was completed, and was only evaluated after the injection, which was performed 3 min after application of the topical anaesthesia (Fig. 1). The patient answered the same questions for the palatal side as for the buccal side, with the exception of the three needle sticks, since they were not performed on the palatal side (Table 1, Fig. 1).

Heart rate

Heart rate (HR) in beats per minute (bpm) was registered by the treating clinician at baseline and before and after each needle stick on the buccal side, and after injection on the buccal and palatal side (Fig. 1). The relative HR change (HR immediately after each intervention divided by HR immediately before each intervention) was used for evaluation of HR change during each intervention (insertion or injection).

After these steps, the premolar was extracted, but the extraction procedure was not evaluated in the study. One week after each treatment, the PI called the patient to ask if there had been any unexpected side effects (Table 2).

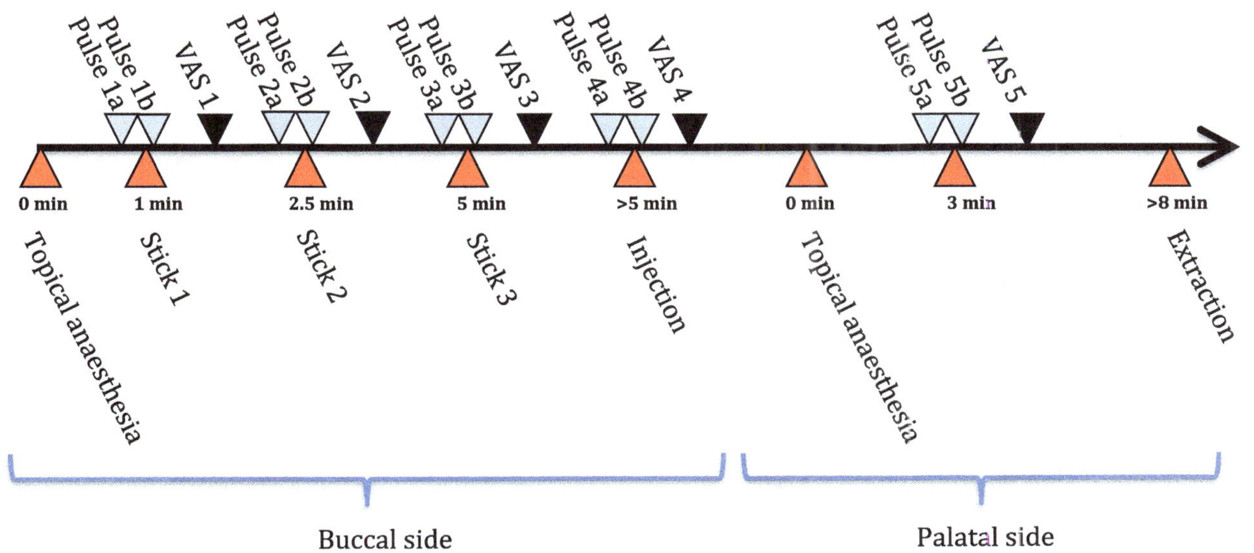

Fig. 1 Flow chart describing the time schedule at each visit. Visual analogue scale (VAS) was used for evaluation of pain and discomfort according to the questionnaire presented in Table 1

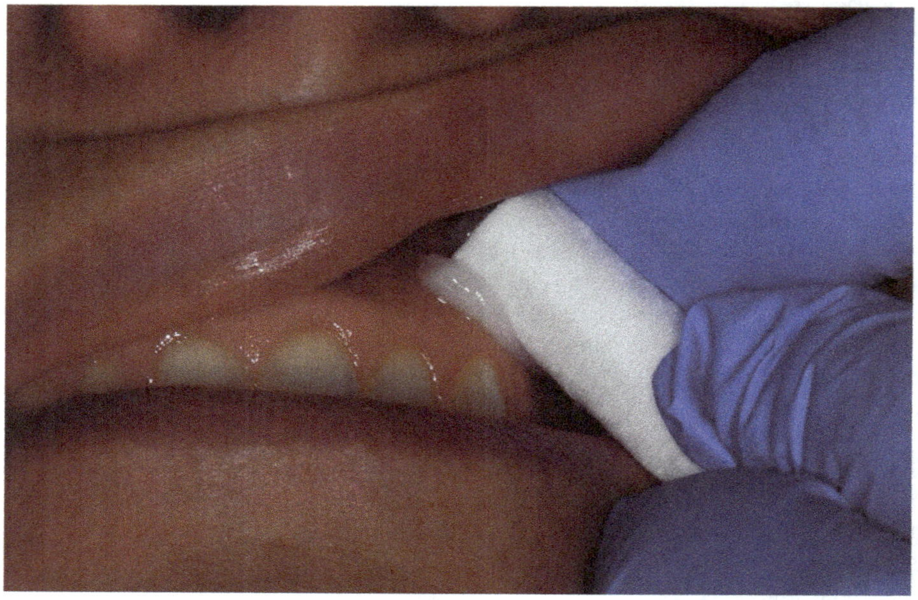

Fig. 2 Lidocaine 5% gel applied on the buccal mucosa

Second appointment

The second appointment was not performed until all symptoms and possible side effects from the first treatment had definitely subsided. A minimum time of 2 weeks between the extractions was applied, to ensure that no confounding pain from the first extraction persisted at the second visit. At the second appointment, the mucosa at the contralateral maxillary premolar was treated with the topical anaesthesia (lidocaine 5% gel or ice) that had not been used at the first appointment. The same protocol was followed for the second appointment. One week after the second treatment, the PI made another phone call to ask about any unexpected side effects of the treatment. This

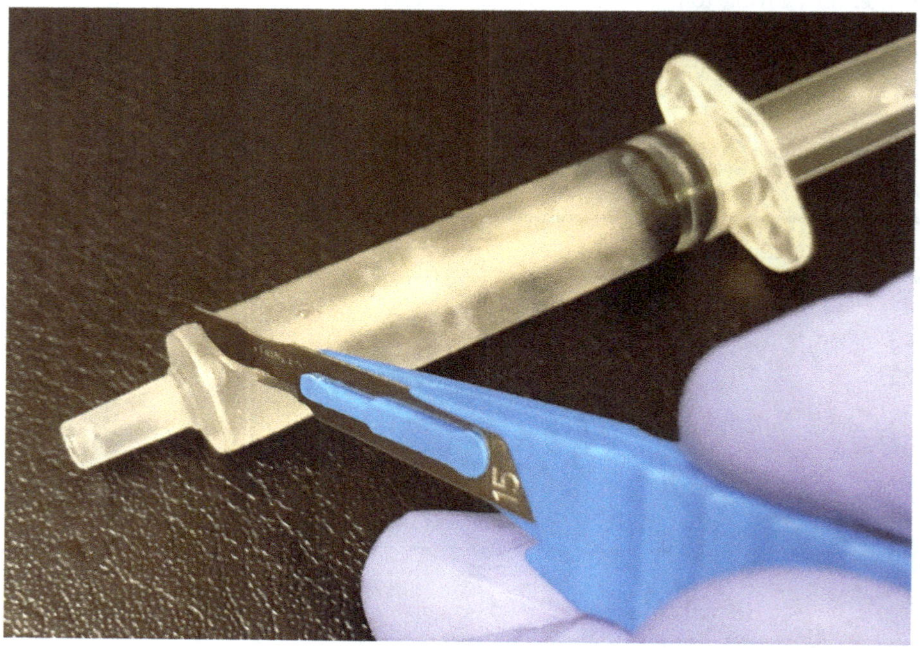

Fig. 3 The 2.5 ml syringe was filled with ordinary tap water which was frozen at the clinic. A scalpel was used to cut off the tip of the syringe

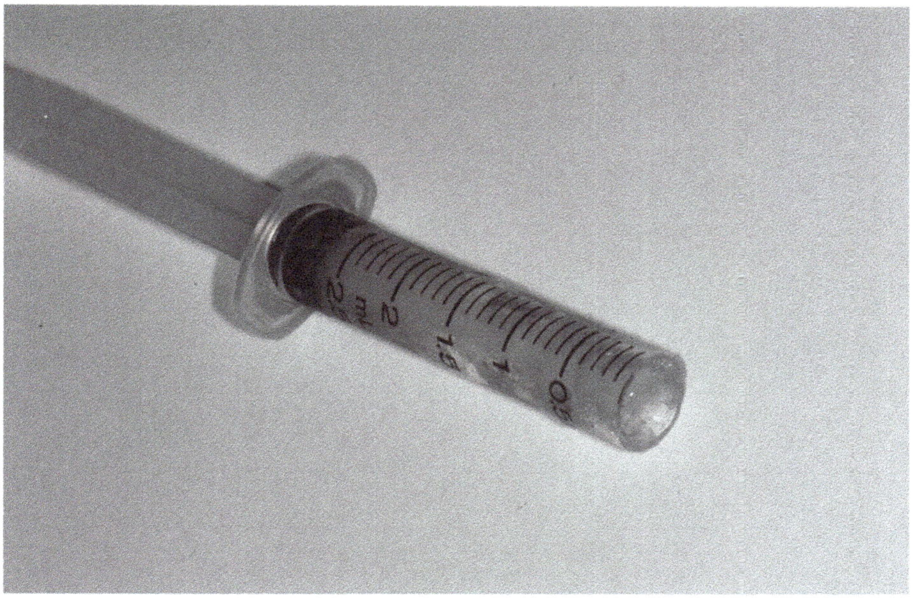

Fig. 4 Ice-filled syringe after cutting off the tip

phone call completed the patient's participation in the study (Table 2).

Statistical methods

The primary outcome was whether ice and lidocaine had similar effects on subjective pain according to the VAS, with effects being considered similar if the mean ± standard deviation (SD) difference, δ, between the methods was 4 ± 6 mm or less. A statistical power calculation based on previous results concluded that 40 patients would be needed to achieve 80% power to detect the primary outcome at the 0.05 level of significance when

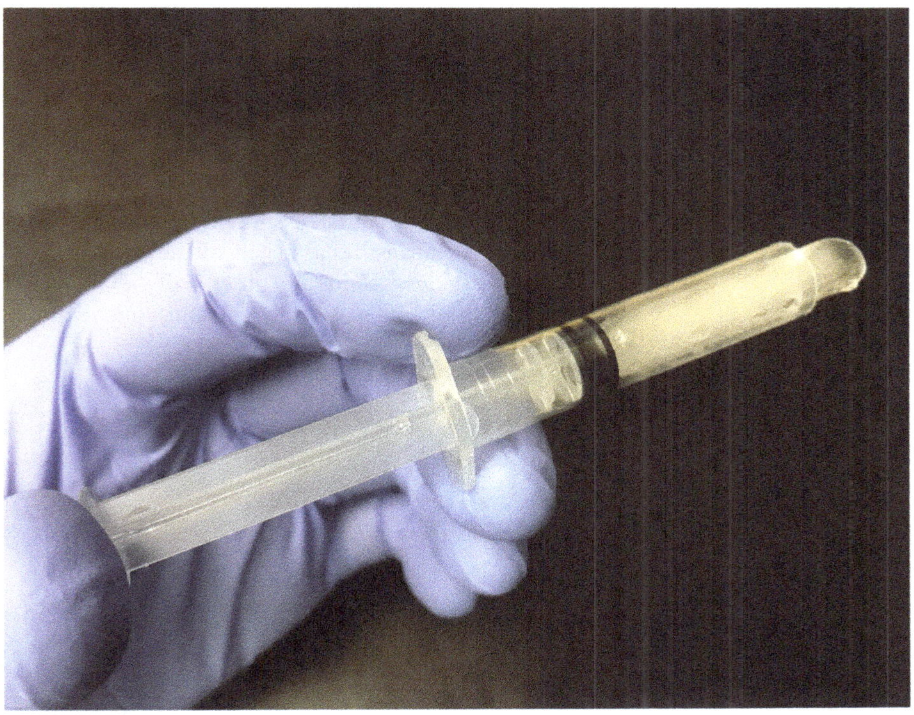

Fig. 5 The ice-filled applicator in the hand of the operator

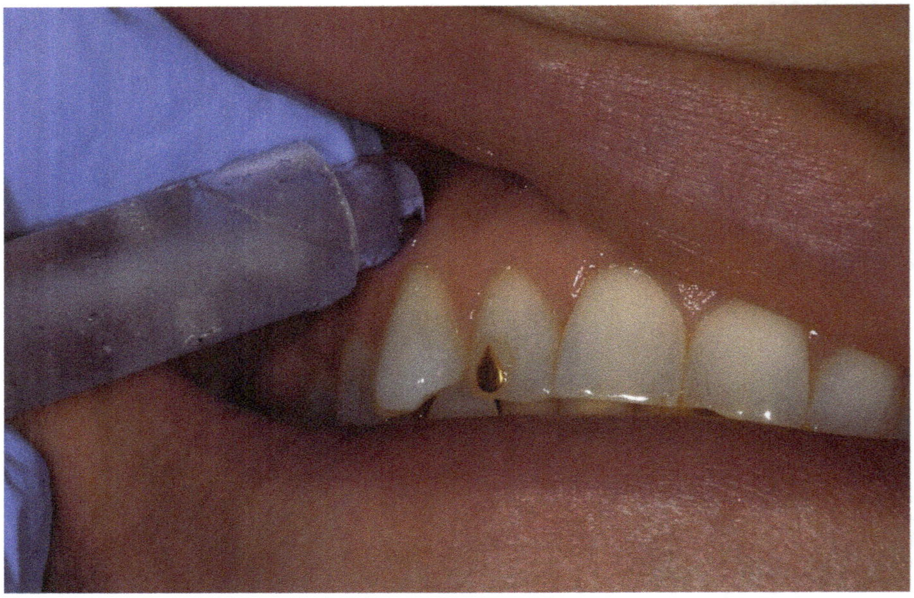

Fig. 6 Ice applied on the buccal mucosa

using the paired t-test to compare mean values. Paired t-test was used for evaluation of repeated measures, a chi^2 test was used for comparison of proportions, and a Pearson correlation test was used for analysis of correlation between variables. Unless stated otherwise, data are expressed as mean ± SD.

Results

Data were collected from 5 August 2014 to 30 August 2016. Of the 42 patients who agreed to participate, one was excluded because the same topical anaesthesia was accidentally used at both visits, and another was excluded because written consent could not be obtained from one of their parents. The remaining 40 (19 M, 21F) participants had an mean age of 15.6 ± 2.2 years (range: 10.7–19.5) when they entered the study. None of the participating patients or guardians denied further participation after entering the study. The HR change measurements from 13 (6 M, 7F) patients could not be evaluated since they only included pulse at the beginning of each visit and measurements *after* each intervention (insertion or injection), but not immediately *before* each intervention. HR change (from before to after each insertion and injection, respectively) could therefore only be evaluated in 27 (13 M, 14F) of the patients.

The first treatment was performed with ice as topical anaesthesia in half of the patients ($n = 20$) and lidocaine 5% gel in the other half ($n = 20$). None of the participants were smokers, and none expressed any dental fear.

Table 1 Questions answered by the patient, following the flowchart presented in Fig. 1. For evaluation of the palatal site, only questions 4–9 were used

1. How painful was the needle stick at 1 min?[a]
2. How painful was the needle stick at 2.5 min?[a]
3. How painful was the needle stick at 5 min?[a]
4. How painful was the injection?[a]
5. How did the topical anaesthesia feel?[b]
6. What's your opinion of the taste of the topical anaesthesia?[c]
7. Did you feel any discomfort or irritation in the area treated with topical anaesthesia?[d]
8. If you answered yes to Question 7, please describe what you felt.
9. Please write something more about what you thought of the pre-treatment with gel or ice.

[a]Answered on a 100 mm visual analogue scale (VAS) with the extremes 'no pain' and 'worst possible pain'
[b]Answered on a 100 mm VAS with the extremes 'no discomfort' and 'worst possible discomfort'
[c]Answered with the alternatives 'very good', 'good', 'no taste', 'bad', 'very bad'
[d]Answered with the alternatives 'yes' or 'no'

Table 2 Actions performed before, during, and after each visit

Visit no:	1[a]		2		3	
Phone call no:		1		2		3
Verbal information	X	X				
Informed consent			X			
Patient history	X					
Inclusion and exclusion criteria	X		X			
Randomization			X			
Treatment			X		X	
Registration of possible adverse events			X	X	X	X

[a]Performed at the orthodontic clinic

VAS ratings

The VAS ratings at the different interventions following application of ice and lidocaine 5% gel are presented in Table 3. When ice was used, buccal VAS pain at 2.5 min was rated higher ($p = 0.016$), buccal injection pain was rated lower ($p = 0.044$), and VAS discomfort was rated higher ($p = 0.001$), in comparison to when lidocaine was used. Palatal VAS data did not differ between the two methods (Table 3).

When comparing VAS pain ratings following needle insertion at different times after application of the topical anaesthesia, there were no differences between ratings at 1 min (ice: 9.7 ± 9.2; gel: 8.5 ± 9.6) and at 2.5 min (ice: 11.8 ± 9.4; gel: 7.3 ± 10.4) for either ice ($p = 0.168$) or lidocaine 5% gel ($p = 0.382$). Similarly, there were no differences between ratings at 1 min and at 5 min (ice: 11.8 ± 13.7; gel: 8.2 ± 7.5) for either ice ($p = 0.242$) or gel ($p = 0.832$).

VAS pain ratings were higher for the palatal injection (ice: 19.1 ± 11.0; gel: 21.4) than for the buccal injection (ice: 12.4 ± 10.6; gel: 16.4 ± 14.5), and according to the paired t-test the difference was significant both when ice was used ($p = 0.000$) and when lidocaine 5% gel was used ($p = 0.008$). When ice was used, the VAS discomfort rating was higher ($p = 0.011$) following buccal injection (9.5 ± 10.7) than following injection on the palatal site (6.5 ± 8.5). When lidocaine 5% gel was used, there was no difference in discomfort between buccal and palatal injection.

There were no correlations between age and either VAS pain or VAS discomfort.

For treatment on the buccal site, a significantly higher proportion of patients ($p = 0.025$; chi^2 test) reported a bad or very bad taste when lidocaine 5% gel was used ($n = 7$; 17.5%) than when ice was used ($n = 1$; 2.5%). The situation was similar on the palatal site, with a significantly higher ($p = 0.018$; chi^2 test) proportion of patients reporting a bad or very bad taste when lidocaine was used ($n = 14$; 35%) than when ice was used ($n = 5$; 12%).

There were no gender differences regarding the prevalence of a bad or very bad taste for either the ice or the gel on the buccal or palatal site. There were also no significant gender differences in VAS ratings, except that girls' VAS pain ratings following injection were higher than boys' for both the buccal (girls: 15.7 ± 13.1; boys: 12.9 ± 12.4; $p = 0.004$) and palatal (girls: 23.1 ± 13.1; boys: 17.2 ± 11.4; $p = 0.032$) sites.

None of the VAS ratings regarding pain, discomfort, or taste differed significantly between the first and second visit.

Heart rate

The initial HR at the start of the first visit was 83 ± 15 bpm and did not differ significantly ($p = 0.14$) between girls (86 ± 15 bpm) and boys (79 ± 13 bpm); it also did not differ significantly ($p = 0.417$) from the initial HR at the second visit (80 ± 15 bpm). There was a negative (Pearson) correlation ($p = 0.001$) between baseline pulse at first visit and age ($r = -0.50$).

The relative HR change at intervention did not differ between lidocaine 5% gel and ice at any of the interventions (insertion of needle or injection) (Table 4).

There was no significant difference ($p = 0.636$) between the relative HR change following injection on the buccal (1.00 ± 0.07) and palatal side (0.99 ± 0.07) following application of ice, while the application of lidocaine 5% gel resulted in a HR change significantly different ($p = 0.010$; paired t-test) between palatal and buccal site, with a relative reduction after palatal injection (0.99 ± 0.06) as compared to a relative increase after buccal injection (1.02 ± 0.08).

Comments from patients

Of the 30 patients who wrote comments in their final questionnaire, seven found the two methods similar, eight preferred the lidocaine 5% gel, and 15 preferred the ice. The preferred method was not correlated with

Table 3 VAS ratings after the different interventions (needle insertion and injection) following application of ice and lidocaine 5% gel ($n = 40$)

Intervention/variable measured (application time)	Ice mean ± SD (mm)	Lidocaine 5% gel mean ± SD (mm)	Paired *t*-test (*p*-value)
VAS pain buccal needle insertion (1 min)	9.7 ± 9.2	8.5 ± 9.6	0.469
VAS pain buccal needle insertion (2.5 min)	11.8 ± 9.4	7.3 ± 10.4	0.016
VAS pain buccal needle insertion (5 min)	11.8 ± 13.7	8.2 ± 7.5	0.079
VAS pain buccal injection	12.4 ± 10.6	16.4 ± 14.5	0.044
VAS discomfort buccal injection	9.6 ± 10.7	3.7 ± 3.7	0.001
VAS pain palatal injection	19.1 ± 11.0	21.4 ± 14.17	0.252
VAS discomfort palatal injection	6.5 ± 8.5	5.9 ± 9.1	0.633

Table 4. Relative heart rate change (heart rate immediately after each intervention divided by heart rate immediately before each intervention) during each intervention (insertion or injection) following application of ice or lidocaine 5% gel ($n = 27$)

Intervention/variable measured (application time)	Ice mean ± SD	Lidocaine 5% gel mean ± SD	Paired *t*-test (*p*-value)
HR change buccal needle insertion (1 min)	0.99 ± 0.04	0.98 ± 0.04	0.665
HR change buccal needle insertion (2.5 min)	0.99 ± 0.06	1.00 ± 0.04	0.506
HR change buccal needle insertion (5 min)	1.00 ± 0.07	1.00 ± 0.04	0.706
HR change buccal injection	1.00 ± 0.07	1.02 ± 0.08	0.210

HR heart rate

the method used at the last appointment. One of the patients who found no difference between the two methods did comment that the ice resulted in more water in the mouth. Five patients, all of whom preferred ice to gel, commented on a bad taste. Four patients found the ice more comfortable than the gel. One said that the treatment time felt shorter when ice was used. Better anaesthetic effect was mentioned by four patients who preferred the lidocaine 5% gel and three who preferred the ice. No unintended side effects were found.

Discussion

Pain has been defined by the International Association for the Study of Pain as "an unpleasant sensory and emotional experience associated with actual or potential tissue damage, or described in terms of such damage" [20]. The purpose of using topical anaesthesia before dental injection is to eliminate or reduce the pain as effectively and non-invasively as possible. Although previous authors have questioned the effect of topical anaesthesia before injection in the oral cavity [7], many studies have shown a good effect [5, 6, 21, 22].

A confounding factor in the study of pain and discomfort is that the sensation and feelings are subjective, leading to difficulties in objectively comparing experiences of pain and discomfort from different individuals [23]. We therefore decided to compare pain from one side to the other in the same patient. Lidocaine 5% gel was used as a control substance to compare with the ice, since its effect has been described earlier [21, 22] and it is commonly used as topical anaesthesia in dentistry [4]. To minimize the discomfort and pain, and to standardise the injection speed, we used a 30-gauge ½ inch needle along with a computerised standardised anaesthetic injection device, The Wand, as described in a previous study [24].

We decided to use pulse change and VAS ratings as indicators of pain and discomfort, as these have been found to be reliable indicators of a patient's response to pain [23, 25] and have also been used for evaluation of discomfort [24, 26]. The study was designed as a randomized split-mouth crossover study, which reduced the risk of bias since each patient received both treatments. This gives more reliable results, since there is a variability between different patients' response to pain [27]. To minimize the risk for bias related to the evaluation of the buccal site, topical anaesthesia on the palatal site was not applied until after the completion of injection and evaluation of the buccal side.

In 2009 Aminabadi and Farahani [14] stated that only one previous study [13] had investigated the effects of local mucosal cooling prior to infiltration of local anaesthesia in dentistry. Even if later published studies have shown results indicating that pre-cooling is effective, the pre-cooling can be administered in many different ways and in combination with various other techniques. An article from 2015 [16] stated that even if the use of cryoanesthesia to reduce injection pain had been reported to be promising, only sparse literature reports exist regarding the clinical efficacy of these agents. Our study is an effort to increase the available publications in this field of knowledge.

Many of the published articles dealing with pre-cooling of oral mucosa prior to dental injection have used ice in combination with pharmaceutical topical anesthetics [28–30], why the genuine effect of the cooling has not been evaluated in those studies, as it was done in our study.

The study design had two main limitations. Firstly, it was unblinded, which always increases the risk of bias. Unfortunately neither patients nor clinicians could have been blinded, since the temperature difference between lidocaine 5% gel and ice, and the different methods of application, made it obvious which method was used. Secondly, although a control group treated with placebo could have made the results even stronger, we felt that ethical considerations ruled this out as an option, since we did not wish to cause any painful experience that could increase the risk of dental anxiety.

The VAS is a frequently used reproducible method for the measurement of painful procedures [23, 31, 32]. The only difference between the genders was that the girls scored the VAS pain at injection higher than boys, which is in accordance with several other reports [2, 24, 33]. Generally speaking, the VAS pain intensity ratings in our study were low, for both ice and lidocaine gel and at all time points, when compared to medical pain ratings [34]. Several previous studies – using ice as a pre-cooling agent before dental injection - have only evaluated a shorter time for application of the cooling agent; usually 1 min [16, 28–30]. In our study the ice was kept in place during 5 min before injection was performed, and evaluation of insertion pain was measured three times during that time. Our results showed that there was no additional reduction of insertion pain after a 1-min application time for either ice or gel, which makes it reasonable to suggest that for both these methods an application time of 1 min is sufficient to reach superficial topical anaesthetic effect before injection using a 30 gauge needle. An earlier study concluded that lidocaine 5% gel might provide a better superficial anaesthesia of the oral mucosa if the application time was extended to 15 min [24], although the recommended application time on the summary of product characteristics is 2–3 min [35]. Our findings suggest that this application time can be reduced to 1 min, but since this is only applicable to the superficial insertion pain, it is necessary to perform the injection gradually and very slowly to avoid pain from tension in the tissue. It is also important to slowly increase the depth of the needle into already anaesthetized tissue before further injection of local anaesthesia can be performed by stages, in order to make the injection as pain-free as possible.

The finding that a palatal injection was more painful than a buccal injection is well known to dental clinicians, and is probably due to the absence of free mucosa on the palatal side. The fact that the mucosa of the hard palate is highly keratinized and very dense and tight [36] makes the injection pain from pressure in the tissue more prominent. Several studies have reported failure to satisfactorily anaesthetize the palatal site [37–40].

Our finding that a significantly higher proportion of the participants reported a bad or very bad taste following treatment with lidocaine 5% gel on the buccal site, in comparison to when ice was used on the same site, confirms that the patient's experience of topical anaesthesia can be improved if a different substance is used or if the method for application is improved. Previous studies have also emphasized the bad taste experience associated with anaesthetic gels [41].

The simple method for topical anaesthesia of oral mucosa (using a plastic syringe filled with frozen water for direct application of ice on the oral mucosa) described in our manuscript has not been published previously, and an evaluation of the comparison between this method and Lidocain 5% gel for topical anaesthesia of the oral mucosa has therefore not been presented heretofore. The methods used by several other authors have included ice incapsulated in plastics [14, 29] or in empty cartridges of glass filled with ice [30] or ice-filled cotton buds [28]. All these mentioned methods have the disadvantage of not having direct contact between the ice and the mucosa. Under such circumstances the plastics or glass will isolate the ice from the surrounding. The superficial part of the ice will melt first and melted water will surround the ice (when covered by plastics or glass), diminishing the temperature effect from the ice on the oral mucosa after a short time of application. When an ice-filled cotton roll or cotton bud is used, the ice on the surface will melt first and after a short time there will be no ice in direct contact with the oral mucosa. The temperature on the oral mucosa will therefore be higher for all those other methods than when ice is in direct contact with the oral mucosa. The method described in our study makes it possible to have direct contact between the ice and the oral mucosa during the entire time of application (Fig. 6).

In a study by Lathval et al. [16] a custom made ice cone was used for topical anaesthesia of the injection site, but the size and shape of the ice cone was not described, neither how the ice cone was kept in place [16]. Jayasuriya et al. [28] stated that a limitation of the method when ice is placed directly on the oral mucosa, is that ice will slip from the operators hand due to wetness and will cool the operators fingers [16]. These problems are, anyhow, not present when our described method is used, since the operator's fingers are only in contact with the plastic syringe and will not touch the ice itself (Figs. 5 and 6).

No previous study has presented the temperature of the ice used for cooling of the oral mucosa. The temperature of the cooling agent is important, since too low temperature or too long application time may cause frostbite to the oral mucosa – especially if other cooling agents than ice are used [16].

The method described for application of ice on oral mucosa is readily available, and according to the dentists in our study is easy to perform. It could therefore be a good alternative to the commercially available lidocaine 5% gel, especially when other types of topical anaesthesia are not available, or if certain pharmacological components should be avoided due to the risk of allergic reactions or intoxication [10, 42].

Regarding heart rate, the negative Pearson correlation between baseline pulse and age confirmed the findings of previous studies that HR decreases with age [43].We chose to evaluate the relative HR change rather than the actual HR change, to avoid bias from diverging HR at baseline. Unfortunately, the HR from 13 patients was not measured immediately before each intervention, and so their values could not be included in the evaluation of relative HR change. The results showed no significant difference in relative HR change between ice and lidocaine 5% gel, meaning that the two methods have a similar effect on HR change. The significantly larger reduction in relative HR when using lidocaine 5% gel after palatal injection, compared to buccal injection, indicates that the gel had a better pain-reducing effect on the palatal mucosa than on the buccal mucosa. When using ice, there was no significant difference in HR change following injection between the buccal and palatal sites, indicating that topical anaesthesia with ice had similar pain-relieving effects on both the buccal and palatal mucosa. A limitation of the HR analysis was that data were only available from 27 of the 40 patients. However, we believe that this is an acceptable number of patients from which to draw conclusions, since previous similar studies have also included around 30 patients [24, 25, 37, 44, 45]. Another limitation is that HR is a very unspecific metric, and that it can e.g. be influenced by memories or emotional reactions, not least related to smell [46].

The individual comments by the patients showed an obvious variety of preferences. While the effectiveness of the topical anaesthesia was important to several patients, comfort was more important to others. This implies that a continuous communication with the patient is important in choosing the best method of topical anaesthesia for each individual.

Conclusions

The described method for the use of ice as topical anaesthesia on oral mucosa before injection has an effect similar to that of lidocaine 5% gel on pain relief at insertion of needle, and the topical anaesthetic effect is present as early as 1 min after application. The taste of lidocaine 5% gel is worse than that of ice. The method described here for administration of ice as topical anaesthesia before injection in oral mucosa is a good, cheap, easy available alternative to the commercially available lidocaine 5% gel.

Abbreviations

BPM: beats per minute; HR: Heart rate; PI: Principal investigator (PI); VAS: Visual Analogue Scale

Acknowledgements

The authors wish to thank Forum Östergötland for helping with the process of application to the medical products agency, as well as for monitoring the study.

Endnotes

This article describes an easy, readily available and non-toxic method for topical anaesthesia of oral mucosa with similar effect as a commonly used commercially available product.

Authors' contributions

MB and NH conceived the ideas and structured the research plan; MB and NH performed the application for ethical approval. MB and NH performed the application to the Swedish Medical Products Agency (SMPA) and the EudraCT-registration. MB and FM made revision (regarding registration of pulse) to the protocol and applied for changes to the Regional Ethical Board and the SMPA. NH (1/4) and FM (3/4) collected the data. FM compiled the data. MB performed statistical analysis together with statistician. All authors (MB, EB, FM and NH) participated substantially in the writing process and approved the final manuscript.

Author details

[1]Department of Ear, Nose, Throat and Maxillofacial Surgery, Zealand University Hospital, Koege, Denmark. [2]Public Dental Service Östergötland, Linköping, Region Östergötland, and Department of Biomedical and Clinical Sciences, Linköping University, Linköping, Sweden. [3]Pain and Rehabilitation Center, and Department of Medical and Health Sciences, Linköping University, Linköping, Sweden. [4]Centre for Orthodontics and Paediatric Dentistry, Norrköping, Public Dental Service Östergötland, Region Östergötland, and Department of Biomedical and Clinical Sciences, Linköping University, Linköping, Sweden.

References

1. Friedman MJ. New advances in local anesthesia. Compend Contin Educ Dent. 2000;1:432–40.
2. Peretz B, Mann J. Dental anxiety among Israeli dental students: a 4-year longitudinal study. Eur J Dent Educ. 2000;4:133–7.
3. Milgrom P, Coldwell SE, Getz T, Weinstein P, Ramsay DS. Four dimensions of fear of dental injections. J Am Dent Assoc. 1997;128:756–66.
4. Ramacciato JG, Meechan JG. Recent advances in local anaesthesia. Dent Update. 2005;32:8–14.
5. Meechan JG. Intra-oral topical anaesthetics: a review. J Dent. 2000;28:3–14.
6. Bhalla J, Meechan JG, Lawrence HP, Grad HA, Haas DA. Effect of time on clinical efficacy of topical anesthesia. Anesth Prog. 2009;56:36–41.
7. Parirokh M, Sadeghi AS, Nakhaee N, Pardakhty A, Abbott PV, Yosefi MH. Effect of topical anesthesia on pain during infiltration injection and success of anesthesia for maxillary central incisors. J Endod. 2012;38:1553–6.
8. Houpt MI, Heins P, Lamster I, Stone C, Wolff MS. An evaluation of intraoral lidocaine patches in reducing needle-insertion pain. Compend Contin Educ Dent. 1997;18:309–16.
9. Hersh EV, Houpt MI, Cooper SA, Feldman RS, Wolff MS, Levin LM. Analgesic efficacy and safety of an intraoral lidocaine patch. J Am Dent Assoc. 1996; 127:1626–34.
10. Amado A, Sood A, Taylor JS. Contact allergy to lidocaine: a report of sixteen cases. Dermatitis. 2007;18:215–20.
11. Silver K, Silver J. The place of James Arnott (1797-1883) in the development of local anaesthesia in dentistry. Br Dent J. 2016;220:249–52.
12. Davoudi A, Rismanchian M, Akhavan A, Nosouhian S, Bajoghli F, Haghighat A, Arbabzadeh F, Samimi P, Fiez A, Shadmehr E, Tabari K, Jahadi S. A brief review on the efficacy of different possible and nonpharmacological techniques in eliminating discomfort of local anesthesia injection during dental procedures. Anesth Essays Res. 2016;10:13–6.
13. Harbert H. Topical ice: a precursor to palatal injections. J Endod. 1989;15:27–8.
14. Aminabadi NA, Farahani RMZ. The effect of pre-cooling the injection site on pediatric pain perception during the administration of local anesthesia. J Contemp Dent Pract. 2009;10:43–50.
15. Ernst E, Fialka V. Ice freezes pain? A review of the clinical effectiveness of analgesic cold therapy. J Pain Symptom Manag. 1994;9:56–9.
16. Lathwal G, Pandit IK, Gugnani N, Gupta M. Efficacy of different precooling agents and topical anesthetics on the pain perception during intraoral injection: a comparative clinical study. Int J Clin Pediatr Dent. 2015;8:119–22.
17. Malanga GA, Yan N, Stark J. Mechanisms and efficacy of heat and cold therapies for musculoskeletal injury. Postgrad Med. 2015;127:57–65.
18. Halar EM, DeLisa JA, Brozovich FV. Nerve conduction velocity. Relationship of skin, subcutaneous and intramuscular temperatures. Arch Phys Med Rehabil. 1980;61:199–203.
19. Sankar A, Johnson SR, Beattie WS, Tait G, Wijeysundera DN. Reliability of the American Society of Anesthesiologists physical status scale in clinical practice. Br J Anaesth. 2014;113:424–35.

20. Merskey H, Bogduk N. Part III: pain terms. A current list with definitions and notes on usage. IASP Task Force on Taxonomy editors. Classification of chronic pain. 2nd ed. Seattle: IASP Press; 1994. p. 209–14.
21. Yaacob HB, Noor GM, Malek SN. The pharmacological effect of xylocaine topical anaesthetic--a comparison with a placebo. Singap Dent J. 1981;6:55–7.
22. Rosivack RG, Koenigsberg SR, Maxwell KC. An analysis of the effectiveness of two topical anesthetics. Anesth Prog. 1990;37:290–2.
23. McGrath PA. An assessment of children's pain: a review of behavioral, physiological and direct scaling techniques. Pain. 1987;31:147–76.
24. Bågesund M, Tabrizi P. Lidocaine 20% patch vs lidocaine 5% gel for topical anaesthesia of oral mucosa. Int J Paediatr Dent. 2008;18:452–60.
25. Kreider KA, Stratman RG, Milano M, Agostini FG, Munsell M. Reducing children's injection pain: lidocaine patches versus topical benzocaine gel. Pediatr Dent. 2001;23:19–23.
26. Mosskull-Hjertton P, Bågesund M. Er:YAG laser or high-speed bur for cavity preparation in adolescents. Acta Odontol Scand. 2013;71:610–5.
27. Kendroud S, Bhimji SS. Physiology, nociceptive pathways. Treasure Island (FL): StatPearls Publishing; 2019. Available from https://www.ncbi.nlm.nih. - gov/books/NBK470255/ (accessed Nov 18, 2019) StatPearls
28. Jayasuriya NSS, Weerapperuma ID, Amarasinghe MGCK. The use of an iced cotton bud as an effective pre-cooling method for palatal anaesthesia: a technical note. Singap Dent J. 2017;38:17–9.
29. Mohiuddin I, Setty JV, Srinivasan I, Desai JA. Topical application of local anaesthetic gel vs ice in pediatric patients for infiltration anaesthesia. J Evol Med Dent Sci. 2015;4:12934–40.
30. Ghaderi F, Banakar S, Rostami S. Effect of pre-cooling injection site on pain perception in pediatric dentistry: "a randomized clinical trial". Den Res J. 22. 2013;10:790–4.
31. Gupta V, Chandrasekar T, Ramani P. Anuja. Determining toothache severity in pediatric patients: a study. J Indian Soc Pedod Prev Dent. 2006;24:140–3.
32. Revill SI, Robinson JO, Rosen M, Hogg MI. The reliability of a linear analogue for evaluating pain. Anaesthesia. 1976;31:1191–8.
33. Dao TT, Le Resche L. Gender differences in pain. J Orofac Pain. 2000;14:169–84.
34. Collins SL, Moore RA, McQuay HJ. The visual analogue pain intensity scale: what is moderate pain in millimetres? Pain. 1997;72:95–7.
35. Produktresumé. Stockholm: APL pharma specials. 2015; Available from: https://aida.apl.se/_layouts/APL_ProduktDokument/PDSPage.aspx?nplId=20030804002454&docType=spc%20 (accessed Nov 18, 2019).
36. Nanci A. Oral Mucosa. In: Nanci A, editor. Ten Cate's oral histology: development, structure, and function. 8th ed. Saint Louis: Elsevier/Mosby; 2012. p. 278–310.
37. Holst A, Evers H. Experimental studies of new topical anaesthetics on the oral mucosa. Swed Dent J. 1985;9:185–91.
38. Svensson P, Petersen JK. Anesthetic effect of EMLA occluded with orahesive oral bandages on oral mucosa. A placebo-controlled study. Anesth Prog. 1992;39:79–82.
39. Al-Melh MA, Andersson L. Reducing pain from palatal needle stick by topical anesthetics: a comparative study between two lidocaine/prilocaine substances. J Clin Dent. 2008;19:43–7.
40. Franz-Montan M, De Paula E, Groppo FC, Silva AL, Ranali J, Volpato MC. Liposomal delivery system for topical anaesthesia of the palatal mucosa. Br J Oral Maxillofac Surg. 2012;50:60–4.
41. Kosaraju A, Vandewalle KS. A comparison of a refrigerant and a topical anaesthetic gel as preinjection anaesthetics: a clinical evaluation. J Am Dent Assoc. 2009;140:68–72.
42. Curtis LA, Dolan TS, Seibert HE. Are one or two dangerous? Lidocaine and topical anesthetic exposures in children. J Emerg Med. 2009;37:32–9.
43. Allen J, Murray A. Age-related changes in peripheral pulse timing characteristics at the ears, fingers and toes. J Hum Hypertens. 2002;16:711–7.
44. Fukayama H, Suzuki N, Umino M. Comparison of topical anesthesia of 20% benzocaine and 60% lidocaine gel. Oral Surg Oral Med Oral Pathol Oral Radiol Endod. 2002;94:157–61.
45. Movassaghian S, Afzalifar R, Alaeddini M. Clinical anesthetic effectiveness of intraoral mucoadhesive tablets of amitriptyline in healthy volunteers. J Oral Maxillofac Surg. 2013;71:23–8.
46. Matsunaga M, Isowa T, Yamakawa K, Kawanishi Y, Tsuboi H, Kaneko H, Sadato N, Oshida A, Katayama A, Kashiwagi M, Ohira H. Psychological and physiological responses to odor-evoked autobiographic memory. Neuro Endocrinol Lett. 2011;32:774–80.

5

Accuracy and trending abilities of finger plethysmographic blood pressure and cardiac output compared to invasive measurements during caesarean delivery in healthy women

Ivar N. Omenås[1], Christian Tronstad[2] and Leiv Arne Rosseland[1,3*]

Abstract

Background: In women presenting for caesarean section under spinal anesthesia, continuous measurement of circulatory aspects, such as blood pressure and cardiac output, is often needed. At present, invasive techniques are used almost exclusively. Reliable non-invasive monitoring would be welcome, as it could be safer, less uncomfortable, and quick and easy to apply. We aimed to evaluate whether a non-invasive, finger plethysmographic device, the ccNexFin monitor, can replace invasively measured blood pressure in the radial artery, and whether cardiac output measurements from this device can be used interchangeably with measurements from the mini-invasive LiDCO monitor currently in use at our institution.

Methods: Simultaneous invasive measurements were compared to ccNexFin in 23 healthy women during elective caesarean section under spinal anesthesia. We used Bland Altman statistics to assess agreement, and polar plot methodology to judge trending abilities with pre-defined limits.

Results: Mean arterial and systolic pressures showed biases (invasive – ccNexFin) of – 4.3 and 12.2 mmHg, with limits of agreement of – 15.9 – 7.4 and – 11.1 – 35.6, respectively. The ccNexFin trending abilities were within the suggested limits for mean pressure but insufficient for systolic pressure compared to invasive measurements. Cardiac output had a small bias of 0.2 L/min, but wide limits of agreement of – 2.6 – 3.0. The ccNexFin trending abilities compared to the invasive estimated values (LiDCO) were unsatisfactory.

Conclusions: We consider the ccNexFin monitor to have sufficient accuracy in measuring mean arterial pressure. The limits of agreement for systolic measurements were wider, and the trending ability compared to invasive measurements was outside the recommended limit. The ccNexFin is not reliable for cardiac output measurements or trend in pregnant women for caesarean delivery under spinal anesthesia.

Keywords: Blood pressure, Cardiac output, Caesarean section, Validation studies, Bland Altman, Polar plot

* Correspondence: l.a.rosseland@medisin.uio.no
[1]Division of Emergencies and Critical Care, Oslo University Hospital, Oslo, Norway
[3]Institute of Clinical Medicine, University of Oslo, Oslo, Norway
Full list of author information is available at the end of the article

Background

In a normal pregnancy, large alterations occur in the circulatory physiology. Blood volume, stroke volume, heart rate, and cardiac output (CO) increase, where blood pressure (BP) and peripheral resistance decrease [1]. During caesarean section (CS), both spinal anesthesia and oxytocin administration can precipitate severe drops in peripheral arterial resistance and BP. Vasopressors and inotropes are administered to counteract the changes in BP and CO [2]. Perioperatively, BP is usually measured intermittently using oscillatory devices, and changes of short duration are mostly unnoticed, even if substantial. In healthy parturients, changes in BP and CO are usually well tolerated and easily corrected, but in patients with pre-eclampsia or cardiac disease, close monitoring of hemodynamic variables is necessary to prevent harm to the mother or fetus. Cardiac disease often goes undiagnosed in pregnant women; of maternal deaths from a cardiac cause in the UK and Ireland in 2009–2014, 77% did not have a known pre-existing cardiac condition [3].

Anesthetists are trained to observe and interpret heartbeat-to-heartbeat variables and often need to see trends and changes over time. In our department, the current standard tool for continuous cardiovascular monitoring is the LiDCOplus monitor (LiDCO Ltd., London, UK). LiDCO offers continuous data on BP, peripheral resistance, and CO, among other variables. However, the monitor requires intra-arterial access and is reserved for delivery in high-risk pregnancies.

It would be of great advantage for research and clinical monitoring of pregnant women if detailed and reliable continuous measurements could be obtained using non-invasive technologies. Advanced monitoring could be established more quickly and easily, and with less risk. For example, the ccNexFin monitor (NexFin Systems, BMEYE, Amsterdan, NL) is non-invasive and easy to apply. There is, however, currently insufficient evidence that non-invasive monitors are reliable for pregnant women.

The objectives of the present study were to assess the agreement and trending abilities for systolic and mean arterial BP between ccNexFin and invasive BP measures, assess the agreement and trending abilities for CO between the ccNexFin and LiDCO monitors, and determine if ccNexFin can replace invasive measurements of BP and CO during CS under spinal anesthesia in healthy, pregnant women. The expected outcome was that the non-invasive measurements and trending abilities of BP are reliable compared to invasive measurements, but we expected CO to be less reliable.

Methods

Ethics approval

The study was approved by the Regional Committee for Medical and Health Research Ethics, Southern Norway (REC ID: 2012/1155 approved 01/02/2013). All participants provided written informed consent. The study followed the Declaration of Helsinki and was conducted according to Good Clinical Practice.

Patient population

Healthy, non-smoking, normotensive women with singleton pregnancies scheduled for elective caesarean delivery under spinal anesthesia were asked to participate in this study. Participants were recruited in collaboration with "The Placenta Project" (REC ID: 2011/2419) and, for this subset of the study population, a common information leaflet was developed. The information was released during the recruitment period and included detailed information about the anticipated pain during arterial cannulation and the extra time needed when establishing both invasive and non-invasive monitoring. As part of the study protocol for "The Placenta Project", all participants received an intra-arterial line used for blood sampling at delivery. The protocol for The Placenta Project and description of the entire recruitment period was published previously [4]. Exclusion criteria were considerable pre-existing morbidity, pregnancy complications, contractions prior to scheduled C-section, and prior Raynaud phenomena, as this is not compatible with use of the ccNexFin monitor. Two women with hypothyroidism, each supplemented with a low dose of L-thyroxine (50 and 75 µg daily) and one woman with mild asthma and occasional use of salbutamol (not taken in the days prior to participation in the study) were included in the study. The inclusion period was from May 2013 to January 2014. Demographics of the study population are given in Table 1.

Monitoring devices

The LiDCOplus monitor (LiDCO Ltd., London, UK, version 4.02.95) is in routine clinical use and has documented accuracy and trending abilities [5]. This monitor provides information about circulatory changes from heartbeat to heartbeat and is used when advanced monitoring is indicated, such as during major surgery, or during interventions on patients with circulatory disorders. Mathematical analysis of the intra-arterial pressure curve is performed with pulse power analysis using the built-in software PulseCO. The LiDCO monitor estimates many

Table 1 Patient demographics

	Mean (SD)	Range
Age, yr.mo	35.10 (3.2)	29.6–42.7
Height, cm	167 (5.0)	160–180
Weight before pregnancy, kg	64.0 (10.7)	50–91
Weight at delivery, kg	78.9 (12.3)	60–105
Length of pregnancy, days	275 (6.5)	260–292

aspects of the circulation and can be used with or without lithium dilution calibration. In this study, we used calibrated CO, aiming for optimal accuracy. This technology has been used in studies of healthy women and pregnant women with heart disease [6], and is the standard method for perioperative monitoring of preeclamptic women at our institution. In the comparison of CO methods, LiDCO serves as the reference.

The ccNexfin monitor (NexFin Systems, BMEYE, Amsterdan, NL, version 1.9.0.1001) is based on the principle of the unloaded vascular wall [7], the Physiocal criteria [8], and a generalized waveform filter to reconstruct brachial pressure from finger pressure [9]. An inflatable cuff is placed around one of the three middle fingers of either hand. An integrated plethysmograph measures the volume of blood under the cuff using an infrared light source and a photosensor. The monitor initially determines a set point for the finger cuff pressure at which most of the venous blood is displaced and the arterial diameter is reduced to no more than 50% of the expanded diameter. The set point is intermittently calibrated according to the Physiocal criteria to account for changes in the vascular state of the finger. The cuff pressure is continuously adjusted to counter the varying intra-arterial BP, keeping the signal from the photosensor and, consequently, the blood volume and arterial diameter under the cuff constant. This way, the artery wall is said to be unloaded, transmural pressure is zero, and the pressure in the cuff represents the intra-arterial pressure. The measured finger BP is transformed to reflect brachial BP. The CO calculations in the ccNexFin are based on pulse contour analysis of the derived arterial pressure curve. The monitor is designed to work without external calibration. Our research group has been involved in several projects using finger plethysmographic monitor technology, including the largest population-based study ever utilizing this technology, The Tromsø Study [10].

Study design

In this prospective observational study, a 20G BD arterial cannula (Becton Dickinson Infusion Therapy Systems, Inc., Utah, USA) was placed in the radial artery after skin infiltration with lidocaine (5–10 mg). The cannula was connected to a Siemens Dräger Infinity Gamma XL hemodynamic monitor (Drägerwerk AG & Co. KgaA, Lübeck, Germany) via a Codan X-trans pressure transducer (CODAN pvb Critical Care GmbH, Forstinning, Germany) and the signal calibrated according to standard departmental procedures. Peripheral IV catheters were placed on both arms.

Intra-arterial BP data was passed through to the LiDCOplus monitor. Invasive heart rate (HR_{inv}), invasive systolic arterial pressure (SAP_{inv}), and invasive mean arterial pressure (MAP_{inv}) were recorded at a rate of one sample per heartbeat. The CO_{LiDCO} estimated by PulseCO was also recorded. A single point calibration of CO was performed. The ccNexFin monitor was applied to one of the three middle fingers on the same arm as the intra-arterial cannula and corresponding variables (HR_{nex}, SAP_{nex}, MAP_{nex}, and CO_{nex}) recorded.

While sitting on the operating table, the subjects received spinal anesthesia with bupivacaine (10 mg) and fentanyl (20 µg) using a 27G pencil point needle. Coloading with intravenous 0.9% NaCl (1000 mL) was started. The parturients were then placed in the supine position with a left lateral tilt using a wedge under the right hip. Immediately after injection of the drugs, an intravenous bolus of phenylephrine (25–50 µg) was given, followed by an infusion starting at 0.25 µg/kg/min and titrated according to invasive BP, aiming for a stable $SAP_{inv} > 90$ mmHg.

Data recording

To acquire synchronous sampling from both monitors, measurements were sampled in real time by the same computer. Samples were acquired through the RS232 port of the LiDCO monitor and the analog output from the ccNexFin monitor using a data acquisition card and software from National Instruments. This setup was evaluated for electrical safety and approved by the appointed committee at Oslo University Hospital.

Time-stamped data for inter-beat interval (IBI), SAP, MAP, and CO from both monitoring devices was recorded to a single dataset per subject, one sample per heartbeat, using software developed in-house using National Instruments LabVIEW®. Events were marked in real time and saved to a file using the same software.

Due to subject movement following spinal anesthesia, placement of a hip wedge, and adjustment of the arterial pressure transducer and the ccNexFin heart reference system, we considered data from the first 2 min after spinal anesthesia as unreliable. The arterial line was used for blood sampling just prior to delivery, causing a pause in our registration, and following delivery there was again more subject movement causing unreliable data. It is also the experience of our group that the LiDCO needs recalibration after delivery [11]. We included the data between 2 and 12 min after spinal anesthesia for our calculations.

Statistical analysis

Due to differences in processing time between the two monitors, the LiDCO samples were ahead of the ccNexFin samples, by approximately two heartbeats on average, though they were sampled synchronously from the outputs of the monitors. For each session, this difference was adjusted by calculating the lag using a cross-covariance analysis of the IBI time-series, which are assumed to be equal between monitors, and then shifting the ccNexFin recording ahead by the calculated lag in order to align the recordings for comparison at equivalent beats. This was performed in Matlab R2014b (Mathworks, Nantick, Massachusetts, USA).

Artefacts were reduced using a previously published method for detecting and removing outliers in continuous BP and CO recordings [12]. Data points for statistical analysis were constructed with 1-min intervals by averaging data over the first 10 s of each minute.

Methods were compared using Matlab and Stata v15 (Statacorp LLC, College Station, Texas, USA). We used the method first described by Bland and Altman to investigate the agreement of the ccNexFin monitor with invasive BP and LiDCO CO measurements [13, 14]. Early versions of this method did not sufficiently consider the structure of the data and could produce too narrow limits of agreement, and too narrow confidence intervals, with repeated measurements per subject. We calculated limits of agreement based on the repeated observations method as described by Zou [15]. Confidence intervals for the limits of agreement were calculated using the MOVER algorithm [15]. This method is preferred when the true value varies, when there is a different number of measurements from each subject, and when the between-subject variance is large with respect to the within-subject variance. The MOVER method also allows the construction of asymmetric CIs. Diagnostic plots suggested by Bland and Altman were inspected to check for underlying assumptions. The high number of repeated measurements increases the information and the statistical power. However, sample size was decided without a formal power calculation.

Polar plots were used to assess trending abilities for both BP and CO [16]. As suggested by Critchley [16], the smallest changes were considered to most likely represent noise and were excluded from the Polar plot analysis. Data points with an average change from the previous measurement of more than 5 mmHg for BP or 0.5 L/min for CO were included.

Results

Of 63 subjects approached to participate in the study, 45 agreed to participate. Of these women, 7 went into labor prior to the CS, and study personnel were not available at the time of the CS for 12. Another two women were excluded due to technical problems with the recording equipment, and in one woman we did not succeed in placing an intra-arterial line. This left us with 23 participants eligible for BP analysis. Two additional women were excluded from the analysis of CO due to unsuccessful calibration of the LiDCO monitor (Fig. 1).

Mean (SD) time from spinal anesthesia to blood sampling was 16.1 (5.5) minutes, with values ranging from 5.6 and 31.7 min. We had some missing data, mostly due to delivery sooner than 12 min after spinal anesthesia, or misalignment of the ccNexFin heart reference system. For the BP analysis, 209 of a theoretical maximum of 230 data points remained (90.9%). For the 21 participants included in the CO analysis, 187 of 210 possible data points remained (89.0%).

The Bland Altman plots and Polar plots are shown in Fig. 2, and the limits of agreement and Polar plot analyses are shown in Table 2.

Discussion

Even though the anesthetist aims to keep the patient as stable as possible during caesarean delivery, rapid and major fluctuations in BP and CO are common. Both spinal anesthesia and injections of oxytocin result in sudden drops in the peripheral resistance, with decreases in BP and concomitant increases in CO [2, 17]. Standard clinical practice is to administer fluids and vasopressors [18]. Surgery, bleeding, anxiety, and discomfort also affect the cardiovascular system. Thus, this clinical setting is challenging for any monitoring device, especially regarding trending abilities. Could inclusion of parturients with pre-eclampsia or cardiac diseases have increased the hemodynamic challenge and added value to the evaluation? Pre-eclamptic patients tolerate spinal anesthesia with less of a change in BP and CO due to peripheral vasoconstriction [19]. Parturients with cardiac disease are another group in which invasive monitoring is indicated and part of standard care in our hospital. The patients usually receive spinal anesthesia, and vasodilation has to be carefully managed throughout the surgery. The hemodynamic response varies a lot depending on cardiac diagnosis and function [6]. Collecting a large sample of patients with invasive monitoring in obstetric anesthesia is challenging. Spinal anesthesia-induced vasodilation and hypotension is common and has a major impact in healthy parturients, and beat-to-beat monitoring is recommended to titrate prophylaxis and the treatment of severe hypotension. Implementing this into practice is important for clinicians who manage parturients with severe cardiac co-morbidity.

Blood pressure varies by measurement site and modality

The definition of a gold standard for BP is debatable. Although auscultatory BP, measured on the upper arm, may still be considered the gold standard, it is too slow and impractical for use in the setting of caesarean delivery. For most patients, intermittent oscillometric measurements are sufficient, but in more challenging cases, continuous measurements are needed. These measurements are usually obtained invasively. For invasive measurements, the gold standard may be the BP in the

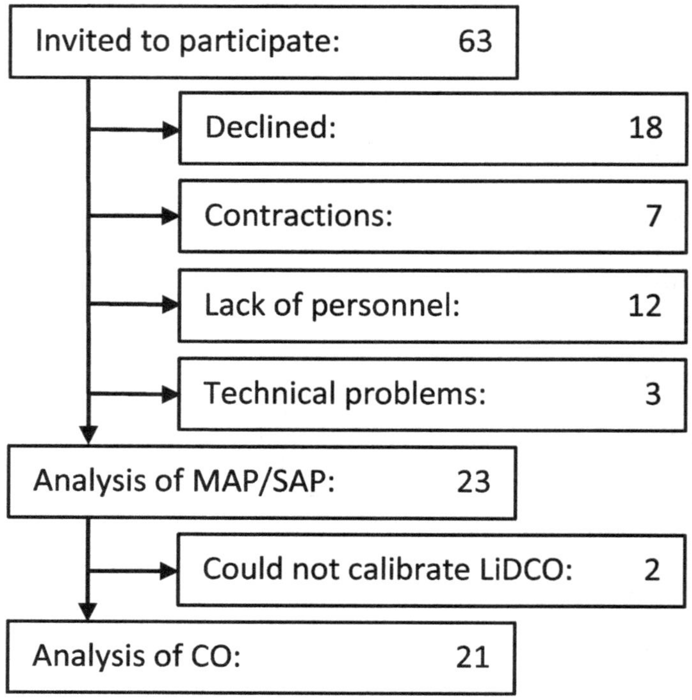

Fig. 1 Flow chart of patient screening, inclusion, and analysis

ascending aorta, but this measurement is not obtainable. The radial artery is the preferred site, as it is conveniently located, easy to cannulate, and the incidence of complications is low [20]. Still, peripherally measured intra-arterial BP is not equal to the central pressure. The pressure curve is modified as it travels along the branches of the arterial tree by both the elastic properties of the central vessels and reflected waves from the periphery.

Oscillometric non-invasive BP measured in the upper arm underestimates high BP and overestimates low BP, whereas mean pressures are similar compared to intra-arterial measurements in the radial artery [21]. In 1990, Gravlee et al. [22], compared intra-arterial BP in the brachial artery measured with four methods of non-invasive BP measurement on the upper arm before, during, and after cardiopulmonary bypass. Averaging overall measurements, they found that the auscultatory method reported lower systolic, but higher mean and diastolic pressures than the invasive measurements, whereas the oscillometric method reported an equal systolic and higher mean and diastolic values compared to invasive measurements. Judging from the graphs, the same is true when considering the first two measurements (i.e. before open chest surgery) separately [22].

In 1951, Wood et al. simultaneously measured the BP in radial and brachial arteries in 17 healthy subjects and found that the SAP in the radial artery was 6 mmHg higher, and MAP and DAP slightly lower (2 and 1 mmHg), than in the brachial artery. For hypertensive subjects, the difference in systolic pressure was increased [23]. Pauca et al. measured pressures in the radial artery and in the ascending aorta during bypass surgery. They found small differences in MAP and DAP, but greater differences between centrally and peripherally measured SAP, with pressures in the radial artery being 12 mmHg higher on average. Systolic values were also found to have much greater variance than the mean and diastolic values [24].

The ccNexFin measures BP in a finger. The waveform is transformed to approximate invasive brachial BP [9] using a model that relies on measurements and assumptions in a group of 53 men, some healthy, and some with varying degrees of hypertension and cardiovascular disease. We found similar MAP values between the monitors, with ccNexFin reporting values an average 4 mm higher than the invasive measurements. Systolic values were approximately 12 mm lower on average. A slightly lower systolic value is expected, as ccNexFin aims to represent a more central pressure, but the difference is larger than can reasonably be explained by this effect. The inaccuracy is small and will likely be of minor importance during caesarean delivery under spinal anesthesia.

Varying definitions of hypotension

An analysis by Klöhr et al. reviewing definitions of hypotension after spinal anesthesia for caesarean delivery

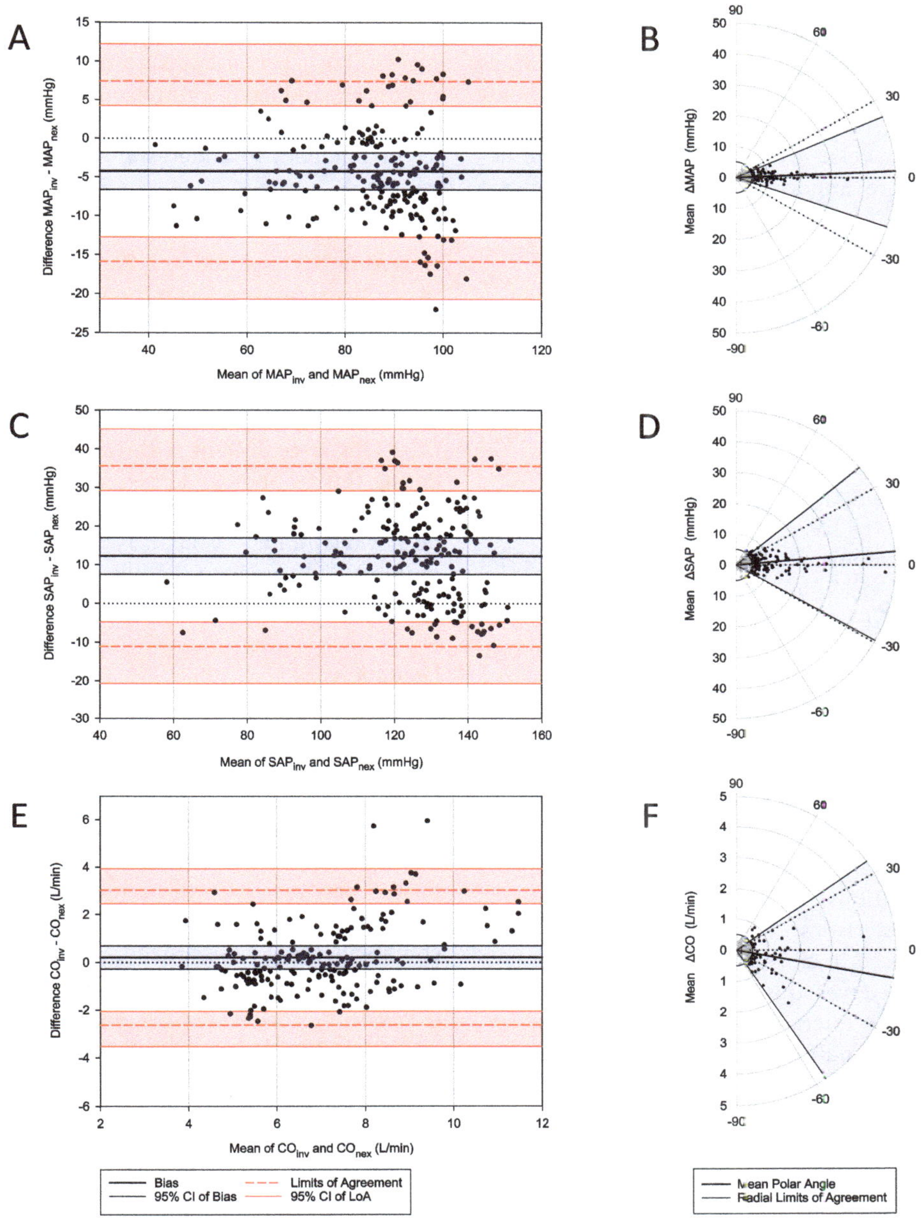

Fig. 2 Comparison of invasive measurements with ccNexFin. **a** Mean arterial pressure (MAP) in a Bland Altman plot and **b** Polar plot. **c** Systolic arterial pressure (SAP) in a Bland Altman plot and **d** Polar plot. **e** Cardiac output (CO) in a Bland Altman plot and **f** Polar plot

Table 2 Bias (invasive – ccNexFin), limits of agreement (LoA), and Polar plot analyses

	Bias (95% CI)	LoA (95% CI)	Mean polar angle (SD)	Radial LoA
MAP	−4.3 mmHg (−6.6, −1,9)	−15.9 (−20.7, − 12.8) to 7.4 (4.2, 12.2)	2.3° (10.0°)	−18.6°, 23.2°
SAP	12.2 mmHg (7.5, 17.0)	− 11.1 (− 20.7, − 4.8) to 35.6 (29.2, 45.2)	5.0° (17.3°)	−29.2°, 39.2°
CO	0.2 L/min (− 0.3, 0.7)	− 2.6 (− 3.5, − 2.0) to 3.0 (2.5, 3.9)	−10.4° (27.2°)	−55.9°, 35.1°

found that, in research, relative limits seem to be more popular than absolute thresholds [25]. This and other papers reference a survey by Burns et al. from 2001 as an argument that anesthetists prefer absolute thresholds in this setting [26], but they actually did not. The authors claimed that a relative rather than an absolute decrease may be more important. They added that, not only the degree of hypotension, but also the duration may be important. Nevertheless, as absolute limits do not require a baseline to be determined, it may be reasonable to assume that this simpler approach would be preferred by many. In a recent consensus document, Kinsella et al. suggested taking a baseline BP measurement before spinal anesthesia using repeated measurements if the BP is not stable, if it is higher than expected, or if the woman is in labor [27]. They recommended aiming for a SAP ≥90% of baseline and to avoid a decrease to < 80% of baseline. The SAP was also suggested to be a less important variable than MAP as a determinant of organ perfusion. Recommended limits are still based on the SAP, as this has been the primary outcome in most of the available research. MAP is unlikely to be used to define hypotension in this clinical setting without more supportive data [27].

Auscultatory, oscillometric, invasive, and finger plethysmographic techniques use different principles to measure or estimate BP. In addition, measurements are made at different anatomic sites. It is important to be aware of the measurement techniques used in scientific studies, their definitions of safe limits for BP, and to consider the characteristics of these methods compared to the ones being used in clinical practice.

From this perspective, the inaccuracy of ccNexFin compared to invasive arterial pressure has a minor impact, and we recommend finger plethysmographic measurement for clinical use and in research.

Trending abilities for blood pressure

The degree to which two monitors agree in their ability to track changes is also crucial. For the Polar plot method we applied, Critchley et al. suggest using a limit of ±5° for angular bias and radial limits of no more than ±30° for good trending abilities [16]. Only the MAP measurements satisfied these limits. The low angular bias suggests that the monitors were in good calibration, and with radial limits well within ±30° the ccNexFin exhibits good trending ability compared to intra-arterial measurements. The SAP had an angular bias on the border of the suggested range, but the radial limits were too wide. Taking into consideration the hemodynamic variations typical for caesarean delivery under spinal anesthesia, this is a challenging model, with larger intra-individual variations than in critical care patients. We recommend finger plethysmographic measurements in clinical settings and for research purposes requiring good BP trending ability, such as repeated measurements. In pre-eclampsia or other settings with pregnancy-induced hypertension, invasive measurements should replace the finger plethysmographic method due to the tendency to underestimate SAP.

Cardiac output

Regarding CO, we did not find sufficient agreement between the monitors. Even though the bias was small, the limits of agreement were wide, more than ±40% of the mean CO. Both the angular bias and radial limits of agreement were far outside recommended limits, suggesting that ccNexFin cannot reliably track changes in CO. This is consistent with the results in a study comparing this technology to echocardiographic estimates of CO [28]. Based on the interpretation of the results, we do not recommend using ccNexFin to measure CO or to monitor CO trends in the clinic or research in pregnant women.

Limitations

In this study, we presented the accuracy (bias) and precision (variability) of agreement between two methods. We calculated limits of agreement and assessed the use of ccNexfin against invasive measurements for BP and the LiDCO monitor for CO. As described by Hapfelmaier et al. [29], the precision of agreement partly depends on the precision of measurement (repeatability) of both devices. For example, the limits of agreement will become wider as a consequence of using an imprecise reference technique. This means that the agreement between a new technique and a reference technique needs to be judged in light of the precision that the techniques themselves are able to achieve [29]. In the present study, it was not possible to determine the repeatability (variation around a true value). Obstetric anesthesia is characterized by constantly changing hemodynamics, and repeated measurements during one constant value of BP or CO within the experiment is impossible. Thus, determining the precision of measurement of the LiDCO per se and the Nexfin technique per se was not possible.

A total of 21 patients were analyzed and a larger sample could have increased the precision and generalizability. However, it is important to take into consideration the large number of repeated measurements per patient and that the analyses included all of these data points to assess trending abilities.

Conclusion

We consider the ccNexFin monitor to have sufficient accuracy in measuring MAP. The limits of agreement for systolic measurements were wider, and the trending ability compared to invasive measurements was outside the recommended limit. The ccNexFin is not reliable for CO measurements or trending ability in pregnant women undergoing caesarean delivery under spinal anesthesia.

Abbreviations

CO: Cardiac output; BP: Blood pressure; HR: Heart rate; SAP: Systolic arterial pressure; MAP: Mean arterial pressure; IBI: Inter-beat interval

Acknowledgements

The authors thank Dr. Ane M. Holme, Dr. Maia B. Holm, and Dr. Hildegunn Horne for valuable collaboration during data collection.

Authors' contributions

INO contributed during planning, data collection, analyses, and interpretation, and manuscript preparation. CT contributed during planning, data collection, analyses, and interpretation, and manuscript preparation. LAR is the principle investigator, contributed during planning, approval of the protocol, data collection, analyses, and interpretation, and manuscript preparation. All authors have read and approved the manuscript.

Author details

[1]Division of Emergencies and Critical Care, Oslo University Hospital, Oslo, Norway. [2]Department of Clinical and Biomedical Engineering, Oslo University Hospital, Oslo, Norway. [3]Institute of Clinical Medicine, University of Oslo, Oslo, Norway.

References

1. Grindheim G, Estensen M-E, Langesaeter E, Rosseland LA, Toska K. Changes in blood pressure during healthy pregnancy: a longitudinal cohort study. J Hypertens. 2012;30:342–50.
2. Langesaeter E, Rosseland L, Stubhaug A. Hemodynamic effects of oxytocin during cesarean delivery. Int J Gynaecol Obstet. 2006;95:46–7.
3. Knight M, Nair M, Tuffnell D, Kenyon S, Shakespeare J, Brocklehurst P, et al.. Saving Lives, Improving Mothers' Care - Surveillance of maternal deaths in the UK 2012–14 and lessons learned to inform maternity care from the UK and Ireland. 2016.
4. Holme AM, Holm MB, Roland MCP, Horne H, Michelsen TM, Haugen G, Henriksen, T. The 4-vessel Sampling Approach to Integrative Studies of Human Placental Physiology In Vivo. J Vis Exp. 2017;(126):e55847. https://doi.org/10.3791/55847.
5. Langesaeter E, Gibbs M, Dyer RA. The role of cardiac output monitoring in obstetric anesthesia. Curr Opin Anaesthesiol. 2015;28:247–53.
6. Langesaeter E, Dragsund M, Rosseland L. Regional anaesthesia for a caesarean section in women with cardiac disease: a prospective study. Acta Anaesthesiol Scand. 2010;54:46–54.
7. Penaz J. Photoelectric Measurement of Blood Pressure, Voluma and Flow in the Finger. Digest of the 10th International Conference on Medical and Biological Engineering - 1973 - Dresden; 1973.
8. Wesseling KH, De Wit B, Van der Hoeven GMA, Van Goudoever J, Settels JJ. Physiocal, calibrating finger vascular physiology for Finapres. Homeostasis. 1995;36:67–82.
9. Gizdulich P, Prentza A, Wesseling KH. Models of brachial to finger pulse wave distortion and pressure decrement. Cardiovasc Res. 1997;33:698–705.
10. Olsen RB, Bruehl S, Nielsen CS, Rosseland LA, Eggen AE, Stubhaug A. Chronic pain and cardiovascular stress responses in a general population: the Tromsø study. J Behav Med. 2014;37:1193–201.
11. Langesaeter E. Is it more informative to focus on cardiac output than blood pressure during spinal anesthesia for cesarean delivery in women with severe preeclampsia? Anesthesiology. 2008;108:771–2.
12. Tronstad C, Omenås IN, Rosseland LA. An improved artifact removal algorithm for continuous cardiac output and blood pressure recordings. 2015 37th Annual International Conference of the IEEE Engineering in Medicine and Biology Society (EMBC). New York City: IEEE; 2015. p. 5968–72.
13. Bland JM, Altman DG. Statistical methods for assessing agreement between two methods of clinical measurement. Lancet. 1986;1:307–10.
14. Bland JM, Altman DG. Agreement between methods of measurement with multiple observations per individual. J Biopharm Stat. 2007;17:571–82.
15. Zou GY. Confidence interval estimation for the Bland-Altman limits of agreement with multiple observations per individual. Stat Methods Med Res. 2013;22:630–42.
16. Critchley LA, Yang XX, Lee A. Assessment of trending ability of cardiac output monitors by polar plot methodology. J Cardiothorac Vasc Anesth. 2011;25:536–46.
17. Langesæter E, Rosseland LA, Stubhaug A. Continuous invasive blood pressure and cardiac output monitoring during cesarean delivery: a randomized, double-blind comparison of low-dose versus high-dose spinal anesthesia with intravenous phenylephrine or placebo infusion. Anesthesiology. 2008;109:856–63.
18. Fitzgerald JP, Fedoruk KA, Jadin SM, Carvalho B, Halpern SH. Prevention of hypotension after spinal anaesthesia for caesarean section: a systematic review and network meta-analysis of randomised controlled trials. Anaesthesia. 2020;75:109–21.
19. Sharwood-Smith G, Drummond GB. Hypotension in obstetric spinal anaesthesia: a lesson from pre-eclampsia. Br J Anaesth Oxford University Press. 2009;102:291–4.
20. Scheer B, Perel A, Pfeiffer UJ. Clinical review: complications and risk factors of peripheral arterial catheters used for haemodynamic monitoring in anaesthesia and intensive care medicine. Crit Care. 2002; 6:199–204.
21. Wax DB, Lin H-M, Leibowitz AB. Invasive and concomitant noninvasive intraoperative blood pressure monitoring: observed differences in measurements and associated therapeutic interventions. Anesthesiology. 2011;115:973–8.
22. Gravlee GP, Brockschmidt JK. Accuracy of four indirect methods of blood pressure measurement, with hemodynamic correlations. J Clin Monit. 1990; 6:284–98.
23. Wood EH, Fuller J, Clagett OT. Intraluminal pressures recorded simultaneously from different arteries in man. Am J Phys. 1951;167:838–9.
24. Pauca AL, Wallenhaupt SL, Kon ND, Tucker WY. Does radial artery pressure accurately reflect aortic pressure? Chest. 1992;102:1193–8.
25. Klöhr S, Roth R, Hofmann T, Rossaint R, Heesen M. Definitions of hypotension after spinal anaesthesia for caesarean section: literature search and application to parturients. Acta Anaesthesiol Scand. 2010; 54:909–21.
26. Burns SM, Cowan CM, Wilkes RG. Prevention and management of hypotension during spinal anaesthesia for elective caesarean section: a survey of practice. Anaesthesia. 2001;56:794–8.
27. Kinsella SM, Carvalho B, Dyer RA, Fernando F, McDonnell N, Mercier FJ, et al. International consensus statement on the management of hypotension with vasopressors during caesarean section under spinal anaesthesia. Anaesthesia. 2018;73:71–92.
28. Duclos G, Hili A, Resseguier N, Kelway C, Haddam M, Bourgoin A, et al. Clearsight™ use for haemodynamic monitoring during the third trimester of pregnancy – a validation study. Int J Obstet Anesth Elsevier Ltd. 2018;36:85–95.
29. Hapfelmeier A, Cecconi M, Saugel B. Cardiac output method comparison studies: the relation of the precision of agreement and the precision of method. J Clin Monit Comput. 2016;30:149–55.

6

Changes in the sublingual microcirculation following aortic surgery under balanced or total intravenous anaesthesia

Silvia Loggi[1], Nicoletta Mininno[1], Elisa Damiani[1], Benedetto Marini[1], Erica Adrario[1], Claudia Scorcella[1], Roberta Domizi[1], Andrea Carsetti[1], Simona Pantanetti[1], Gabriele Pagliariccio[2], Luciano Carbonari[2] and Abele Donati[1*]

Abstract

Background: In vascular surgery with aortic cross-clamping, ischemia/reperfusion injury induces systemic haemodynamic and microcirculatory disturbances. Different anaesthetic regimens may have a varying impact on tissue perfusion. The aim of this study was to explore changes in microvascular perfusion in patients undergoing elective open abdominal aortic aneurysm repair under balanced or total intravenous anaesthesia.

Methods: Prospective observational study. Patients undergoing elective open infrarenal abdominal aortic aneurysm repair received balanced (desflurane + remifentanil, $n = 20$) or total intravenous anaesthesia (TIVA, propofol + remifentanil using target-controlled infusion, $n = 20$) according to the clinician's decision. A goal-directed haemodynamic management was applied in all patients. Measurements were obtained before anaesthesia induction (baseline) and at end-surgery and included haemodynamics, arterial/venous blood gases, sublingual microvascular flow and density (incident dark field illumination imaging), peripheral muscle tissue oxygenation and microcirculatory reactivity (thenar near infrared spectroscopy with a vascular occlusion test).

Results: The two groups did not differ for baseline characteristics, mean aortic-clamping time and requirement of vasoactive agents during surgery. Changes in mean arterial pressure, systemic vascular resistance index, haemoglobin and blood lactate levels were similar between the two groups, while the cardiac index increased at end-surgery in patients undergoing balanced anaesthesia. The sublingual microcirculation was globally unaltered in the TIVA group at end-surgery, while patients undergoing balanced anaesthesia showed an increase in the total and perfused small vessel densities (from 16.6 ± 4.2 to 19.1 ± 5.4 mm/mm^2, $p < 0.05$). Changes in microvascular density were negatively correlated with changes in the systemic vascular resistance index. The area of reactive hyperaemia during the VOT increased in the balanced anaesthesia group (from 14.8 ± 8.1 to 25.6 ± 14.8%*min, $p < 0.05$). At end-surgery, the tissue haemoglobin index in the TIVA group was lower than that in the balanced anaesthesia group.

Conclusions: In patients undergoing elective open abdominal aortic aneurysm repair with a goal-directed hemodynamic management, indices of sublingual or peripheral microvascular perfusion/oxygenation were globally preserved with both balanced anaesthesia and TIVA. Patients undergoing balanced anaesthesia showed microvascular recruitment at end-surgery.

(Continued on next page)

* Correspondence: a.donati@univpm.it
[1]Anaesthesia and Intensive Care Unit, Department of Biomedical Sciences and Public Health, Università Politecnica delle Marche, via Tronto 10/a, 60126 Torrette di Ancona, Italy

(Continued from previous page)

Keywords: Aortic surgery, Ischemia/reperfusion injury, Anaesthesia, Haemodynamics, Microcirculation

Background

Ischemia/reperfusion (I/R) injury is common in patients undergoing aortic clamping for vascular surgery and leads to systemic inflammation and organ dysfunction [1–3]. The production of pro-inflammatory molecules and oxidative stress increase especially in the reperfusion phase and are responsible for microvascular alterations similar to those observed during sepsis [4–6]. These include an impairment in blood flow, capillary shunting with reduction in microcirculatory density and increased perfusion heterogeneity, resulting in a mismatch between oxygen delivery and consumption [4, 5]. The severity of microcirculatory dysfunction increases along with the duration of the ischemic phase [2, 3, 7].

A number of studies explored how drugs can modulate microvascular perfusion in different disease states. In septic patients with impaired blood flow auto-regulation, vasoactive agents may have limited potential for microvascular recruitment [8]: the use of norepinephrine titrated to reach a mean arterial pressure (MAP) > 65 mmHg was unable to improve microcirculatory perfusion during septic shock [9, 10]. Dobutamine increased intestinal microvascular blood flow in animal models of sepsis [11] but failed to restore capillary perfusion in patients with septic shock [12]. Conversely, after cardiac surgery a rise in MAP by norepinephrine infusion induced an increase in splanchnic oxygen extraction without altering the intestinal mucosal perfusion, possibly because of autoregulation phenomenon [13–15].

Anaesthetics can affect microvascular perfusion as well. Propofol causes vasodilation by stimulating nitric oxide production: this may result in microvascular shunting with reduction in capillary density, increased blood flow heterogeneity and reduced tissue oxygen delivery [16–18]. Volatile anaesthetics also cause dose-dependent vasodilation [19, 20]. In anesthetised dogs, desflurane, unlike isoflurane and halothane, was able to maintain myocardial, hepatic, intestinal and skeletal muscle blood flow [21]. In patients undergoing thoracoscopic surgery, desflurane-remifentanil anaesthesia was associated with better microvascular perfusion as compared to propofol-remifentanil anaesthesia [22]. In female patients undergoing breast surgery, the use of sevoflurane, unlike propofol, was associated with a significant decrease in the capillary filtration coefficient, suggesting a lower risk of interstitial oedema and tissue perfusion alteration [23]. Microcirculatory dysfunction was found in different surgical settings despite the optimization of systemic hemodynamic parameters [24] and was associated with the development of post-operative complications [25].

We aimed to verify whether desflurane might have a better impact on the microcirculation as compared to propofol in patients at risk for I/R injury due to aortic surgery. The goal of this study was to explore changes in sublingual and peripheral muscle microcirculation in patients undergoing elective open abdominal aortic aneurysm repair under balanced or total intravenous anaesthesia (TIVA).

Methods

The study was approved by our local ethic committee of Azienda Ospedaliera Universitaria "Ospedali Riuniti" of Ancona in Italy (ClinicalTrials.gov identifier: NCT03510793, www.clinicaltrials.gov, principal investigator: Prof. Abele Donati, date of registration: April 27th 2018, retrospectively registered). A written informed consent was obtained from all patients before enrolment. This was designed as a prospective observational study on 40 patients undergoing elective open infrarenal abdominal aortic aneurysm repair with prosthetic aorto-aortic or aorto-bisiliac bypass under general anaesthesia. The study was performed at Vascular Surgery of the Azienda Ospedaliera Universitaria "Ospedali Riuniti" of Ancona in Italy between September 2013 and November 2017.

Inclusion criteria were: elective infrarenal abdominal aortic open repair; use of a protocol of intraoperative hemodynamic goal-directed therapy; American Society of Anaesthesiology (ASA) class ≤ III. Exclusion criteria were: age < 18 years, pregnancy, endovascular aneurysm repair, presence of infections, trauma, emergency surgery.

Patients received balanced anaesthesia or TIVA based on the attending physician's decision, resulting in two study groups of 20 patients each. The choice of the anaesthetic regimen was based exclusively on the physician preference and was taken before and independently of the patient's enrolment, the anaesthesiologist was unaware of baseline microcirculatory measurements. The patients' distribution between the two groups was initially due to chance; the enrolment was then stopped in the balanced anaesthesia group once the required sample size ($n = 20$) had been reached, in order to achieve the same number of patients in the TIVA group. Patients undergoing balanced anaesthesia received desflurane (with an inspiratory oxygen fraction of 0.4–0.5) and remifentanil, administered as a target-controlled infusion (Minto model). TIVA was performed with a target-controlled infusion of propofol (Schnider model) and remifentanil (Minto model). In all patients, anaesthetic depth was monitored with spectral entropy and the anaesthetic dose was titrated in order to maintain a state entropy value of 35 to 45%, resulting in an age-adjusted minimum alveolar concentration of 0.8 for desflurane and an estimated effect-site target concentration (Ce) of 2–4 mcg/ml and 2.5–5 ng/ml for propofol and remifentanil, respectively. Neuromuscular blockade was achieved with a bolus of 0.6 mg/kg rocuronium at anaesthesia induction; additional boluses (10 mg) were provided based on train-of-four neuromuscular monitoring. Haemodynamic parameters were monitored in all patients with Flotrac/Vigileo (Edwards Lifesciences); arterial and central venous blood gases were monitored according to routine clinical practice. A protocol of intraoperative goal-directed therapy was applied in all patients for haemodynamic optimization, according to standard care in our unit [26]. This includes: first, stroke volume optimization by fluid therapy (targeting an increase in stroke volume < 10% after a 200 ml fluid bolus over 5 min); second maintenance of a MAP > 70 mmHg by titrated vasopressor administration; third, maintenance of a cardiac index (CI) ≥2.5 ml/kg per m^2 by titrated inotropic therapy [26].

Measurements were collected at baseline (before induction of anaesthesia) and at end-surgery (before anaesthesia discontinuation) and included haemodynamic parameters, arterial and central venous blood gases and assessment of the sublingual microcirculation and peripheral muscle tissue oxygenation and microvascular reactivity.

Evaluation of the sublingual microcirculation

The sublingual microcirculation was assessed with incident dark field (IDF) imaging that is incorporated into a handheld video microscope (CytoCam, Braedius, Amsterdam, The Netherlands) and enables a real time visualisation of microvascular blood flow. Details on this technique have been described elsewhere [27]. After gentle removal of saliva and other secretions with a gauze, the probe was applied on the sublingual mucosa. Three videos of 10 s' duration were recorded on three different areas with adequate focus and contrast. All efforts were made to avoid pressure artifacts. Videos were analysed offline with a dedicated software (Automated Vascular Analysis v3.0, Microvision Medical, Amsterdam, The Netherlands). For small (diameter < 20 μm) and medium (diameter 20–50 μm) vessels, we calculated the Total Vessel Density (TVD), Perfused Vessel Density (PVD), De Backer score, Percentage of Perfused Vessels (PPV), Microvascular Flow Index (MFI) and Flow Heterogeneity Index (FHI), as previously described [28].

Evaluation of tissue oxygenation and microvascular reactivity

Near-infrared spectroscopy (NIRS) (InSpectra™ Model 650, Hutchinson Technology Inc., Hutchinson, MN, USA) was applied on the thenar eminence with a 15-mm sized probe to measure peripheral muscle tissue oxygen saturation (StO_2) and tissue haemoglobin index (THI) [29] before and during a vascular occlusion test (VOT), as described previously [30]. This was performed by inflating a sphygmomanometer cuff placed on the forearm to 50 mmHg above the systolic blood pressure. Arterial inflow was arrested until the StO_2 decreased to 40%. StO_2 was recorded during the ischemic and the reperfusion phases until stabilization [31]. NIRS-derived parameters were calculated by using a software package (version 3.02 InSpectra Analysis Program; Hutchinson Technology Inc.). The StO_2 downslope was calculated from the regression line of the StO_2 decay after occlusion, providing an index of tissue oxygen extraction rate [31]. The desaturation slope may vary during the ischaemic phase of the VOT, becoming more or less steep before reaching the 40% StO_2 threshold: the inflection point was identified and the downslope was calculated separately for the first and the last part of the desaturation curve (downslope 1 and downslope 2, respectively), as previously described [32]. Whenever a change in the slope was not observed, the desaturation curve was divided into two halves for the calculation of the two downslope values. The delta-downslope was calculated as the difference between the last and the first part of the desaturation slope (downslope 2 - downslope1), so that a positive value indicated a flattening in the second part of the slope (slower StO_2 decay) [32]. The StO_2 upslope during the reperfusion phase and the area under the curve of the StO_2 (AUC StO_2) during the hyperaemic response were calculated as indices of microcirculatory reactivity [31].

Statistical analysis

The analysis was performed using Graphpad Prism 6 (GraphPad Software, La Jolla, CA, USA). The Kolmogorov-Smirnov test was used to check the normality of distribution. Data were expressed as mean ± standard deviation or median [1st-3rd quartile], as appropriate. A chi-square test or Student's t test (or Mann Whitney U test) were applied for between-group comparisons of nominal or continuous variables, as appropriate. A two-way analysis of variance (ANOVA) with the Sidack's multiple comparison test was used whenever possible. Alternatively, the Wilcoxon and Mann-Whitney U test were used for non-normally distributed variables for comparisons between the two time points in the same group and between the two groups at the same time point. The Spearman rho was calculated to evaluate the correlation between variables. A (two-sided) p value < 0.05 was used to indicate statistical significance. For sample size calculation, we considered a difference in MFI at end-surgery of 0.4 (standard deviation 0.4) as clinically relevant [28]. A sample size of 16 patients per group was sufficient to detect such a difference with a power of 80% and an alpha error of 0.05. We included 40 patients (20 per group) to allow for missing data or dropouts.

Results

Figure 1 shows the study flow diagram, with details on the number of patients evaluated for eligibility and reasons for exclusion. The two groups did not differ for age, gender distribution, comorbidities, ASA score, and intraoperative data including clamping time, fluid balance at end-surgery and vasoactive agent requirements (Table 1). Changes in haemodynamics and blood gases from baseline to end-surgery are reported in Table 2. MAP and systemic vascular resistance index (SVRI) decreased in both groups. The CI increased in patients undergoing balanced anaesthesia, while it remained substantially stable in the TIVA group. The two groups showed similar changes in haemoglobin (Hb), central venous oxygen saturation ($ScvO_2$), arterial lactate levels and arterial base excess.

Changes in microcirculatory and NIRS-derived parameters are shown in Table 3. The TVD and PVD for small vessels increased at end-surgery in the balanced anaesthesia group, while the small vessel MFI and PPV remained unaltered in both groups (Fig. 2). At both time points, the TVD and PVD for medium vessels were lower in the TIVA group as compared to those in the balanced anaesthesia group (Table 3). Changes in microvascular density were negatively correlated with changes in SVRI (TVD for small vessels: $r = -0.479$ $p = 0.002$; PVD for small vessels: $r = -0.451$ $p = 0.003$). These correlations remained if considering the two groups separately, although appearing weaker in the TIVA group (TVD for small vessels: $r = -0.453$ $p = 0.045$, PVD for small vessels: $r = -0.362$ $p = 0.116$) as compared to those observed the balanced anaesthesia group (TVD for small vessels: $r = -0.526$ $p = 0.017$, PVD for small vessels: $r = -0.515$ $p = 0.020$). No correlation was found between microvascular parameters and CI, MAP or mean norepinephrine dose during surgery. In all patients, a negative correlation was found between changes in SVRI and mean norepinephrine dose ($r = -0.387$, $p = 0.022$).

The StO_2 did not vary from baseline to end-surgery in either group (Fig. 3). The StO_2 downslope 1 increased in the TIVA group at end-surgery (indicating a slower desaturation rate in the initial part of the ischemic phase), while it remained stable in the balanced anaesthesia group (Fig. 3). The StO_2 downslope 2, delta-downslope and StO_2 upslope did not vary in either group (Table 3). The AUC StO_2 increased at end-surgery in the balanced anaesthesia group (Fig. 3). The THI tended to decrease and was significantly lower at end-surgery in the TIVA group, while it remained stable in the balanced anaesthesia group (Fig. 4).

Discussion

In this prospective observational study on 40 patients undergoing elective open abdominal aortic aneurysm repair with an intraoperative goal-directed haemodynamic optimization, we aimed to explore whether different anaesthetic regimens could have a varying impact on microvascular perfusion in a condition of potential I/R

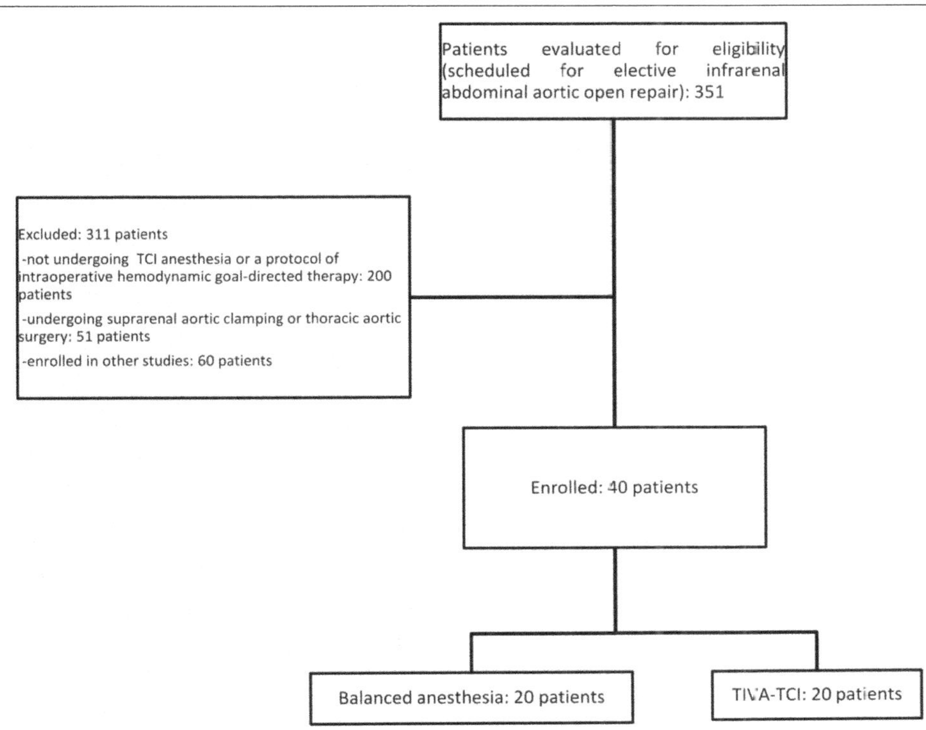

Fig. 1 Study flow diagram

Table 1 General and intraoperative data for the two groups of patients receiving balanced anaesthesia or total intravenous anaesthesia

	Balanced anaesthesia	TIVA	*p*
Age (years)	75 ± 7	74 ± 6	0.464
Gender (nr, % of males)	16, 80%	18, 90%	0.376
ASA score (nr, %)			0.127
2	13, 65%	18, 90%	
3	7, 35%	2, 10%	
Comorbidities (nr, %)			
Arterial hypertension	20, 100%	18, 90%	0.149
Cardiopathy	6, 30%	10, 50%	0.197
Renal Failure	3, 15%	5, 25%	0.429
COPD	12, 60%	8, 40%	0.206
Dyslipidaemia	10, 50%	10, 50%	0.999
Vasculopathy (lower limbs or carotid)	10, 50%	8, 40%	0.525
Clamping time (min)	65 ± 29	69 ± 31	0.691
Fluid balance (ml)	−200 [− 1100 − + 150]	− 195 [−670 − + 300]	0.657
Norepinephrine			
number, %	20, 100%	20, 100%	0.999
mean dosage (mcg/kg/min)	0.15 [0.08–0.20]	0.12 [0.09–0.15]	0.466
Dobutamine			
number, %	13, 65%	16, 80%	0.288
mean dosage (mcg/kg/min)	2.00 [1.23–3.00]	2.39 [1.67–3.92]	0.416
Esmolol (nr, %)	14, 70%	10, 50%	0.197
Levosimendan (nr, %)	3, 15%	5, 25%	0.429
Blood transfusions			
number, %	10, 50%	10, 50%	0.999
average amount (ml)	540 [450–1060]	580 [450–780]	0.837

Data are expressed as mean ± standard deviation or median [1st-3rd quartile], as appropriate
Cardiopathy was defined by the presence of echocardiographic alterations including left ventricular hypertrophy and valvulopathy, or a history of coronary artery disease and/or heart failure and reduced left ventricular ejection fraction. Renal failure was defined by the presence of an estimated glomerular filtration rate lower than 60 ml/min/1.73mq
TIVA total intravenous anaesthesia, *ASA* American Society of Anesthesiology, *COPD* chronic obstructive pulmonary disease

injury. Our first finding is that both balanced anaesthesia and TIVA were associated with overall maintenance of microvascular perfusion and tissue oxygenation. Patients receiving balanced anaesthesia showed an increase in microvascular density, which was inversely related to a reduction in systemic vascular resistance. In patients undergoing TIVA we observed a minor reduction in the skeletal muscle tissue oxygen extraction rate during a VOT and lower THI at end-surgery as compared to that observed in the balanced anaesthesia group. Balanced anaesthesia was associated with an increase in microvascular reactivity, as reflected by a greater area of hyperaemia after the VOT as compared to that seen at baseline.

The activation of the inflammatory response may occur early during aortic surgery [33] with maximal production of oxygen free radicals within 5 min of lower-limb reperfusion [34]. Previous studies showed that oxidative stress during supraceliac or infrarenal aortic cross clamping and reperfusion leads to distributive alterations in microvascular oxygenation and perfusion of splanchnic organs [35]. Heterogeneous flow distribution is characterized by capillaries with stagnant blood cells next to capillaries with normal flow [36] and can be found in microvascular beds far from the site of direct ischemic damage [37]. In rats subjected to I/R injury of the small bowel, the intestinal microvascular blood flow was reduced early in the first 10 min of reperfusion and failed to normalize in the first 2 h [38]. Microcirculatory disturbances during I/R injury may occur independently of changes in macro-haemodynamics and tissue hypo-perfusion may persist despite a normalisation of systemic cardiocirculatory parameters due to a loss of haemodynamic coherence [39]. In our study, we did not find an impairment in microvascular perfusion at end-surgery. We hypothesize that intraoperative hemodynamic

Table 2 Changes in haemodynamics and blood gases from baseline to end-surgery in the two groups of patients receiving balanced anaesthesia or total intravenous anaesthesia

	Balanced anaesthesia		TIVA		p for interaction (2-way ANOVA)
	baseline	end-surgery	baseline	end-surgery	
MAP (mmHg)	94 ± 18	86 ± 13*	92 ± 14	81 ± 12**	0.642
HR (bpm)	67 ± 13	71 ± 11	70 ± 13	71 ± 14	0.521
CI (ml/m^2/min)	2.4 ± 0.7	3.2 ± 0.6***	2.6 ± 0.5	2.8 ± 0.7	0.005
SVRI (dyn*s*cm^{-5})	2800 [2352–3224]	1839 [1691–2085]***	2488 [2203–2952]	2119 [1754–2350]***	–
pH	7.42 [7.39–7.47]	7.40 [7.38–7.43]	7.43 [7.42–7.44]	7.41 [7.37–7.45]	–
PaO_2 (mmHg)	70 [62–88]	159 [145–207]**	72 [63–166]	194 [134–235]***	–
$PaCO_2$ (mmHg)	38 ± 4	38 ± 4	37 ± 3	39 ± 5*	0.027
Base excess (mEq/l)	0.5 [−0.3, + 2.5]	− 0.4 [− 3.2, + 1.2]**	0.5 [− 1.4, + 1.2]	− 0.4 [− 1.9, + 2.4]	–
$ScvO_2$ (%)	72 [69–78]	90 [82–92]***	79 [70–90]#	91 [86–94]**	–
Lactate (mmol/l)	0.6 [0.6–0.8]	1.3 [1.1–1.9]***	0.7 [0.6–1.0]	1.3 [1.0–1.5]***	–
Hb (g/dl)	13.3 ± 2.0	11.8 ± 0.8***	13.4 ± 1.6	11.8 ± 1.3***	0.793
Glucose (mg/dl)	96 [86–107]	121 [105–131]***	102 [95–112]	125 [106–141]***	–

*$p < 0.05$ **$p < 0.01$ ***$p < 0.001$ versus baseline, #$p < 0.05$ versus time-matched balanced anaesthesia. Two-way Analysis of Variance (ANOVA) with Sidack's multiple comparisons test or Wilcoxon and Mann-Whitney U test, as appropriate. Data are expressed as mean ± standard deviation or median [1st-3rd quartile], as appropriate. *TIVA* total intravenous anaesthesia, *MAP* mean arterial pressure, *HR* heart rate, *CI* cardiac index, *SVRI* systemic vascular resistance index, *PaO_2* arterial oxygen tension, *$PaCO_2$* arterial carbon dioxide tension, *$ScvO_2$* central venous oxygen saturation, *Hb* haemoglobin

Table 3 Changes in sublingual microcirculation and NIRS-derived parameters from baseline to end-surgery in the two groups of patients receiving balanced anaesthesia or total intravenous anaesthesia

	Balanced anaesthesia		TIVA		p for interaction (2-way ANOVA)
	Baseline	end-surgery	baseline	end-surgery	
MFI (small vessels) [AU]	2.67 [2.50–2.75]	2.83 [2.37–2.98]	2.75 [2.58–2.90]	2.67 [2.42–2.81]	–
Abnormal MFI[a] (n, %)	9, 45%	6, 30%	7, 35%	9, 45%	–
FHI [AU]	0.15 [0.00–0.29]	0.18 [0.02–0.36]	0.23 [0.09–0.28]	0.19 [0.10–0.38]	–
TVD (small) (mm/mm2)	18.4 ± 3.8	21.0 ± 4.7*	19.8 ± 4.0	20.7 ± 4.5	0.216
TVD (medium) (mm/mm2)	1.5 [0.9–2.2]	1.2 [1.1–1.5]	0.8 [0.6–1.1]##	0.5 [0.1–0.8]###	–
PVD (small) (mm/mm2)	16.6 ± 4.2	19.1 ± 5.4*	18.1 ± 4.2	19.2 ± 4.9	0.302
PVD (medium) (mm/mm2)	1.5 [0.9–2.2]	1.2 [1.1–1.5]	0.8 [0.6–1.1]##	0.5 [0.1–0.8]###	–
PPV (small, %)	91 [83–97]	91 [82–97]	96 [93–98]	95 [90–97]	–
StO_2 (%)	83 ± 5	86 ± 7	82 ± 6	85 ± 9	0.975
StO_2 Downslope 1 (%/min)	−8.0 [−10.8, −6.8]	−7.8 [− 10.4, − 6.9]	− 8.3 [− 12.0, − 7.8]	−8.1 [− 11.1, − 5.9]**	–
StO_2 Downslope 2 (%/min)	−8.2 ± 3.3	− 8.0 ± 4.8	−8.2 ± 2.8	− 8.0 ± 3.4	0.962
Delta Downslope (2–1) (%/min)	1.1 [− 0.5, 2.4]	−0.1 [− 1.6, 1.8]	0.9 [− 0.8, 3.9]	−0.7 [− 1.4, 1.0]	–
StO_2 Upslope (%/min)	226 ± 64	206 ± 103	264 ± 84	247 ± 77	0.900
AUC StO_2 (%*min)	14.8 ± 8.1	25.6 ± 14.8*	20.4 ± 6.0	26.1 ± 19.1	0.359
THI [AU]	15.2 ± 2.0	15.3 ± 3.1	14.6 ± 3.3	12.8 ± 3.6#	0.140

*$p < 0.05$ **$p < 0.01$ versus baseline, #$p < 0.05$ ##$p < 0.01$ ###$p < 0.001$ versus time-matched balanced anesthesia. Two-way Analysis of Variance (ANOVA) with Sidack's multiple comparisons test or Wilcoxon and Mann-Whitney U test, as appropriate. Data are expressed as mean ± standard deviation or median [1st-3rd quartile], as appropriate

[a]An abnormal MFI was defined as an MFI lower than 2.6 [25]

NIRS near infrared spectroscopy, *TIVA* total intravenous anaesthesia, *MFI* microvascular flow index, *AU* arbitrary unit, *FHI* flow heterogeneity index, *TVD* total vessel density, *PVD* perfused vessel density, *PPV* percentage of perfused vessels, *StO_2* tissue oxygen saturation, *AUC StO_2* area under the curve of StO_2, *THI* tissue haemoglobin index

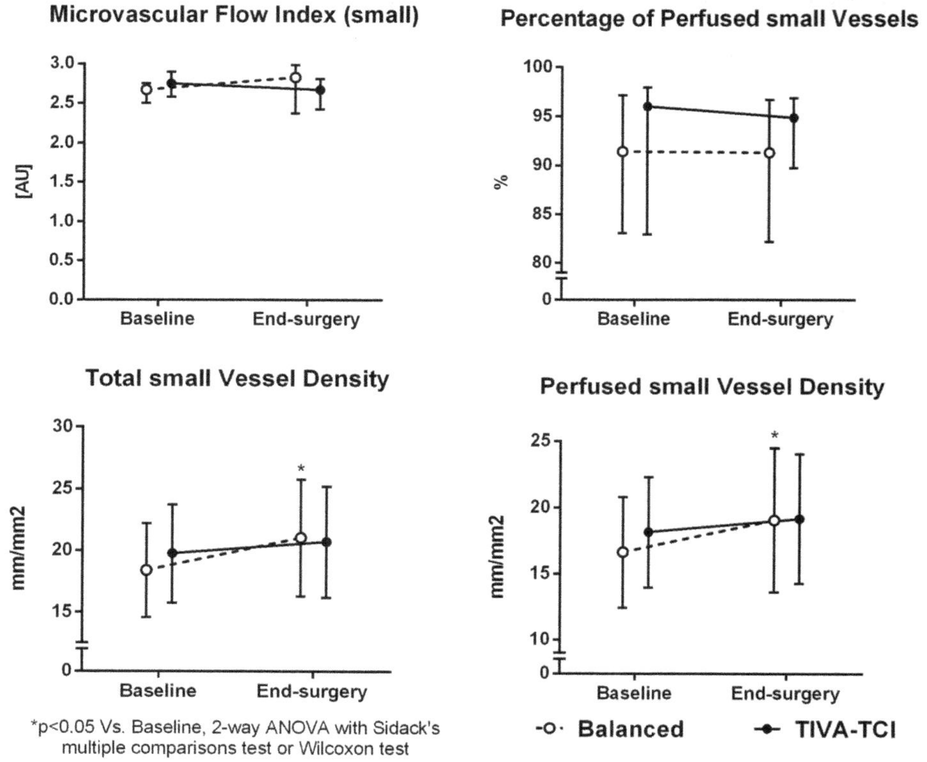

Fig. 2 Changes in sublingual microvascular parameters from baseline to end-surgery in the two groups of patients receiving balanced anaesthesia or total intravenous anaesthesia (TIVA)

optimization with the routine use of a protocol of goal-directed therapy prevented the development of microvascular derangements. In pigs subjected to colon anastomosis, a goal-directed colloid administration was able to improve microvascular perfusion and oxygenation of healthy and perianastomotic colon [40]. Although we could not find any correlation with MAP or CI, changes in sublingual capillary density were inversely related with changes in systemic vascular resistance, reflecting a certain degree of coherence between the macro- and micro-haemodynamic responses in our population [41].

Sublingual microvascular density increased at end-surgery in patients receiving balanced anaesthesia, while it remained unaltered in the TIVA group. It cannot be excluded that the microvascular changes observed were the effect of vasodilating metabolites (e.g. adenosine monophosphate, hypoxanthine) released during reperfusion, however we would expect this reactive hyperaemia to disappear in a late reperfusion phase at end-surgery [3]. Even if the observational design of our study prevents to define cause-effect relationships, the between-group homogeneity in baseline and intraoperative characteristics (including clamping time, fluid balance, blood losses, type and dose of vasoactive agents) would corroborate the hypothesis of direct and separate actions of desflurane and propofol on the microcirculation.

Previous studies showed that both propofol and sevoflurane can exert a protective effect towards I/R injury by modulating the inflammatory response, reducing oxidative stress and tissue apoptosis [42]. Halogenated anaesthetics induce peripheral vasodilation [43] and reduce vascular permeability [23], thus favouring microvascular recruitment and tissue oxygen diffusion. On the other hand, propofol can modulate the inflammatory response and oxidative stress [44], thus increasing tolerance to hypoxia also in tissues far from those directly exposed to ischemia [45]. In this study, desflurane may have been responsible for vasodilation and vascular recruitment in the balanced anaesthesia group due to dilation of resistive arterioles. The increased area of hyperaemia after the VOT would also be consistent with a greater microvascular recruitment following the ischemic challenge in the balanced anaesthesia group.

The rationale of evaluating the microcirculatory response to therapies is that improving microvascular perfusion will guarantee tissue oxygenation and prevent the development of organ dysfunction. In a previous study in patients undergoing abdominal aortic aneurysm surgery, we showed that portal lactate, intramucosal sigmoid pH and arterial-sigmoid

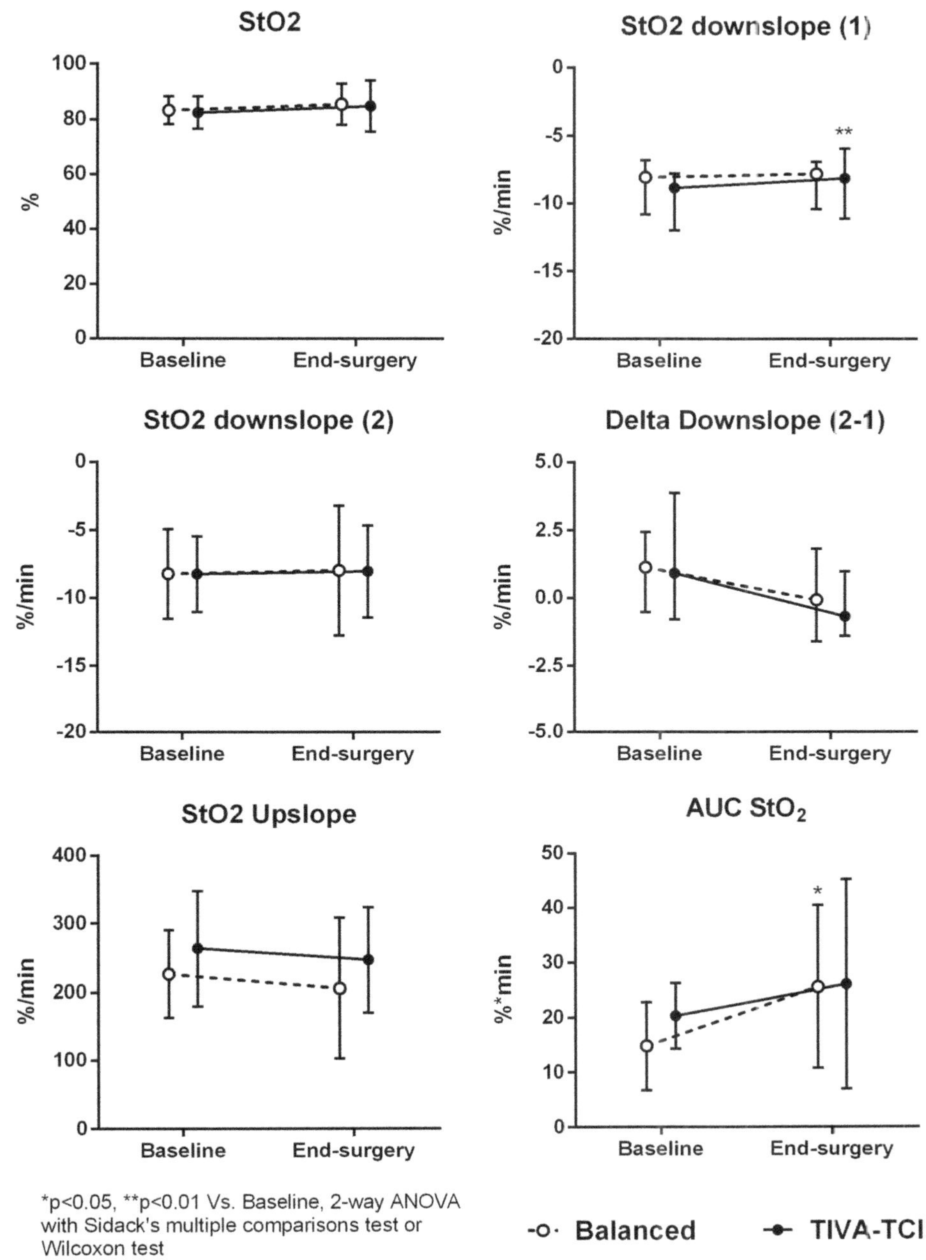

Fig. 3 Changes in NIRS-derived parameters from baseline to end-surgery in the two groups of patients receiving balanced anaesthesia or total intravenous anaesthesia (TIVA). *StO_2* tissue oxygen saturation, *AUC StO_2* area under the curve of StO_2 (area of hyperaemia)

delta pCO_2 (as indices of splanchnic hypo-perfusion) were able to predict the occurrence of post-operative complications [46]. In the present study, we could not show a better impact on anaerobic metabolism of desflurane or propofol, as a clinically relevant hyper-lactataemia was not found in either group at end-surgery. This was consistent with the absence of major microcirculatory alterations in both the balanced anaesthesia and the TIVA groups.

While the StO_2 remained stable in both groups, the desaturation rate in the first part of the ischemic challenge decreased at end-surgery in patients undergoing TIVA. This may result from a reduction in peripheral microvascular density and would be consistent with the lower THI at end-surgery as compared to that seen in the balanced anaesthesia group, which seems to be related to a lower tissue perfusion rather than to a reduction in Hb levels as these remained similar in the two groups. Baseline differences in StO_2 downslope between the groups, although not significant, could also explain our results: the observed variation may only depend

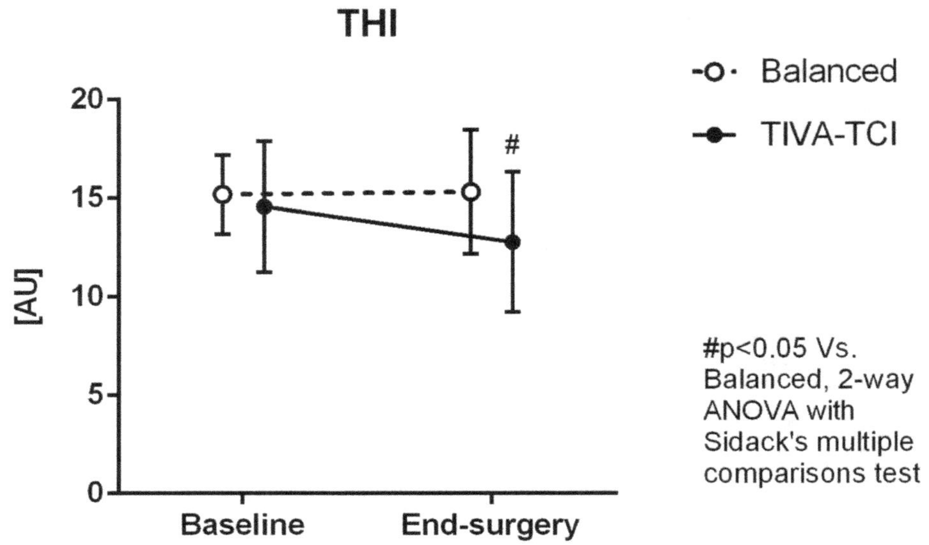

Fig. 4 Changes in the tissue haemoglobin index (THI) from baseline to end-surgery in the two groups of patients receiving balanced anaesthesia or total intravenous anaesthesia (TIVA)

upon a rebalance in the metabolic pattern in the TIVA group without a dysfunctional meaning. In critically ill patients, we showed that a decrease in the desaturation rate in the last part of the ischaemic phase of the VOT is associated with worse outcome and could suggest impaired microcirculatory auto-regulation [32]. In this study, the StO_2 downslope was again similar between the groups in the final part of vascular occlusion and the delta-downslope did not differ between the two groups. Therefore, the type of anaesthesia may not significantly affect peripheral microcirculatory auto-regulation.

Limitations of the study

First, the observational design does not allow drawing any cause-effect relationship between the type of anaesthesia and the microvascular changes observed. Moreover, lack of randomization and the relatively small sample size prevented to control for possible confounding factors. This study was designed as a preliminary exploratory analysis with the aim to detect any possible influence of different anaesthetic regimens on microvascular perfusion alterations during aortic surgery. Future randomized trials are needed to confirm our findings. Second, we cannot exclude that baseline differences in some parameters influenced our results. Even if the main haemodynamic parameters were similar between the groups at baseline, the lower $ScvO_2$ in the balanced anaesthesia group, as well as differences in baseline microvascular medium vessel density, may indicate a higher initial tissue O_2 demand/consumption. However, baseline microvascular small vessel density and NIRS-derived parameters were similar between the two groups, suggesting a similar pattern of tissue perfusion. Third, a relevant number of patients among those assessed for eligibility was excluded, therefore we cannot exclude the presence of a selection bias. Lastly, the microcirculation was globally preserved in both groups, suggesting an overall low prevalence of I/R injury syndrome in our sample. Our study may have been underpowered to detect significant microvascular derangements following aortic surgery. Moreover, monitoring of the sublingual microcirculation may not be sensitive enough to detect tissue perfusion alterations in splanchnic organs [47]. Unfortunately, we did not evaluate the incidence of organ dysfunction or post-operative complications.

Conclusions

In patients undergoing open abdominal aortic aneurysm repair under general anaesthesia with a protocol of intraoperative hemodynamic goal-directed therapy, microvascular perfusion and peripheral tissue oxygenation were generally preserved, however the use of balanced anaesthesia was associated with increased microvascular density and reactivity, while these remained unaltered with TIVA. Further studies are needed to clarify whether the choice of different anaesthetic regimens may contribute to prevent I/R injury in aortic surgery.

Abbreviations

ASA: American Society of Anaesthesiology; *AUC StO_2*: Area under the hyperaemic phase; *CI*: Cardiac index; *Cp*: Plasma target concentration; *FHI*: Flow heterogeneity index; *Hb*: Haemoglobin; *I/R*: Ischemia/reperfusion; *IDF*: Incident Dark Field; *MAP*: Mean arterial pressure; *MFI*: Microvascular flow index; *NIRS*: Near infrared spectroscopy; *PPV*: Percentage of perfused vessels; *PVD*: Perfused vessel density; *$ScvO_2$*: Central venous oxygen saturation; *StO_2*: Tissue oxygen saturation; *SVRI*: Systemic vascular resistance index; *THI*: Tissue haemoglobin index; *TIVA*: Total intravenous anaesthesia; *TVD*: Total vessel density; *VOT*: Vascular occlusion test

Acknowledgements

The authors wish to thank the medical and nurse staff of the operating room of the Unit of Vascular Surgery of Ancona (Italy) for the cooperation in the realization of this work.

Authors' contributions

SL contributed to the study design, acquisition of the data, interpretation of the results and drafted the manuscript. NM, ED collected the data and drafted the manuscript. BM, EA, CS, RD, AC, SP and GP participated in the acquisition and analysis of the data and revised the manuscript. LC and AD contributed to the study design and interpretation of the results and revised the manuscript critically for important intellectual content. All authors read the manuscript and gave final approval of the version to be published. All authors agree to be accountable for all aspects of the work in ensuring that questions related to the accuracy or integrity of any part of the work are appropriately investigated and resolved.

Author details

[1]Anaesthesia and Intensive Care Unit, Department of Biomedical Sciences and Public Health, Università Politecnica delle Marche, via Tronto 10/a, 60126 Torrette di Ancona, Italy. [2]Unit of Vascular Surgery, Azienda Ospedaliera Universitaria "Ospedali Riuniti Umberto I – Lancisi – Salesi" of Ancona, Ancona, Italy.

References

1. Norwood MG, Bown MJ, Sutton AJ, Nicholson ML, Sayers RD. Interleukin 6 production during abdominal aortic aneurysm repair arises from the gastrointestinal tract and not the legs. Br J Surg. 2004;91:1153–6.
2. Wahlberg E, Dimuzio PJ, Stoney RJ. Aortic clamping during elective operations for infrarenal disease: the influence of clamping time on renal function. J Vasc Surg. 2002;36:13–8.
3. Siegemund M, van Bommel J, Stegenga ME, Studer W, van Iterson M, Annaheim S, et al. Aortic cross-clamping and reperfusion in pigs reduces microvascular oxygenation by altered systemic and regional blood flow distribution. Anesth Analg. 2010;111:345–53.
4. De Backer D, Ospina-Tascon G, Salgado D, Favory R, Creteur J, Vincent JL. Monitoring the microcirculation in the critically ill patient: current methods and future approaches. Intensive Care Med. 2010;36:1813–25.
5. De Backer D, Donadello K, Taccone FS, Ospina-Tascon G, Salgado D, Vincent JL. Microcirculatory alterations: potential mechanisms and implications for therapy. Ann Intensive Care. 2011;1:27.
6. Maksimenko AV, Turashev AD. No-reflow phenomenon and endothelial glycocalyx of microcirculation. Biochem Res Int. 2012;2012:859231.
7. Peerless JR, Alexander JJ, Pinchak AC, Piotrowski JJ, Malangoni MA. Oxygen delivery is an important predictor of outcome in patients with ruptured abdominal aortic aneurysms. Ann Surg. 1998;227:726–34.
8. Boerma EC, Ince C. The role of vasoactive agents in the resuscitation of microvascular perfusion and tissue oxygenation in critically ill patients. Intensive Care Med. 2010;36:2004–18.
9. Krejci V, Hiltebrand LB, Sigurdsson GH. Effects of epinephrine, norepinephrine, and phenylephrine on microcirculatory blood flow in the gastrointestinal tract in sepsis. Crit Care Med. 2006;34:1456–63.
10. Dubin A, Pozo MO, Casabella CA, Palizas F Jr, Murias G, Moseinco MC, et al. Increasing arterial blood pressure with norepinephrine does not improve microcirculatory blood flow: a prospective study. Crit Care. 2009;13:R92.
11. Ospina-Tascón GA, García Marin AF, Echeverri GJ, Bermudez WF, Madrinàn-Navia H, Valencia JD, et al. Effects of dobutamine on intestinal microvascular blood flow heterogeneity and O2 extractionduring septic shock. J Appl Physiol (1985). 2017;122:1406–17.
12. De Backer D, Creteur J, Dubois MJ, Sakr Y, Koch M, Verdant C, et al. The effects of dobutamine on microcirculatory alterations in patients with septic shock are independent of its systemic effects. Crit Care Med. 2006;34:403–8.
13. Nygren A, Thorén A, Ricksten SE. Effects of norepinephrine alone and norepinephrine plus dopamine on human intestinal mucosal perfusion. Intensive Care Med. 2003;29:1322–8.
14. Nygren A, Thorén A, Ricksten SE. Vasopressors and intestinal mucosal perfusion after cardiac surgery: norepinephrine vs. phenylephrine. Crit Care Med. 2006;34:722–9.
15. Thorén A, Jakob SM, Pradl R, Elam M, Ricksten SE Takala J. Jejunal and gastric mucosal perfusion versus splanchnic blood flow and metabolism: an observational study on postcardiac surgical patients. Crit Care Med. 2000;28:3649–54.
16. Petros AJ, Bogle RG, Pearson JD. Propofol stimulates nitric oxide release from cultured porcine aortic endothelial cells. Br J Pharmacol. 1993;109:6–7.
17. Bazin JE, Dureuil B, Danialou G, Vicaut E, Aubier M, Desmonts JM, et al. Effects of etomidate, propofol and thiopental anaesthesia on arteriolar tone in the rat diaphragm. Br J Anaesth. 1998;81:430–5.
18. Koch M, De Backer D, Vincent JL, Barvais L, Hennart D, Schmartz D. Effects of propofol on human microcirculation. Br J Anaesth. 2008;101:473–8.
19. Tanaka K, Kawano T, Nakamura A, Nazar H, Kawahito S, Oshita S, et al. Isoflurane activates sarcolemmal adenosine triphosphate-sensitive potassium channels in vascular smooth muscle cells: a role for protein kinase a. Anesthesiology. 2007;106:984–91.
20. O'Riordan J, O'Beirne HA, Young Y, Bellamy MC. Effects of desflurane and isoflurane on splanchnic microcirculation during major surgery. Br J Anaesth. 1997;78:95–6.
21. Hartman JC, Pagel PS, Proctor LT, Kampine JP, Schmeling WT, Warltier DC. Influence of desflurane, isoflurane and halothane on regional tissue perfusion in dogs. Can J Anaesth. 1992;39:877–87.
22. Cho YJ, Bae J, Kim TK, Hong DM, Seo JH, Bahk JH, et al. Microcirculation measured by vascular occlusion test during desflurane-remifentanil anesthesia is superior to that in propofol-remifentanil anesthesia in patients undergoing thoracic surgery: subgroup analysis of a prospective randomized study. J Clin Monit Comput. 2017;31:989–97.
23. Bruegger D, Bauer A, Finsterer U, Bernasconi P, Kreimeier U, Christ F. Microvascular changes during anesthesia: sevoflurane compared with propofol. Acta Anaesthesiol Scand. 2002;46:481–7.
24. Vellinga NAR, Ince C, Boerma EC. Microvascular dysfunction in the surgical patient. Curr Opin Crit Care. 2010;16:377–83.
25. Jhanji S, Lee C, Watson D, Hinds C, Pearse RM. Microvascular flow and tissue oxygenation after major abdominal surgery: association with post-operative complications. Intensive Care Med. 2009;35:671–7.
26. Feldheiser A, Conroy P, Bonomo T, Cox B, Garces TR, Spies C. Anaesthesia working Group of the Enhanced Recovery after Surgery (ERAS®) society; enhanced recovery after surgery society. Development and feasibility study of an algorithm for intraoperative goalcirected haemodynamic management in noncardiac surgery. J Int Med Res. 2012;40:1227–41.
27. Aykut G, Veenstra G, Scorcella C, Ince C Boerma C. Cytocam-IDF (incident dark field illumination) imaging for bedside monitoring of the microcirculation. Intensive Care Med Exp. 2015;3:40.
28. Ince C, Boerma EC, Cecconi M, De Backer D, Shapiro NI, Duranteau J, et al. Second consensus on the assessment of sublingual microcirculation in critically ill patients: results from a task force of the European Society of Intensive Care Medicine. Intensive Care Med. 2018;44:281–99.
29. Gómez H, Mesquida J, Simon P, Kim HK, Puyana JC, Ince C, et al. Characterization of tissue oxygen saturation and the vascular occlusion test: influence of measurement sites, probe sizes and deflation thresholds. Crit Care. 2009;13(Suppl 5):S3.
30. Myers D, McGraw M, George M, Mulier K, Beilman G. Tissue hemoglobin index: a non-invasive optical measure of total tissue hemoglobin. Crit Care. 2009;13(Suppl 5):S2.
31. Gómez H, Torres A, Polanco P, Kim HK, Zenker S, Puyana JC, et al. Use of non-invasive NIRS during a vascular occlusion test to assess dynamic tissue O(2) saturation response. Intensive Care Med. 2008;34:1600–7.
32. Donati A, Damiani E, Domizi R, Scorcella C, Carsetti A, Tondi S, et al. Near-infrared spectroscopy for assessing tissue oxygenation and microvascular reactivity in critically ill patients: a prospective observational study. Crit Care. 2016;20:311.
33. Katseni K, Chalkias A, Kotsis T, Dafnios N, Arapoglou V, Kaparos G, et al. The effect of perioperative ischemia and reperfusion on multiorgan dysfunction following abdominal aortic aneurysm repair. Biomed Res Int. 2015;2015:598980.
34. Thompson MM, Nasim A, Sayers RD, Thompson J, Smith G, Lunec J, et al. Oxygen free radical and cytokine generation during endovascular and conventional aneurysm repair. Eur J Vasc Endovasc Surg. 1996;12:70–5.
35. Nemeth N, Kiss F, Klarik Z, Toth E, Mester A. Furka I, et al. Simultaneous investigation of hemodynamic, microcirculatory and arterio-venous micro-rheological parameters in infrarenal or suprarenal aortic cross-clamping model in the rat. Clin Hemorheol Microcirc. 2014;57:339–53.
36. Elbers PW, Ince C. Mechanisms of critical illness--classifying microcirculatory flow abnormalities in distributive shock. Crit Care. 2006;10:221.
37. Neary P, Redmond HP. Ischaemia-reperfusion injury and the systemic inflammatory response syndrome. In: Grace PA, Mathie RT, editors. Ischaemia-reperfusion injury. Blackwell science, London; 1999. p. 123–36.

38. Gordeeva AE, Sharapov MG, Tikhonova IV, Chemeris NK, Fesenko EE, Novoselov VI, et al. Vascular pathology of ischemia/reperfusion injury of rat small intestine. Cells Tissues Organs. 2017;203:353–64.
39. Ince C. Hemodynamic coherence and the rationale for monitoring the microcirculation. Crit Care. 2015;19(Suppl 3):S8.
40. Kimberger O, Arnberger M, Brandt S, Plock J, Sigursson GH, Kurz A, et al. Goal-directed colloid administration improves the microcirculation of healthy and perianastomotic colon. Anesthesiology. 2009;110:496–504.
41. Carsetti A, Watson X, Cecconi M. Haemodynamic coherence in perioperative setting. Best Pract Res Clin Anaesthesiol. 2016;30:445–52.
42. Xu Z, Yu J, Wu J, Qi F, Wang H, Wang Z, et al. The effects of two anesthetics, Propofol and sevoflurane, on liver ischemia/reperfusion injury. Cell Physiol Biochem. 2016;38:1631–42.
43. Ogawa Y, Iwasaki K, Shibata S, Kato J, Ogawa S, Oi Y. Different effects on circulatory control during volatile induction and maintenance of anesthesia and total intravenous anesthesia: autonomic nervous activity and arterial cardiac baroreflex function evaluated by blood pressure and heart rate variability analysis. J Clin Anesth. 2006;18:87–95.
44. Gan X, Xing D, Su G, Li S, Luo C, Irwin MG, et al. Propofol attenuates small intestinal ischemia reperfusion injury through inhibiting NADPH oxidase mediated mast cell activation. Oxidative Med Cell Longev. 2015;2015:167014.
45. Bellanti F, Mirabella L, Mitarotonda D, Blonda M, Tamborra R, Cinnella G, et al. Propofol but not sevoflurane prevents mitochondrial dysfunction and oxidative stress by limiting HIF-1α activation in hepatic ischemia/reperfusion injury. Free Radic Biol Med. 2016;96:323–33.
46. Donati A, Cornacchini O, Loggi S, Caporelli S, Conti G, Falcetta S, et al. A comparison among portal lactate, intramucosal sigmoid Ph, and deltaCO2 (PaCO2 - regional PCo2) as indices of complications in patients undergoing abdominal aortic aneurysm surgery. Anesth Analg. 2004;99:1024–31.
47. Edul VS, Ince C, Navarro N, Previgliano L, Risso-Vazquez A, Rubatto PN, et al. Dissociation between sublingual and gut microcirculation in the response to a fluid challenge in postoperative patients with abdominal sepsis. Ann Intensive Care. 2014;4:39.

7

Anesthetic management of a patient with a continuous-flow left ventricular assist device for video-assisted thoracoscopic surgery

Shihoko Iwata*, Sumire Yokokawa, Mihoshi Sato and Makoto Ozaki

Abstract

Background: As patients with left ventricular assist device (LVAD) have long expected survival, the incidence of noncardiac surgery in this patient population is increasing. Here, we present the anesthetic management of a patient with a continuous-flow LVAD who underwent video-assisted thoracic surgery (VATS).

Case presentation: A 37-year-old man with LVAD was scheduled to undergo VATS because of repeated spontaneous pneumothorax. Generally, patients with these devices have marginal right heart function; therefore, it is important to avoid factors that worsen pulmonary vascular resistance (PVR). However, VATS requires one-lung ventilation (OLV) and it tends to cause increase in PVR, leading to right heart failure.

In the present case, when the patient was set in a lateral decubitus position and progressive hypoxia was observed during OLV, transesophageal echocardiography demonstrated a dilated right ventricle and a temporally flattened interventricular septum, and the central venous pressure increased to approximately 20 mmHg. Because we anticipated deterioration of right heart function, dobutamine and milrinone were administered and/or respirator settings were changed to decrease PVR for maintaining LVAD performance. Finally, resection of a bulla was completed, and the patient was discharged in stable condition on postoperative day 37.

Conclusions: The anesthetic management of a patient with LVAD during VATS is challenging because the possible hemodynamic changes induced by hypoxia associated with OLV affect LVAD performance and right heart function. In our experience, VATS that requires OLV will be well tolerated in a patient with LVAD with preserved right heart function, and a multidisciplinary approach to maintain right heart function will be needed.

Keywords: One-lung ventilation, Left ventricular assist device, Transesophageal echocardiography, Pneumothorax, Video-assisted thoracoscopic surgery

Background

Left ventricular assist devices (LVADs) are gaining popularity as a viable treatment, and patients with LVADs survive for many years; consequently, such patients who require noncardiac surgery are becoming increasingly common [1, 2]. The management of LVAD-supported patients for noncardiac surgery presents many challenges, and case reports of patients with LVADs who underwent several different types of noncardiac surgeries have been published [3–10]. However, none of these cases reported the perioperative management of video-assisted thoracic surgery (VATS). Here, we present the case of a patient with a continuous-flow LVAD in whom VATS and resection of a bulla were successfully completed.

Case presentation

A 37-year-old man (weight 61 kg, height 183 cm) was diagnosed with Becker muscular dystrophy-associated cardiomyopathy. Eventually, he received implantation of EVAHEART® (Sun Medical Technology Research Corporation, Nagano, Japan), which is an implantable centrifugal

* Correspondence: shk_wt_0204@ybb.ne.jp
Department of Anesthesiology, Tokyo Women's Medical University Hospital, 8-1 Kawada-cho, Shinjuku-ku, Tokyo 162-8666, Japan

LVAD, in addition to tricuspid annuloplasty (TAP) and patent foramen ovale closure surgery. One month later and 2 months after LVAD implantation, he developed spontaneous right-sided pneumothorax. Chest radiography and computed tomography (CT) revealed right-sided pneumothorax (Figs. 1 and 2, respectively). Moreover, bullae of the right pulmonary apex with moderately retained pleural effusion were observed on CT images. Subsequently, the patient was scheduled for VATS.

Prior to surgery, the patient's body weight decreased due to loss of appetite. He was hydrated with crystalloids at the request of the cardiac surgery team to prevent occurrence of the sucking phenomenon and the formation of thrombi. Consequently, he gained 3.5 kg of body weight in 4 days, exceeding his target body weight by 1 kg. However, a preoperative chest radiograph showed a dilated cardiac shadow and pulmonary congestion. The patient was routinely administered aspirin (100 mg) each day and warfarin to maintain the prothrombin time-international normalized ratio (PT-INR) at approximately 2.5–3.5 for systemic anticoagulation. The patient bridged from warfarin to intravenous heparin 3 days preoperatively. On the day of the operation, heparin administration was discontinued 3 h before surgery. Routine laboratory test results were within the normal limits except for anemia and coagulation abnormalities: prothrombin time: 17 s, activated partial thromboplastin time (APTT): 52.9 s (APTT control: 32.9 s), and PT-INR: 1.51.

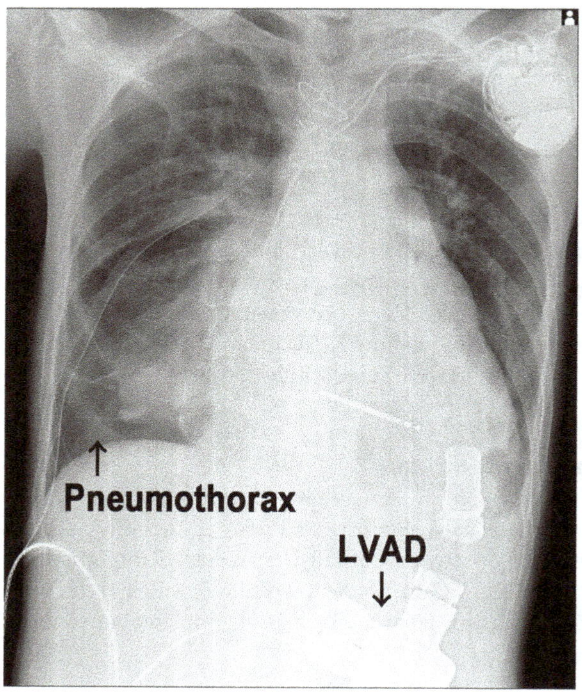

Fig. 1 Chest radiograph. Chest radiograph showing the right-side pneumothorax with a chest tube. LVAD: left ventricular assist device

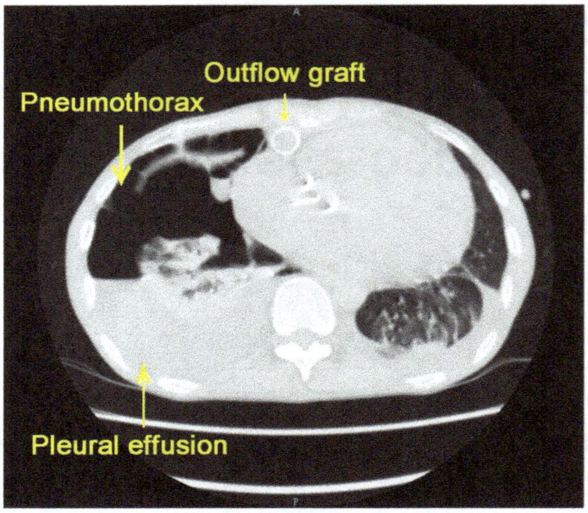

Fig. 2 A computed tomography image of the chest in lung window. Computed tomography showing the right-side pneumothorax with moderately retained pleural effusion

The patient was transported to the operating room, and monitors were placed according to the Standard American Society of Anesthesiologists. An arterial catheter was inserted in the left radial artery before general anesthesia induction using an ultrasound-guided technique. The pump speed was set at 1700 rpm, pump power consumption was 2.8 W, and the mean arterial blood pressure (ABP) was approximately 80 mmHg.

Anesthetic induction was achieved with midazolam 2 mg, remifentanil 0.2 μg/kg/min, and a propofol target blood concentration at 2 μg/ml using the target-controlled infusion system, with maintenance doses of remifentanil at 0.2–0.5 μg/kg/min and propofol at 2–2.5 μg/ml. To facilitate endotracheal intubation using a left-sided double lumen tube Broncho-Cath™ (Mallinckrodt Medical, Athlone, Ireland), 50 mg of rocuronium bromide was administered. We did not administer additional muscle relaxants except when a 10 mg maintenance dose of rocuronium bromide was used just after the patient was placed into the left lateral decubitus position, and 20 mg rocuronium bromide was administered just before the first incision. The train-of-four was measured for neuromuscular monitoring throughout the operation. A central line was inserted in the right jugular vein. The patient's ABP and central venous pressure (CVP) were continuously monitored using invasive means. Electrocardiography showed the sinus rhythm supported by the pacemaker, but the mode was changed from DDD to DOO at the heart rate of 80 bpm to avoid interference of electrocautery. Defibrillator pads were attached because implantable cardioverter defibrillator detection was inactivated. A transesophageal echocardiography (TEE) probe was placed for monitoring the performance of the LVAD and to determine intraoperative cardiac function. Initial findings included severely dilated left ventricle (LV) and right ventricle (RV), bowing of the intraventricular septum into the RV (Fig. 3), reduced LV and RV wall motion [RV-fractional area change (FAC) 16.8%], severe mitral regurgitation, continuous closed aortic valves, no aortic regurgitation, and trivial tricuspid regurgitation (TR) after TAP. The inflow cannula, anastomosed to the apex of the LV, and the outflow cannula, attached to the ascending aorta, of the LVAD were unobstructed with low flow velocities of 90.2 cm/s and 87.3 cm/s on pulse wave and color Doppler analyses, respectively. The right ventricular systolic pressure (RVSP) was estimated at 21 mmHg by measuring the TR jet maximum velocity. First, arterial gas analysis showed the following results: pH 7.437, pCO_2 31.1 mmHg, pO_2 225 mmHg, BEecf 2.7, lactate 0.7 mmol/L, SaO_2 99% and Hb 9.2 g/dL at FiO_2 of 0.5.

When the patient was placed in the left lateral decubitus position, the CVP increased from 12 mmHg to 20 mmHg despite maintaining a mean ABP of 80 mmHg (Fig. 4 (A)). The external portion of driveline was not kinked. As the patient was coughing slightly, 10 mg rocuronium bromide was administered, and the dose of remifentanil was increased. TEE examination revealed an almost akinetic LV, free wall RV, and a flattened intraventricular septum. The inflow and outflow cannulas of the LVAD were noted to be in the proper position with a pulsatile flow of approximately 60 cm/s and 110 cm/s, respectively. We assessed that the patient needed inotropic support, and hence, the administration of dobutamine (3.3 μg/kg/min) and milrinone (0.2 μg/kg/min) was initiated. Gradually, the CVP returned to 12 mmHg, and TEE showed improved LV and RV motions, with rightward shift of the intraventricular septum. At the beginning of OLV, the pressure-controlled ventilation mode was adjusted; peak inspiratory pressure and positive end-expiratory pressure were changed from 17 cmH_2O to 28 cmH_2O and from 5 cmH_2O to 7 cmH_2O, respectively, to maintain saturation of percutaneous oxygen (SpO_2) above 90%. After insertion of the access ports, SpO_2 decreased to 91% at FiO_2 of 1.0, pump power consumption increased to 3.5 watts, and the CVP reached 20 mmHg, when the mean ABP was maintained at approximately 85 mmHg (Fig. 4 (B)). TEE showed severely reduced RV motion, and the intraventricular septum had again shifted slightly to the left side. The RVSP was calculated at 35 mmHg, whereas the RV-FAC was calculated at 17.7% and appeared to be near the pre-OLV level. For further support of right heart function, continuous intravenous infusion of milrinone was increased to 0.4 μg/kg/min. Arterial blood gas analysis at this time revealed the following results: pH 7.357, pCO2 42.9 mmHg, pO2 67.9 mmHg, BEecf − 1.4, lactate 0.6 mmol/L, SaO2 96.7% and Hb 10.2 g/dL at FiO2 1.0. After a couple of min, TEE examination showed that the LV and RV motions had slightly improved, and the intraventricular septum had shifted toward the RV. Reflecting gradually improved RV wall motion, the RV-FAC was found to be 33.8%. With the increase in urine output, oxygenation improved and CVP decreased to 10 mmHg. The TEE findings did not change, and the mean ABP was maintained at 64–85 mmHg. The pulsatile waveforms were maintained on ABP and SpO_2 throughout the operation. Intraoperatively, the EVAHEART® monitor showed that the pump speed was set at 1700 rpm; the pump power consumption was 2–4 W. The VATS was completed successfully with stable hemodynamic conditions.

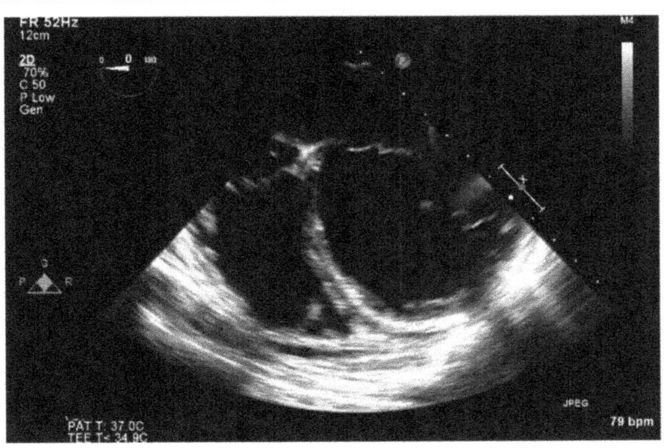

Fig. 3 A transesophageal echocardiographic image. Mid-esophageal 4-chamber view showing the severely dilated right and left ventricles. The intraventricular septum was bowing into the right ventricle

Intraoperatively, the total administration of fentanyl was 450 μg. For postoperative pain control, a single intercostal nerve block (ICNB) was applied by the thoracic surgeons from the inside whilst closing the chest, and an intravenous patient control system (fentanyl 20 μg/h, lock-out time 10 min, 20 μg/one demanded dose) was used. The total OLV time was 3 h 6 min, with an operation time of 3 h 5 min, necessitating a fluid input of 1320 ml crystalloids. The total urine output and blood loss measured were 2550 ml and 23 ml, respectively. Before recovery from general anesthesia, the TEE findings and LVAD parameters showed unremarkable changes in the supine position. The neuromuscular blockade was reversed with sugammadex sodium. After extubation, the patient did not experience pain and could breathe deeply. The patient was transferred to the intensive care unit in stable condition. However, he needed temporary bilevel positive airway pressure support after several hours. Moreover, postoperative pneumonia was suspected on postoperative day 2, and a change in the antibiotic protocol was needed. Finally, he recovered in 1 week and was discharged from our hospital in stable condition on postoperative day 37.

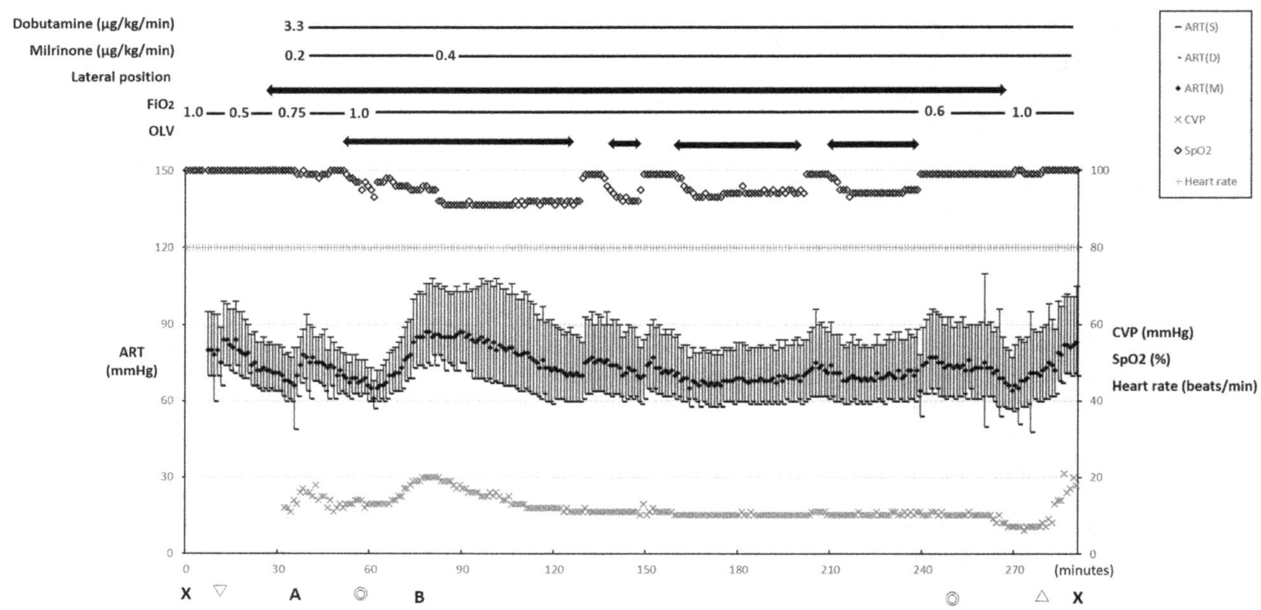

Fig. 4 Anesthetic record. The pulsatile waveforms were maintained on ABP. When the patient was placed in the left lateral decubitus position, CVP increased from 12 mmHg to 20 mmHg (A). After insertion of the access ports, SpO2 decreased to 91% at FiO2 of 1.0, and the CVP reached 20 mmHg, although the mean ABP was maintained at approximately 85 mmHg (B). ABP: arterial blood pressure, CVP: central venous pressure, SpO2: saturation of percutaneous oxygen, FiO2: fraction of inspiratory oxygen, OLV: one-lung ventilation. X: start and completion of anesthesia, ◎: start and completion of surgery, ▽: intubation, △: extubation

Discussion and conclusions

For patients with LVAD, the right heart function is frequently marginal; hence, it is important to avoid factors that worsen PVR (e.g., hypoxia, hypercarbia, and light anesthesia) and overfilling the RV with fluid [11–13]. However, OLV could lead to higher PVR, induced by possible complications such as hypoxemia and hypercarbia, where the RV encounters sudden changes in afterload, preload, and contractility [14]. Therefore, based on the findings of previous studies [3–10], the management of LVAD-supported patients for VATS may be more challenging than that of LVAD-supported patients undergoing noncardiac surgeries, as there may be sudden OLV-associated, deteriorative RV function.

Generally, medical therapy for acute right heart failure starts with meticulous volume optimization. Subsequent management strategies involve inotropes to reduce the cardiac filling pressures (dobutamine and phosphodiesterase III inhibitors) and further measures for afterload reduction [inhaled nitric oxide (iNO)] [15, 16]. NO is administered as a pharmacological intervention to treat right heart failure caused by pulmonary hypertension [15, 16]. However, it remains controversial whether iNO is effective in hypoxia during OLV. Therefore, routine use of iNO to treat hypoxemia during OLV is not recommended [17, 18].

In our present case, relatively preserved right heart function (trivial TR and low CVP and RVSP) could tolerate an increase in PVR caused by OLV-induced hypoxia with administration of dobutamine and milrinone and/or adjustment of the ventilator.

In fluid therapy of a patient with LVAD undergoing noncardiac surgery, hypovolemia can compromise not only the perfusion of vital organs but also LVAD performance, although excessive fluid administration may lead to overload in the interstitial space, with increased pulmonary complications, delayed recovery, hypoxia, induced pulmonary hypertension, and right heart failure [12].

After LVAD implantation, the patient's clinical course was hemodynamically stable. However, it was difficult to maintain the body weight constant due to excessive urination caused by diuretic administration and high or low intake of water, salt, and food. The body weight was controlled by discontinuing the administration of diuretics and adjusting the intake of food, salt, and water. However, pneumothorax recurred, and the body weight was decreased by loss of appetite. Consequently, the patient lost body weight preoperatively, and needed volume load to avoid occurrence of the sucking phenomenon and thrombus formation.

According to Shah et al., at left ventricular internal diastolic dimension (LVIDD) 7 cm, the hazard ratio for axial configuration device thrombosis, compared with the centrifugal configuration device, was 1.61 and continued to rise as the LVIDD increased. It was considered that the patient potentially had higher thrombotic risk because the preoperative LVIDD of the patient was measured at 7.7 cm, although EVAHEART® is a centrifugal LVAD. Conversely, in multivariable models, the hazard of stroke was higher with the CC device regardless of LVIDD [19]. In addition, interruption of anticoagulation due to the bleeding risk associated with an elective procedure may also lead to an elevated risk of thromboembolism, even if heparin bridging is implemented. A recent study recommended an extended personalized approach that incorporates the extent of the patient's underlying risk for thrombosis and bleeding [20].

In LVAD patients, severe right heart failure is a thrombotic risk factor [20] and may be induced by hypovolemia. Therefore, preoperative volume management with anticoagulation therapy is important to avoid thrombus formation.

Consequently, the patient had been hydrated with crystalloids, and a weight gain of 3.5 kg in 4 days was achieved before the VATS, exceeding his target body weight by 1 kg, as the optimal volume management to compensate for body weight loss. Hemodynamic stability was achieved at anesthesia induction, although we had to manage deteriorative desaturation during OLV. Finally, the total fluid balance was minus 1253 ml, and oxygenation during OLV gradually improved, accompanied with an increase in the volume of urine, which was drained continuously.

EVAHEART®, i.e., the patient's LVAD, acts as an implantable centrifugal blood pump. It is used for bridge-to-transplantation and has a gentle-slope pressure-flow characteristic and an extremely high pump flow capacity of 15–20 l/min during systole [21]. Continuous-flow LVADs generate flow that may present pulsatility because of the residual LV function of the assisted heart. Indeed, the presence of pulsatility on pump signals has been used as an anecdotal "marker" of the myocardial contractile state in the clinical realm [11, 21–24]. Therefore, it is anticipated that the pump flow for patient management does not need to be known if the pulsatility is maintained on an arterial line and/or SpO_2. Intraoperatively, in the present case, the pump flow pattern was completely pulsatile at a constant speed of 1700 rpm, with a stable pump power consumption at 2–4 W.

Monitoring of CVP and pulmonary artery catheter (PAC) placement should be considered on a case-by-case basis [4, 12, 13]. In this case, we considered that a PAC was not necessary because the patient showed no evidence of pulmonary hypertension and his right heart function was sufficiently preserved to resist the increase in PVR associated with OLV. In addition, TEE was anticipated to replace PAC because TEE can provide quantification of pulmonary artery systolic pressure by the trans-tricuspid pressure gradient, which is a reliable method compared to PAC [15]. Practically, in conjunction with CVP, TEE was useful to assess the deteriorative hemodynamic changes following OLV and change in patient position and to guide fluid therapy and inotropic drug administration. However, PAC should be considered in cases of pulmonary hypertension and/or highly predictable hemodynamic instability during surgery because of progressive right heart failure, for example, for a LVAD patient with low PAP and high CVP [13] .

A change to the lateral decubitus position could also possibly affect LVAD performance because of decrease in preload [3, 12, 13]. In the current case, we suspected insufficient anesthesia, as a change of the patient position to the lateral decubitus position resulted in a transient increase in PVR. In addition to rocuronium bromide and remifentanil, dobutamine and milrinone were administered to improve right heart function and LVAD performance. Eventually, hemodynamic stability was achieved.

Regarding postoperative analgesia, there is no gold standard for regional analgesia for VATS. In contrast, thoracic epidural analgesia and paravertebral block are established analgesic gold standards for open surgery such as thoracotomy [25]. Recently, several types of regional analgesia have been reported for VATS such as multilevel and single-shot paravertebral blocks, interpleural infusion, long thoracic nerve block [25], retrolaminar block, erector spinae plane block [26], and continuous and single-shot serratus plane blocks [27]. These procedures may be applied even for LVAD patients who require anticoagulation. However, no study has examined the frequency and severity of hemorrhagic complications after plexus or peripheral block in patients receiving anticoagulation therapy. For patients undergoing deep plexus or deep peripheral block, recommendations regarding neuraxial techniques should be similarity applied [28].

In our case, for postoperative pain control, intravenous patient-controlled analgesia with fentanyl was used and a single shot of ICNB was applied by the thoracic surgeons before closing the chest; this was favored due to the lower incidence of serious adverse events such as epidural hematoma, despite poorer pain control than that after thoracic epidural anesthesia [29].

The type of anesthesia (inhalational versus total intravenous anesthesia) by itself does not affect oxygenation during OLV [14, 17], although intravenous anesthetic drugs have a limited effect on hypoxic pulmonary vasoconstriction, which is attenuated by inhaled anesthetics [30]. Because the patient was diagnosed with Becker type muscular dystrophy, we chose total intravenous anesthesia to avoid the potential risk of malignant hyperthermia, although controversial results have been reported regarding whether malignant hyperthermia is caused by administration of succinylcholine rather than volatile anesthetic agents [31, 32]. We believe that it is not crucial to select the type of anesthesia in LVAD patients that require OLV.

The anesthetic management of a patient with LVAD in VATS is challenging because the possible hemodynamic changes induced by hypoxia associated with OLV affect LVAD performance and right heart function.

In our experience, VATS that requires OLV will be well tolerated in a patient with LVAD with preserved right heart function, and a multidisciplinary approach to maintain right heart function will be needed.

Abbreviations

ABP: Arterial blood pressure; APTT: Activated partial thromboplastin time; CT: Computed tomography; CVP: Central venous pressure; FAC: Fractional area change; ICNB: Intercostal nerve block; iNO: inhaled nitric oxide; LV: Left ventricle; LVAD: Left ventricular assist device; LVIDD: Left ventricular internal diastolic dimension; OLV: One-lung ventilation; PAC: Pulmonary artery catheter; PT-INR: Prothrombin time-international normalized ratio; PVR: Pulmonary vascular resistance; RV: Right ventricle; RVSP: Right ventricular systolic pressure; SpO2: Saturation of percutaneous oxygen; TAP: Tricuspid annuloplasty; TEE: Transesophageal echocardiography; TR: Tricuspid regurgitation; VATS: Video-assisted thoracic surgery

Acknowledgements

The authors would like to thank Dr. Takako Matsumoto (thoracic surgeon) for useful discussions. We also appreciate the company named Editage (www.editage.jp) for English language editing.

Authors' contributions

SI was the principal author and principal investigator. SY, MS and MO helped in writing the case report as co-authors. All authors have read and approved the manuscript.

References

1. Nelson EW, Heinke T, Finley A, Guldan GJ, Gaddy P, Toole JM, et al. Management of LVAD patients for noncardiac surgery: a single-institution study. J Cardiothorac Vasc Anesth. 2015;29:898–900.
2. Mathis MR, Sathishkumar S, Kheterpal S, Caldwell MD, Pagani FD, Jewell ES, et al. Complications, risk factors, and staffing patterns for noncardiac surgery in patients with left ventricular assist devices. Anesthesiology. 2017;126:450–60.
3. Goldstein DJ, Mullis SL, Delphin ES, el-Amir N, Ashton RC Jr, Gardocki M, et al. Noncardiac surgery in long-term implantable left ventricular assist-device recipients. Ann Surg. 1995;222:203–7.
4. Stone ME, Soong W, Krol M, Reich DL. The anesthetic considerations in patients with ventricular assist devices presenting for noncardiac surgery: a review of eight cases. Anesth Analg. 2002;95:42–9.
5. Oleyar M, Stone M, Neustein SM. Perioperative management of a patient with a nonpulsatile left ventricular-assist device presenting for noncardiac surgery. J Cardiothorac Vasc Anesth. 2010;24:820–3.
6. Ficke DJ, Lee J, Chaney MA, Bas H, Vidal-Melo MF, Stone ME. Case 6-2010: noncardiac surgery in patients with a left ventricular assist device. J Cardiothorac Vasc Anesth. 2010;24:1002–9.
7. Kartha V, Gomez W, Wu B, Tremper K. Laparoscopic cholecystectomy in a patient with an implantable left ventricular assist device. Br J Anaesth. 2008; 100:652–5.
8. Chacon MM, Hattrup EA, Shillcutt SK. Perioperative management of two patients with left ventricular assist devices presenting for noncardiac surgery in the prone position. A A Case Rep. 2014;2:70–3.
9. Sathishkumar S, Kodavatiganti R, Plummer S, High K. Perioperative management of a patient with an axial-flow rotary ventricular assist device for laparoscopic ileo-colectomy. J Anaesthesiol Clin Pharmacol. 2012;28:101–5.
10. Nayak JG, White CW, Nates W, Sharda R, Home D, Kaler K, et al. Laparoscopic nephroureterectomy in a patient with a left ventricular assist device. Can Urol Assoc J. 2013;7:E640–4.
11. Chung M. Perioperative management of the patient with a left ventricular assist device for noncardiac surgery. Anesth Analg. 2018;126:1839–50.
12. Slininger KA, Haddadin AS, Mangi AA. Perioperative management of patients with left ventricular assist devices undergoing noncardiac surgery. J Cardiothorac Vasc Anesth. 2013;27:752–9.
13. Dalia AA, Cronin B, Stone ME, Turner K, Hargrave J, Vidal-Melo MF, et al. Anesthetic management of patients with continuous-flow left ventricular assist devices undergoing noncardiac surgery: an update for anesthesiologists. J Cardiothorac Vasc Anesth. 2018;32:1001–12.
14. Rana M, Yusuff H, Zochios V. The right ventricle during selective lung ventilation for thoracic surgery. J Cardiothorac Vasc Anesth. 2019;33: 2007–16.
15. Harjola VP, Mebazaa A, Čelutkienė J, Bettex D, Bueno H, Chioncel O, et al. Contemporary management of acute right ventricular failure: a statement from the heart failure association and the working group on pulmonary circulation and right ventricular function of the European society of cardiology. Eur J Heart Fail. 2016;18:226–41.
16. Lin W, Poh AL, Tang WHW. Novel insights and treatment strategies for right heart failure. Curr Heart Fail Rep. 2018;15:141–55.
17. Karzai W, Schwarzkopf K. Hypoxemia during one-lung ventilation: prediction, prevention, and treatment. Anesthesiology. 2009;110:1402–11.
18. Campos JH, Feider A. Hypoxia during one-lung ventilation: a review and update. J Cardiothorac Vasc Anesth. 2018;32:2330–8.
19. Shah P, Birk S, Maltais S, Stulak J, Elmi A, Pagani FD, et al. Left ventricular assist device outcomes based on flow configuration and pre-operative left ventricular dimension: an interagency registry for mechanically assisted circulatory support analysis. J Heart Lung Transplant. 2017;36:640–9.
20. Shah P, Tantry US, Bliden KP, Gurbel PA. Bleeding and thrombosis associated with ventricular assist device therapy. J Heart Lung Transplant. 2017;36:1164–73.
21. Yamazaki K, Saito S, Kihara S, Tagusari O, Kurosawa H. Completely pulsatile high flow circulatory support with a constant-speed centrifugal blood pump: mechanisms and early clinical observations. Gen Thorac Cardiovasc Surg. 2007;55:158–62.
22. Ferreira AL, Wang Y, Gorcsan J 3rd, Antaki JF. Assessment of cardiac function during mechanical circulatory support: the quest for a suitable clinical index. Conf Proc IEEE Eng Med Biol Soc. 2011;2011:223–6.
23. Moazami N, Fukamachi K, Kobayashi M, Smedira NG, Hoercher KJ, Massiello A, et al. Axial and centrifugal continuous-flow rotary pumps: a translation from pump mechanics to clinical practice. J Heart Lung Transplant. 2013;32:1–11.
24. Lim HS, Howell N, Ranasinghe A. The physiology of continuous-flow left ventricular assist devices. J Card Fail. 2017;23:169–80.
25. Steinthorsdottir KJ, Wildgaard L, Hansen HJ, Petersen RH, Wildgaard K. Regional analgesia for video-assisted thoracic surgery: a systematic review. Eur J Cardiothorac Surg. 2014;45:959–66.
26. Onishi E, Toda N, Kameyama Y, Yamauchi M. Comparison of clinical efficacy and anatomical investigation between retrolaminar block and erector spinae plane block. Biomed Res Int. 2019;2019:2578396.
27. Allain PA, Carella M, Agrafiotis AC, Burey J, Assouad J, Hafiani EM, et al. Comparison of several methods for pain management after video-assisted thoracic surgery for pneumothorax: an observational study. BMC Anesthesiol. 2019;19:120.
28. Horlocker TT. Regional anaesthesia in the patient receiving antithrombotic and antiplatelet therapy. Br J Aaesth. 2011;107:i96–i106.
29. Umari M, Falini S, Segat M, Zuliani M, Crisman M, Comuzzi L, et al. Anesthesia and fast-track in video-assisted thoracic surgery (VATS): from evidence to practice. J Thorac Dis. 2018;10:S542–54.
30. Lumb AB, Slinger P. Hypoxic pulmonary vasoconstriction: physiology and anesthetic implications. Anesthesiology. 2015;122:932–46.
31. Cripe LH, Tobias JD. Cardiac considerations in the operative management of the patient with Duchenne or Becker muscular dystrophy. Paediatr Anaesth. 2013;23:777–84.
32. Segura LG, Lorenz JD, Weingarten TN, Scavonetto F, Bojanić K, Selcen D, et al. Anesthesia and Duchenne or Becker muscular dystrophy: review of 117 anesthetic exposures. Paediatr Anaesth. 2013;23:855–64.

8

Acute cerebral infarction in a patient with an epidural catheter after left upper lobectomy

Asuka Kitajima[1], Yuji Otsuka[1], Alan Kawarai Lefor[2] and Masamitsu Sanui[1*]

Abstract

Background: There are several recent reports that left upper lobe lung resection is a risk factor for the development of postoperative thromboembolism. Although administering epidural analgesia is common in thoracic surgery, anesthesiologists should be alert when administering epidural analgesia to a patient undergoing left upper lobectomy, considering the increased risk of postoperative thromboembolism and the potential need for anticoagulation or fibrinolytic therapy in the immediate postoperative period.

Case presentation: A seventy-one-year-old female with a metastatic lung lesion developed a cerebral infarction approximately 30 h after video-assisted thoracoscopic left upper lobectomy. Cerebral intravascular therapy was indicated and the epidural catheter was removed immediately to avoid formation of an epidural hematoma. Approximately four hours after onset, reperfusion was successfully established by aspiration of endovascular thrombi. She recovered with mild residual paralysis of the left upper extremity and was transferred to a rehabilitation facility.

Conclusions: We present a patient with a cerebral infarction after left upper lobectomy. Left upper lobectomy is associated with an increased risk of postoperative thromboembolism. Although the exact mechanism of thrombosis after left upper lobectomy is unclear, a judicious decision should be made regarding epidural catheter placement for postoperative analgesia.

Keywords: Epidural anesthesia, Postoperative complication, Cerebral infarction, Thoracic surgery

Background

Paraplegia due to acute spinal epidural hematoma after the placement or removal of epidural catheters is very rare, but once a hematoma develops, the prognosis is often devastating. Known risk factors for acute spinal epidural hematomas include thrombocytopenia, anti-coagulant or antiplatelet therapy, and being an elderly female.

There are several recent reports that left upper lobe (LUL) lobectomy is a risk factor for the development of postoperative cerebral thromboembolism [1–3]. The mechanism of cerebral infarction after LUL lobectomy may include stasis of blood flow in the stump of the left upper pulmonary vein because the left upper pulmonary vein stump may be longer than other pulmonary vein remnants for anatomical reasons [2]. Although administering epidural analgesia is common in thoracic surgery, anesthesiologists should be alert when administering epidural anesthesia to a patient undergoing LUL lobectomy, considering the risk of postoperative cerebral thromboembolism and potential need for anticoagulation or fibrinolysis therapy in the immediate postoperative period. We present a patient who underwent LUL lobectomy, complicated by the development of a postoperative cerebral thrombo-embolism. The epidural catheter was immediately re-moved to allow urgent administration of intravascular therapy. A neuraxial hematoma did not develop.

Case presentation

A 71-year-old female with a pulmonary metastasis from primary sigmoid colon cancer presented for video-assisted thoracoscopic LUL lobectomy. She

* Correspondence: msanui@mac.com
[1]Department of Anesthesiology and Critical Care Medicine, Jichi Medical University Saitama Medical Center, 1-847 Amanumacho, Omiyaku, Saitama 330-8503, Japan

underwent resection of sigmoid colon cancer (Stage-IIA T3N0M0) five years previously. She did not receive adjuvant chemotherapy. Recent computed tomography scan revealed a mass in the left upper lobe of the lung, and she was admitted to undergo video-assisted thoracoscopic LUL lobectomy. She had a history of hypertension and osteoporosis, treated with raloxifen, alfacalcidol, fexofenadine hydrochloride, pseudoephedrine and esomeprazole magnesium hydrate. She smoked two packs of cigarettes per day for 45 years. Physical examination on admission was unremarkable. Preoperative electrocardiogram showed sinus rhythm with an incomplete right bundle branch block. After placement of an epidural catheter between the fifth and sixth vertebrae, general anesthesia was induced with remifentanil and propofol. Tracheal intubation was accomplished using rocuronium bromide. Combined epidural and general anesthesia was maintained with remifentanil, desflurane and ropivacaine. The LUL lobectomy proceeded without difficulty with an operating time of 157 min. No arrhythmias or severe hypotension were detected during the surgery. She was transferred to a general ward after extubation in the operating room.

The postoperative course was uncomplicated with no episodes of atrial fibrillation on the first postoperative day. On the evening of the second postoperative day, she was seen to lean suddenly to the left after urinating. She developed left hemiparesis, right conjugate deviation and dysarthria. She underwent emergency magnetic resonance imaging after immediate removal of the epidural catheter. Cerebral magnetic resonance angiography revealed cessation of blood flow in the right internal carotid artery (Fig. 1). An acute cerebral infarction was diagnosed and she was transferred to another hospital to receive intravascular therapy. Initially, 4000 units of heparin were given intravenously. Four hours after onset of arterial occlusion, extensive dark brown thrombi were removed though the intravascular catheter, and cerebral perfusion was reestablished. She received protamine at the end of procedure. Anticoagulation therapy was delayed until postoperative day 21 because a minimal hemorrhagic infarction developed. She recovered with only mild paralysis of the left upper extremity and was transferred to a rehabilitation facility on postoperative day 37.

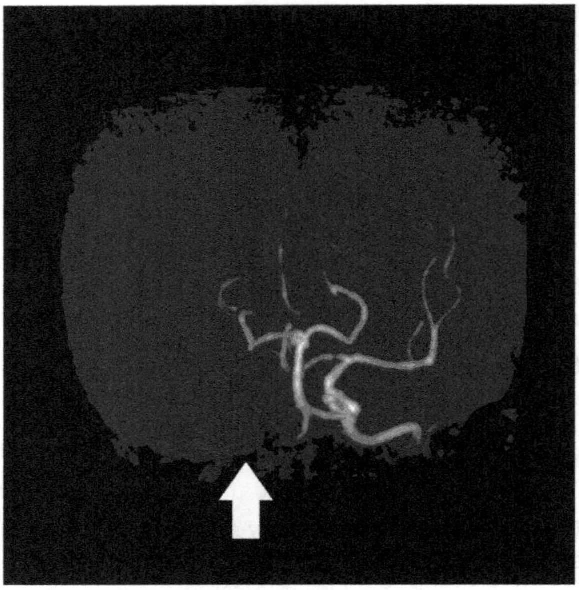

Fig. 1 Cerebral magnetic resonance angiography. Cerebral magnetic resonance angiography performed 30 h after left upper lobe resection demonstrates interruption of blood flow in the right internal carotid artery

Discussion

The incidence of cerebral infarction after pulmonary lobectomy or segmentectomy is reported to be just 0.6% [4]. This incidence is similar to that after other types of operations such as general surgery, cardiac surgery, etc. However, it has been recently reported that the incidence of cerebral infarction following LUL lobectomy is as high as 4.5% [1]. The mechanism of cerebral infarction after LUL lobectomy may include stasis of blood flow in the stump of the left upper pulmonary vein [2]. The left upper pulmonary vein stump may be longer than other pulmonary vein remnants for anatomical reasons [2]. Theoretically, a thrombus may easily be generated in a long vein remnant due to stasis [3]. In the present patient, a potential embolic source may have been in the left upper pulmonary vein remnant since the patient had no features consistent with perioperative atrial fibrillation, or a plaque in the aorta or carotid arteries. The thrombi retrieved by intravascular aspiration appeared relatively fresh, suggesting that they were formed during or immediately after surgery. For these reasons, the left upper pulmonary vein stump is a likely source of the emboli. Therefore, early postoperative anticoagulation may be indicated to prevent thrombus formation.

In the present patient, we removed the epidural catheter immediately after recognizing the cerebral infarction to maximize the time from removal until initiating the planned intravascular treatment for the cerebral embolism. Approximately four hours after removing the epidural catheter, intravascular thrombus aspiration was performed. Although 4000 units of heparin were administered intravenously at the beginning of the intravascular procedure, no thrombolytic medication was used. A four-hour interval between epidural catheter removal and administration of intravenous heparin may be sufficient. The American Society of Regional Anesthesia and Pain Medicine guideline states that a one-hour interval between needle placement and intravenous heparin administration decreases the risk of significant bleeding [5]. Early detection and selective intravascular therapy may have contributed to the good outcome.

Cerebral infarction can occur in patients undergoing LUL lobectomy even when perioperative intravenous heparinization is performed [1, 3]. To prevent thrombus formation, prophylactic subcutaneous heparin injection is probably insufficient and therapeutic systemic heparinization should be considered postoperatively. However, it is not recommended to remove the epidural catheter in patients undergoing continuous intravenous heparinization, since that may increase the risk of epidural hematoma formation. An epidural catheter can be kept in place while a patient is undergoing anticoagulation therapy as long as the acute pain service maintains close observation of the patient. However, migration or spontaneous removal of the catheter can happen. Clinically significant movement of catheters was reported in approximately 30% of patients with postoperative epidural catheters [6, 7], while accidental removal was reported in approximately 17% of catheters [8]. Fibrinolytic therapy may be needed in specific situations. Although this patient was expeditiously given intravascular therapy, this intervention is not ubiquitously available. In facilities where intravascular therapy is not available, it is reasonable to perform fibrinolytic therapy in patients with postoperative cerebral infarction [9]. Nevertheless, the safety of epidural analgesia for patients who have the potential to receive fibrinolytic therapy has been debated. It is reasonable to use other treatment modalities other than epidural analgesia because a patient who underwent LUL lobectomy may develop thromboembolism with increased likelihood and may need early postoperative anticoagulation or fibrinolytic therapy.

In our institution, we have implemented routine intravenous systemic heparinization for three days in patients following LUL lobectomies after having the experience of treating this patient. Along with this protocol for postoperative anticoagulation therapy, we changed postoperative analgesia from the routine placement of epidural catheters to intercostal nerve blocks with intravenous patient-controlled analgesia. After these policy changes, approximately one hundred LUL lobectomies have been performed, and no postoperative thromboembolic events have occurred. In contrast to previous reports [1, 3], this experience suggests that early postoperative intravenous systemic heparinization may be effective to prevent postoperative thromboembolism, although a randomized controlled study with longer follow-up and a larger sample size is necessary to determine the efficacy, safety and optimal duration of this practice.

Conclusions

We present a patient who developed a cerebral infarction after a LUL lobectomy. Although the exact mechanism of thrombosis after LUL lobectomy has been not elucidated, a judicious decision should be made regarding epidural catheter placement for postoperative analgesia. In the future, prophylactic anticoagulation may be indicated depending on the specific type of pulmonary resection.

Abbreviations

LUL: left upper lobe

Acknowledgements

The authors thank to Dr. D. Kakimoto, T. Goto and M. Sekiguchi for their helping for management of the patient.

Authors' contributions

AK performed the literature review, compiled the case report and discussion, reviewed and selected the relevant images and drafted the manuscript. YO helped developing the conception of the case report, and critically revised the manuscript. MS and AL helped drafting the manuscript and critically revised the manuscript. All authors read and approved the final manuscript.

Author details

[1]Department of Anesthesiology and Critical Care Medicine, Jichi Medical University Saitama Medical Center, 1-847 Amanumacho, Omiyaku, Saitama 330-8503, Japan. [2]Department of Surgery, Jichi Medical University, 1-3311 Yakusiji, Shimono, Tochigi, Saitama 329-0498, Japan.

References

1. Yamamoto T, Suzuki H, Nagato K, Nakajima T, Iwata T, Yoshida S, et al. Is left upper lobectomy for lung cancer a risk factor for cerebral infarction? Surg Today. 2016;46:780–4.
2. Ohtaka K, Hida Y, Kaga K, Kato T, Muto J Nakada-Kubota R, et al. Thrombosis in the pulmonary vein stump after left upper lobectomy as a possible cause of cerebral infarction. Ann Thorac Surg. 2013;95:1924–8.
3. Ohtaka K, Takahashi Y, Uemura S, Shoji Y, Hayama S, Ichimura T, et al. Blood stasis may cause thrombosis in the left superior pulmonary vein stump after left upper lobectomy. J Cardiothorac Surg. 2014;9:159–65.
4. Bateman BT, Schumacher HC, Wang S, Shaefi S, Berman MF. Perioperative acute ischemic stroke in noncardiac and nonvascular surgery: incidence, risk factors, and outcomes. Anesthesiology. 2009;110:231–8.
5. Horlocker TT, Vandermeulen E, Kopp SL, Gogarten W, Leffert LR, Benzon HT. Regional anesthesia in the patient receiving antithrombotic or thrombolytic therapy: American Society of Regional Anesthesia and Pain Medicine evidence-based guidelines (fourth edition). Reg Anesth Pain Med. 2018;43:263–309.
6. Burstal R, Wegener F, Hayes C, Lantry G. Subcutaneous tunnelling of epidural catheters for postoperative analgesia to prevent accidental dislodgement: a randomized controlled trial. Anaesth Intensive Care. 1998; 26:147–51.
7. Chadwick VL, Jones M, Poulton B, Fleming BG. Epidural catheter migration: a comparison of tunnelling against a new technique of catheter fixation. Anaesth Intensive Care. 2003;31:518–22.
8. Jabaudon M, Chabanne R, Sossou A, Bertrand PM, Kauffmann S, Chartier C, et al. Epidural analgesia in the intensive care unit: an observational series of 121 patients. Anaesth Crit Care Pain Med. 2015;34:217–23.
9. Voelkel N, Hubert ND, Backhaus R, Haberl RL, Hubert GJ. Thrombolysis in postoperative stroke. Stroke. 2017;48:3034–9.

9

Impact of brief prewarming on anesthesia-related core-temperature drop, hemodynamics, microperfusion and postoperative ventilation in cytoreductive surgery of ovarian cancer

L. Kaufner[1*], P. Niggemann[1], T. Baum[1], S. Casu[2], J. Sehouli[3], A. Bietenbeck[4], M. Boschmann[5], C. D. Spies[1], A. Henkelmann[1] and C. von Heymann[2]

Abstract

Background: General (GA)- and epidural-anesthesia may cause a drop in body-core-temperature (BCT_{drop}), and hypothermia, which may alter tissue oxygenation (StO_2) and microperfusion after cytoreductive surgery for ovarian cancer. Cell metabolism of subcutaneous fat- or skeletal muscle cells, measured in microdialysis, may be affected. We hypothesized that forced-air prewarming during epidural catheter placement and induction of GA maintains normothermia and improves microperfusion.

Methods: After ethics approval 47 women scheduled for cytoreductive surgery were prospectively enrolled. Women in the study group were treated with a prewarming of 43 °C during epidural catheter placement. BCT (Spot on®, 3 M) was measured before (T_1), after induction of GA (T_2) at 15 min (T_3) after start of surgery, and until 2 h after ICU admission (T_{ICU2h}). Primary endpoint was BCT_{drop} between T_1 and T_2. Microperfusion-, hemodynamic- and clinical outcomes were defined as secondary outcomes. Statistical analysis used the Mann-Whitney-U- and non-parametric-longitudinal tests.

Results: BCT_{drop} was 0.35 °C with prewarming and 0.9 °C without prewarming ($p < 0.005$) and BCT remained higher over the observation period ($\Delta T_4 = 0.9$ °C up to $\Delta T_7 = 0.95$ °C, $p < 0.001$). No significant differences in hemodynamic parameters, transfusion, arterial lactate and dCO_2 were measured. In microdialysis the ethanol ratio was temporarily, but not significantly, reduced after prewarming. Lactate, glucose and glycerol after PW tended to be more constant over the entire period. Postoperatively, six women without prewarming, but none after prewarming were mechanical ventilated ($p < 0.001$).

Conclusion: Prewarming at 43 °C reduces the BCT_{drop} and maintains normothermia without impeding the perioperative routine patient flow. Microdialysis indicate better preserved parameters of microperfusion.

Keywords: Prewarming, Ovarian cancer, Microperfusion, Normothermia

* Correspondence: lutz.kaufner@charite.de
[1]Department of Anaesthesiology and Operative Intensive Care Medicine (CCM, CVK), Charité-Universitätsmedizin Berlin, Corporate Member of Freie Universität Berlin, Humboldt-Universität zu Berlin, and Berlin Institute of Health, Campus Virchow-Klinikum, Augustenburger Platz 1, 13353 Berlin, Germany

Background

The incidence of inadvertent perioperative hypothermia in surgery, defined as a body core temperature (BCT) below 36 °C, is still high [1, 2]. A shift of thresholds for vasoconstriction and shivering as well as sympathicolysis-related vasodilatation caused by epidural anesthesia (EDA) result in a redistribution of warm blood from the body core to the periphery [3]. Furthermore, the induction of general anesthesia (GA) aggravates redistribution hypothermia up to 1.5 °C [4]. Cytoreductive surgery for ovarian cancer is characterized by maximum extent of tumour debulking including deperitonea-lisation and massive volume shifts and losses [5]. Stabilisation of the BCT, therefore, requires forced air warming and administration of warmed infusions and transfusions. However, maintainance of normothermia is jeopardized by an anesthesia-reduced base metabolic rate and heat production [5]. Perioperative hypothermia may affect coagulation by altered platelet function [6, 7] and increase intraoperative blood loss [8]. Furthermore, hypothermia-related vasoconstriction may impair microperfusion and reduce the oxygen partial pressure and oxygen saturation (StO_2) in peripheral tissues [9]. As a result of impaired microperfusion cell metabolism of subcutaneous fat- or skeletal muscle cells, measured in microdialysis (MD), may be affected [10].

Preoperative forced-air warming (prewarming) of 10 to 60 min at 43 °C [11–15] before induction of GA has been shown to reduce the temperature gradient between body core and periphery [16] in order to alleviate redistribution hypothermia [3, 16] and to maintain intraoperative normothermia [17] in minor surgery (without EDA) [11] or major abdominal surgery with EDA [12]. However, these studies required holding areas to realize prewarming and a timely patient flow. From a surgical point of view, in major cytoreductive surgery with a duration of more than 180 min it still remains unclear whether a brief prewarming during insertion of EDA is effective to maintain intra- and postoperative normothermia and to improve intraoperative hemodynamics and microperfusion as well as to reduce postoperative shivering and ventilation [18].

We hypothesized that a forced-air prewarming interval of 30 min at 43 °C during epidural catheter placement and induction of GA without any changes of the perioperative patient flow (e.g. no treatment in a preoperative holding area) is effective to maintain perioperative normothermia and improve microperfusion during cytoreductive surgery for ovarian cancer.

Methods

This single-center prospective randomized clinical trial was conducted at the Departments of Anesthesiology and Intensive Care Medicine and Gynecology of the Charité-Universitätsmedizin Berlin, Germany. Ethics approval was obtained from the institutional ethics committee (EA1/348/14, ClinicalTrials.govID: NCT02364219). Women were enrolled if they were of age (> 18 years), mentally healthy, American Society of Anesthesiologists physical status Class I–III and scheduled to undergo elective major cytoreductive surgery in primary or secondary ovarian cancer under combined epidural and general anesthesia. Exclusion criteria were: heart failure (left ventricular ejection fraction (LV-EF) < 30%), chronic obstructive pulmonary disease (GINA-Classification > 3), renal failure (glomerular filtration rate (GFR) < 50 ml/min) or dialysis, participation in another clinical trial and contraindication of EDA including non-eligibility due to refusal of neuraxial anesthesia.

After written informed consent and before surgery, women were prospectively randomized into prewarming (prewarm) and standard group (standard) using a computer-generated block randomization (Excel, Microsoft Corporation, Redmont, WA, USA). Additionally, a subgroup of the standard- and the prewarm group were randomly assigned for microdialysis (MD) measurements. The randomization was concealed. Randomization was blinded, the anesthesist during surgery was not randomized and the data evaluation took place independently from the surgery anesthesist.

According to randomization, women in the prewarming group received forced-air warming at 43 °C, during the establishment of epidural anesthesia. Prewarming was applied using a forced air warming gown (Bair Paws™ Flex Warming Gown, 3 M™, St. Paul, MN, USA) connected to a forced air warmer (Bair Hugger™, Model 750, 3 M™, St. Paul, MN, USA), which warms the front of the body including upper arms (Fig. 1a). In the standard treatment group, patients were covered by a cotton blanket for passive insulation without active warming during the insertion of the epidural catheter.

The perioperative anesthetic setting in both groups was based on the clinical practice and standard operating procedures of the Department. Upon arrival in the operating room (OR), a peripheral vein cannula was inserted and an infusion of balanced crystalloid solution was started under standard monitoring. Body core temperature was taken by using the SpotOn™ temperature system (3 M™; St. Paul, MN, USA) in both groups and throughout the observation period [19]. Perioperative body core temperatures were manually recorded in the case reporting form (CRF) at admission to the OR (T_1), insertion of epidural catheter and induction of GA (T_2) as well as after 15 min (T_3), 60 min (T_4), 120 min (T_5), 180 min (T_6), at the end of operation (T_7), on admission to the ICU (T_{ICU}) and 2 h postoperatively (T_{ICU2h}). In both groups, a thoracic epidural catheter was inserted in the sitting position (Fig. 1a). After induction of GA, EDA was established by a bolus followed by a continuous rate of ropivacaine/

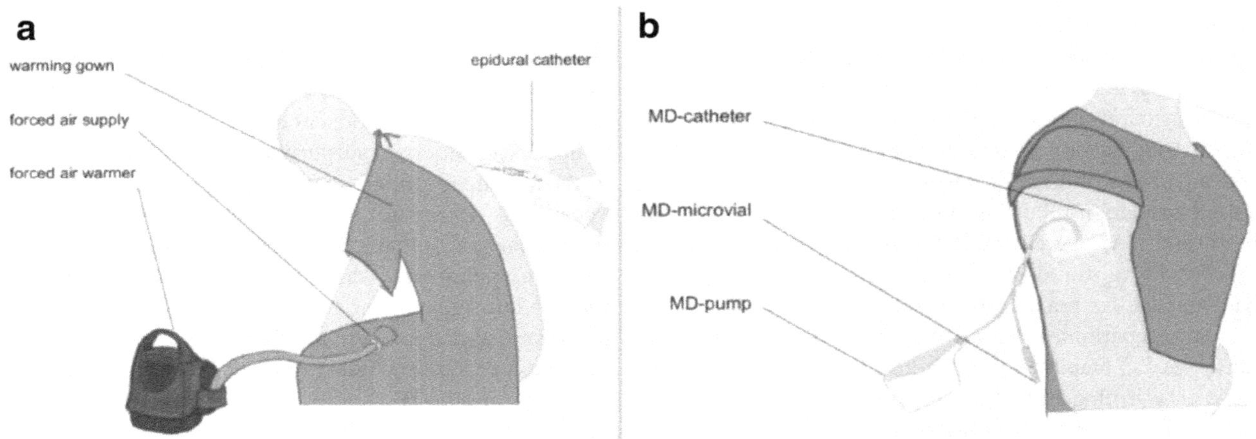

Fig. 1 a) Forced air prewarming during insertion of the epidural catheter; **b**) subcutaneous microdialyses in the upper arm

sufentanil (CADD™ Solis pump, Smiths Medical, St. Paul, MN, USA). GA was induced using propofol, fentanyl and rocuronium for endotracheal intubation and maintained with sevoflurane with a minimum inspired oxygen concentration of 40% and an end-tidal CO_2 concentration of 35 to 40 mmHg. Anaesthesia and muscle relaxation was maintained with repetitive bolusses of fentanyl and rocuronium. A central venous line (Arrow Medical Limited, Kington, UK) was placed into the internal jugular vein and blood pressure was measured by an arterial line (Vygon, Ecouen, France). During surgery, all intravenous (i.v.) fluids were infused using an active warming device (Level 1, Hot Line™, Smiths Medicals, St. Paul, MN, USA). Women were warmed by forced air warming of the upper part of the body (Standard-group: 3M™ Bair Hugger™ Intraoperative Blanket; PW-group: 3M™Bair Paws™ Flex Warming Gown) at 43 °C until end of anesthesia. Forced air warming was shortly paused in both groups during disinfection of the belly before surgery. Postoperatively, women were transferred to the post-anesthesia care unit (PACU). If patients showed clinical signs of hypovolemia (such as heart rate (HR) > 100 bpm, mean arterial pressure (MAP) < 60 mmHg, increased pulse pressure variation (PPV)) as well as hypovolemic changes in the hemodynamic monitoring (stroke volume variation (SVV), stroke volume (SV) and CO; Flo-Trac™, Edwards Lifesciencess, Irvine, CA, USA) and in case of intraoperative volume- and blood loss, crystalloid infusion, gelatine infusion (500–1000 ml Gelafundin™ 4% BBraun, Melsungen, Germany) and, if needed, fresh frozen plasma (FFP) and red blood cell concentrates (RBC) were given according to the transfusion- and hemodynamic algorithm of the standard operating procedures (SOP) of the Department of Anesthesiology and Intensive Care Medicine [20]. During surgery, StO_2 was measured by near-infrared spectroscopy (InSpectra Spot Check, M300™, Hutchinson, MN, USA) on the thenar of the right hand. Central venous and arterial blood gas analysis to determine dCO_2, lactate and hemoglobin (Hb) were performed every 30 min. Patients were extubated when spontaneous breathing was sufficient, body core temperature > 35.5 C and no clinical symptoms of hypovolemia or hemodynamic instability. Postoperative pain relief was achieved using a patient-controlled epidural analgesia (PCEA) and women were transferred to PACU for at least 24 h after operation [20].

For MD, a 60 mm (inlet tubing diameter 1 mm) flexible catheter (63 MD catheter, molecular weight cut-off of 2kD, M Dialysis AB, Stockholm, Sweden) was placed into the subcutaneous fat tissue below the right deltoid muscle after local anesthesia (Fig. 1b). After perfusion with isotonic sterile fluid (perfusion fluid T1, M Dialysis AB) at a rate of 1 μl/min (MD Pump 106, M Dialysis AB) a dialysate was collected every 30 min (first sample at T_3) in a 200 μl microvial (M Dialysis AB) and stored at − 20 °C until analysis. At the end of surgery, the catheter was removed while the patient was still unconscious. All MD analysis were performed by the Experimental & Clinical Research Center (ECRC) of the Franz-Volhard-Centrum, Charité-Universitätsmedizin Berlin, Campus Berlin-Buch.

The primary endpoint was defined as body core temperature drop (BCT_{drop}) from before epidural catheter placement (T_1) and after induction of GA (T_2) in the pre-warming or standard group. Intra- and postoperative change of BCT up to 2 h after ICU admission, StO_2 and hemodynamic parameters (PPV, SVV, SV), MAP, HR, norepinephrine usage, intraoperative transfusion rates (FFP, RBC), arterial lactate as well as the ethanol ratio, the glucose-, lactate- and glycerol concentration via MD were defined as secondary endpoints. In addition, the central venous-arterial dCO_2, which depends on the CO_2 production of the tissues and CO, were measured as a marker for microperfusion [21]. Postoperatively, shivering and postoperative ventilation were obtained.

Sample size calculation was based on the assumption of a minimal difference of 0.5 °C in body core temperature after prewarming compared to no prewarming (standard) [11]. A sample size of totally 48 patients, divided into two groups, was calculated to provide 80% power for detecting statistically significant difference at a two-tailed significance level of 0.05 (nQuery Advisor™, Release 7.0, Stat. Solutions Ltd. & South Bank, Crosse's Green, Cork, Ireland). A dropout rate of 10% of patients not eligible for data sampling was included.

Data are reported as arithmetic mean [standard deviation (SD)] or median [25, 75% percentile] (after rejection of normal distribution) or frequencies (%). In order to assess differences in body core temperature as the primary outcome at timepoints T_1-T_7 the nonparametric (exact) Mann-Whitney-U test was used. Differences between the groups in terms of patient characteristics as well as secondary outcomes were compared with paired or unpaired t-test and chi-squared test. Frequencies were tested by the exact Mantel-Haenszel test (for ordered categories) or the exact Chi-square test (for unordered categories). A two-tailed p-value of < 0.05 was considered statistically significant.

For MD subgroup analysis a sample size of 7 patients for each group was defined according to the study of Rosdahl et al. [10].

All calculations were performed with R software (version 3.3; R Foundation for Statistical Computing, Vienna, Austria).

The reporting of this RCT follows the updated guidelines for reporting parallel group randomized trials (CONSORT 2010 statement).

Results

During January 2015 and December 2017 133 women were screened for eligibility. 85 patients did not meet the inclusion criteria (Fig. 2) and were excluded before randomization, leaving 48 women for randomization (Fig. 2). Data of 47 women were analyzed, as one woman had to be excluded due to termination of the procedure out of surgical reasons (Fig. 2).

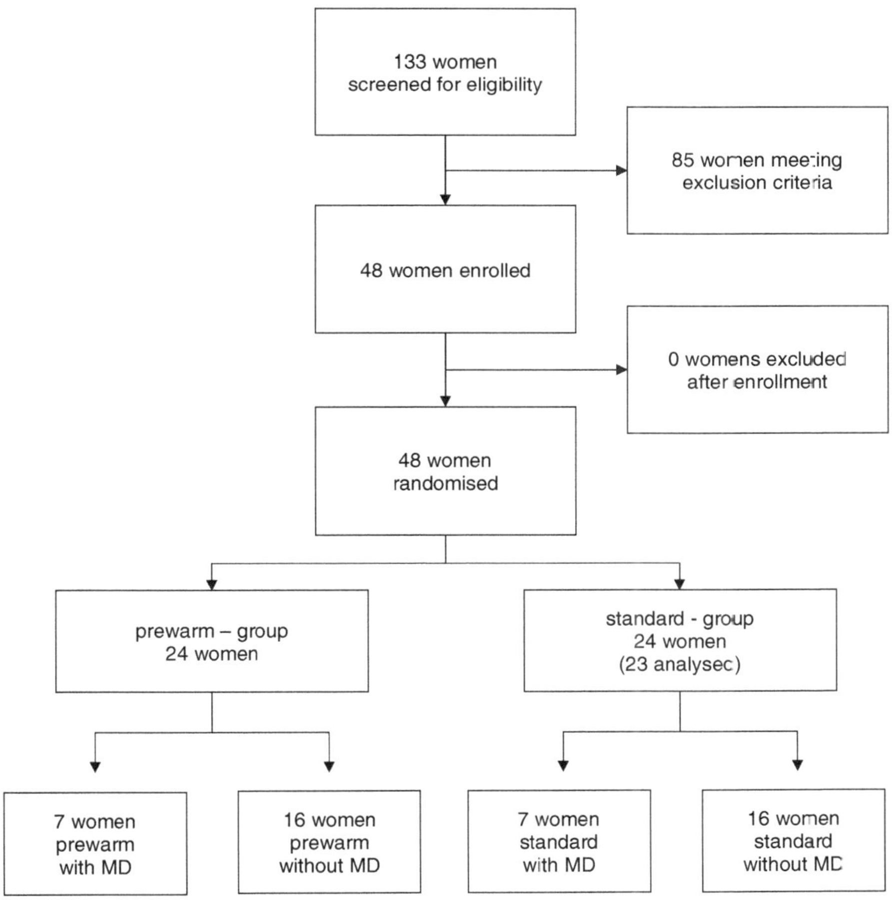

Fig. 2 CONSORT flow diagram

Besides a slight difference in height ($p = 0.047$), patient baseline characteristics, comorbidities and the duration of surgery did not differ significantly between the groups (Table 1). In multivariable linear regressions with group and BMI, group and age or group, BMI, and age as independent variables only group showed a significant relationship ($p < 0.05$) with body core temperature change.

Regarding the primary endpoint, the body core temperature change from T_1 (before) to T_2 amounted to 0.35 °C in the prewarm group and 0.9 °C in the standard group (Fig. 3) with a significant difference (ΔT) at $T_2 = 0.55$ °C ($p < 0.005$) between both groups (Fig. 3). No significant difference in baseline body core temperature (T_1) was measured (Fig. 4). After a further decrease of the BCT between T_2 and T_3 with a significant ΔT_3 of 0.85 °C ($p < 0,001$) (Fig. 4) the BCT increased in both groups during the operation (Fig. 4). The core temperature remained higher in the prewarm

Table 1 Patient baseline characteristics, comorbidities and duration of surgery

	prewarm *n*=24		standard *n*= 23	
Age (Years, mean±SD)	54,4	(±11,7)	61,3	(12,1)
Weight (kg, mean±SD)	73,6	(17,6)	67,8	(10,3)
Height (cm, mean±SD)	167	(4,9)	164,0	(6,1)*
BMI (mean±SD)	26,3	(5,8)	25,4	(4,1)
FIGO stage (n, %)				
I	1	(4)	0	(0)
II	0	(0)	0	(0)
III	17	(68)	14	(64)
IV	5	(20)	4	(18)
Residual tumor after surgery (n, %):				
0 cm	18	(72)	17	(77)
0-1 cm	5	(20)	4	(18)
1-2 cm	1	(4)	1	(5)
>2 cm	2	(8)	0	(0)
Preoperative fasting (Liquids in hrs, mean±SD)	11,3	(4,2)	11,6	(3,8)
Preoperative fasting (Solid in hrs, mean±SD)	16,7	(4,7)	16,2	(4,8)
Coronary artery disease (n,%)	0	(0)	1	(4,4)
Heart failure (n,%)	0	(0)	0	(0)
Diabetes mellitus (n,%)	1	(4,2)	1	(4,4)
Hypothyroidism (n,%)	1	(4,2)	4	(17.4)
Renal failure (n,%)	0	(0)	1	(4,4)
Arterial hypertension (n,%)	5	(20,8)	7	(30,4)
Peripheral arterial vascular disease (n,%)	1	(4,2)	1	(4,4)
COPD (n,%)	1	(4,2)	1	(4,4)
Asthma (n,%)	3	(12,5)	2	(8,7)
Thrombosis (n,%)	3	(12,5)	1	(4,4)
Hyperthyroidism (n,%)	1	(4,2)	1	(4,4)
Nicotine abuse (n,%)	0	(0)	1	(4,4)
Hyperlipoproteinemia (n,%)	0	(0)	3	(13)
ASA Classification (n,%):				
1	4	(16,7)	3	(13)
2	12	(50)	14	(60,9)
3	8	(33,3)	6	(26,1)
Duration of surgery[§] (min, mean ± SD)	334	±114	364	±134

*$p < 0.05$; [§] incision to suture; *SD* Standard deviation, *BMI* body mass index, *FIGO* International Federation of Gynecology and Obstetrics, *COPD* chronic obstructive pulmonary disease, *ASA* American Society of Anesthesiologists

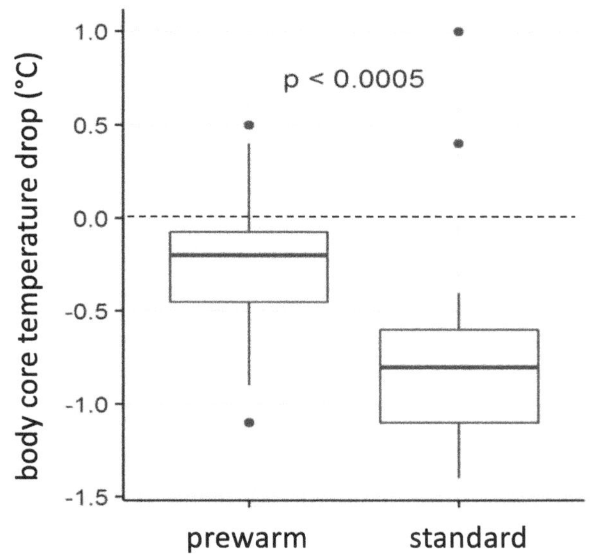

Fig. 3 Primary endpoint: Body core temperature drop between T_1 and after induction of general anesthesia T_2 with (prewarm) or without (standard) prewarming [median and quartile (25%; 75%)]

group over the entire observation period with a significant ΔT at all time points from (ΔT_4 = 0.9 °C up to ΔT_7 = 0.95 °C, p < 0,001, Fig. 4). At T_{ICU} and at T_{ICU2h} the body core temperatures in the PREWARM group were also higher than in the standard group (Fig. 5). One woman in the prewarm group suffered from hypothermia (< 36 °C) temporarily while 17 women in the standard group were hypothermic at one time point and/or over the entire intraoperative observation period (p < 0,001). At T_{ICU} six women in the standard group, but none in the prewarm group were subject to postoperative ventilation (p < 0.001) due to hypothermia at a median core temperature of 34.9 °C (34.8; 35.0). Three women in the standard group at T_{ICU} only, but none in the PREWARM group experienced postoperative shivering (p > 0.05).

StO_2 increased from 86% (T_3) to 88% (T_7) in the prewarm group and was slightly, but not significantly, higher compared to 82% (T_3) and 85% (T_7) in the standard group. In both groups, the dCO_2 did not change intraoperatively (median: prewarm 6.25 mmHg; standard 6.15 mmHg). Hemodynamic parameters such as SVV, SV and PPV as well as MAP, HR and norepinephrine concentration varied temporarily, depending on the volume changes in both groups, but without any significant differences between both groups at T_3, T_4 and T_5 (Table 2). FFP- and RBC transfusion were used in both groups with a non-significant difference between the groups (Table 2). The intraoperative arterial lactate concentration varied within the scope of 6 mg/dl (T_3) to 7.5 mg/dl (T_7) without significant differences between both groups.

For the ethanol ratio, the glucose-, lactate- and glycerol concentration [median (25. quartile/75. quartile)] measured by MD from T_3 to T_7, no significant differences were detectable between the groups. On closer view, the ethanol ratio (Fig. 6) was temporarily reduced in the prewarm compared to the standard group, with comparable results at the end of surgery (T_6). The glucose concentration deferred from 2.05 (0.36/0.36) mmol/l in the prewarm group versus 1.02 (0.42/0.59) mmol/l in the standard group at T_3 and proceeded almost similar in both groups between 1.51 (0.44/0.87) and 2.1 (1.35/0.35) mmol/l from T_4 to T_7. The glycerol concentration decreased continuously from 315 (163/278) µmol/l at T_3 to 191 (21/185) µmol/l at T_7 in the prewarm group and from 245 (106/187) µmol/l at T_3 to 119 (52/131) µmol/l at T_7 in the standard group. The lactate concentration of 0.66 (0.17/0.07) mmol/l at T3 in the prewarm group was higher compared to 0.48 (0.25/0.18) mmol/l in the standard group and both concentrations aligned at 0.6 (0.17/0.02) mmol/l at T_6.

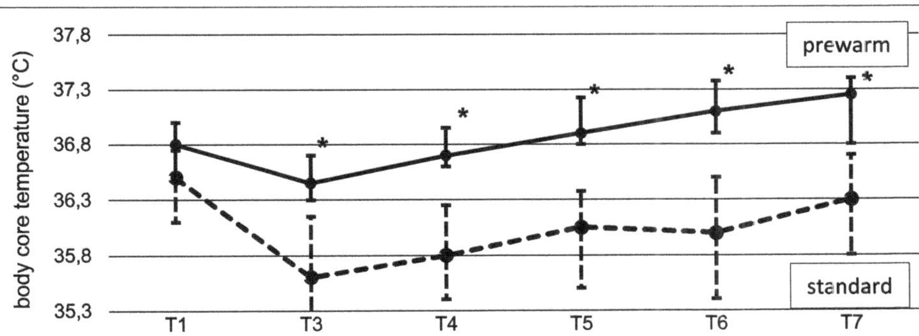

	T1	T3	T4	T5	T6	T7
prewarm	36,80	36,45	36,70	36,90	37,10	37,25
standard	36,50	35,60	35,80	36,05	36,00	36,30
Δ T	0,30	0,85	0,90	0,85	1,10	0,95

Fig. 4 Secondary endpoints: Body core temperature before prewarming (T_1) and during operation (T_3 to T_6) and at the end of surgery (T_7) [median and quartile (25%; 75%)]; * p < 0,001]

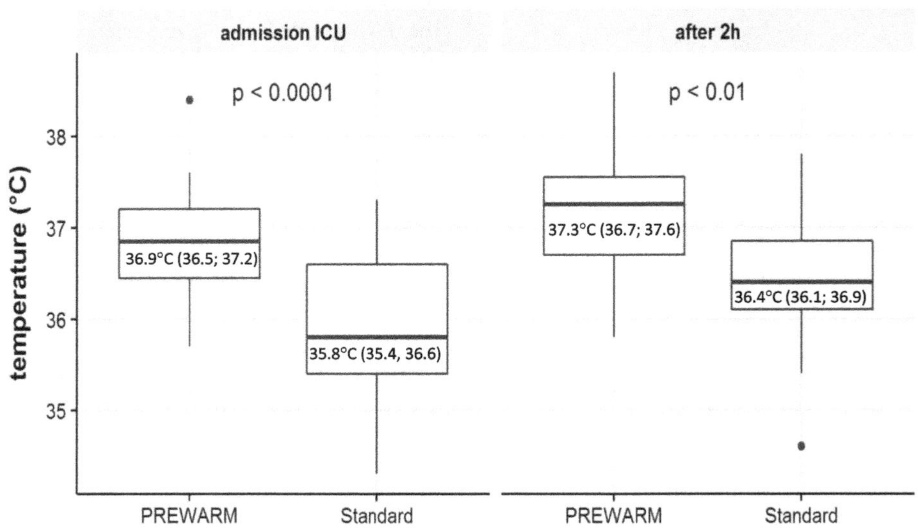

Fig. 5 Secondary endpoints: Body core temperature at T_{ICU} and T_{ICU2h}

Discussion

In this study a forced-air prewarming interval at 43 °C during epidural catheter placement and induction of GA showed efficacy to reduce core temperature drop and to maintain intraoperative normothermia during cytoreductive surgery not only throughout extended surgery but also at ICU admission and two hours thereafter. Furthermore, prewarming reduced the risk of postoperative ventilation due to hypothermia at the end of surgery. Microdialysis and StO_2 showed better results for the prewarming group, however, this did not reach statistical significance. A reason for this may have been, that all hemodynamic parameters, transfusion rates, and dCO_2 were not different in either study group. Nevertheless, small sample size for secondary outcomes should be taken into account for further discussions.

In a prospective randomized trial in 99 patients undergoing major abdominal surgery, Horn et al. [12] analyzed the effects of prewarming over 15 min before and after EDA versus 15 min after EDA or no prewarming. In contrast to our study, forced-air prewarming was performed at 44 °C in a preoperative care unit before and after EDA, which requires higher logistical and staff demands than our approach [12]. Nevertheless, despite pre- and intraoperative forced-air warming the drop in body core temperature with induction of GA still occurs, which can be significantly alleviated by prewarming, which is in line with earlier results [12, 22].

At ICU admission only six women of the standard group but none in the prewarming group were mechanically ventilated on ICU because of hypothermia. These findings are in line with the findings of Horn et al. who measured a 34% postoperative ventilation rate in non-prewarmed patients, which indicates the importance of temperature management for ventilation times after surgery. Even 2 h after ICU admission prewarmed women of our study had a higher body core temperature without any shivering. Our data suggest, that the greater body core temperature drop after induction of GA in the standard seems to be irreversible in spite of all intraoperative approaches, such as intraoperative forced air warming, warm fluids etc., to warm up the patients during surgery effectively.

We hypothesized that StO_2, dCO_2, arterial lactate and parameters of MD may be useful as surrogate parameters to measure an improved microperfusion in prewarmed and normothermic patients. These markers did not differ significantly, but showed a trend in favor of the prewarm group, which may indicate the need for further studies powered to detect a difference in microcirculation parameters.

We measured a non-significant difference in StO_2 in favor of the prewarmed patient group. It still remains unclear if this effect is caused by mild hypothermia-induced vasoconstriction and consecutive hypoperfusion and could be prevented by measures to maintain normothermia [23].

Our MD data could suggest that the tendency of a temporarily reduced ethanol ratio in prewarmed women after induction of GA and during the first hours of operations may represent an improved tissue perfusion [10]. After normothermia is reestablished due to intraoperative forced-air- warming and warmed transfusion/iv-fluids, the ethanol ratios showed similar values. This is consistent with the other microdialysis parameters. In 13 healthy volunteers, Rosdahl et al. demonstrated that the availability of glucose as a substrate for cell metabolism in subcutaneous fat tissue is dependent on tissue perfusion [10].

Table 2 Secondary endpoints: Intraoperative hemodynamic parameters at T_{3-5} and total amount of transfusion at the end of surgery

	prewarm [mean; (SD)]		standard [mean; (SD)]	
MAP (mmHg)				
T_3	80	(±12)	77	(±18)
T_4	77	(±10)	74	(±17)
T_5	78	(±9)	75	(±17)
HR (bpm)				
T_3	62	(±13)	60	(±15)
T_4	68	(±12)	65	(±15)
T_5	72	(±16)	71	(±19)
SVV (%)				
T_3	9	(±3)	8	(±3)
T_4	9	(±3)	9	(±3)
T_5	9	(±3)	9	(±3)
SV (ml)				
T_3	69	(±12)	67	(±16)
T_4	74	(±18)	73	(±21)
T_5	81	(±21)	77	(±24)
PPV (%)				
T_3	7	(±3)	7	(±3)
T_4	9	(±3)	8	(±3)
T_5	9	(±5)	9	(±5)
Norepinephrine (µg/kg/min)				
T_3	0.03	(± 0.02)	0.03	(±0.02)
T_4	0.06	(±0.04)	0.06	(±0.04)
T_5	0.07	(±0.05)	0.07	(±0.04)
Transfusion (ml)				
FFP at T_7	3500	(±2300)	3700	(±2200)
RBC at T_7	1000	(±600)	1000	(±900)

*$p < 0.05$; *MAP* mean arterial pressure, *HR* heart rate, *SVV* Stroke volume variation, *SV* Stroke volume, *PPV* pulse pressure variation, *FFP* fresh frozen plasma, *RBC* red blood cells concentrates

Therefore, the glucose recovery rate in MD acts approximately inverse to the ethanol ratio [10]. This might explain the increased glucose concentration in the prewarmed group at the beginning of surgery when perfusion may be improved due to the higher body core temperature compared to the standard group. Moreover, an increase of the lactate concentration in MD represents hypoperfusion and oxygen deficit in the subcutaneous tissue, as Bahlmann et al. demonstrated after 15–60 min of aortic clamping [24]. Potential hypoperfusion of the subcutaneous tissue due to reduced body core temperature did not result in an increase of the lactate concentration in the standard group with MD. On the other hand, the glycerol concentration in MD represents increased metabolic stress and lipolytic activity in the standard group [24]. Unfortunately and similar to lactate, the concentration remained without significant changes and differences between the groups. It may be hypothesized that mild hypothermia or reduced body core temperature are not very likely to result in a detectable increase of lactate and glycerol in MD. Nevertheless, the MD parameters give a first impression of temperature-related effects on microperfusion and that MD may be a promising technique to identify surrogate parameters for the impact of hypothermia. So far, no comparable data of MD in dependence of changes in body core temperature are published.

Limitations

Our study has a few limitations: Firstly, the study was powered in regards to primary outcome. In terms of secondary outcome, the study was not powered to detect significant changes, but may allow for an estimation of the number of patients needed for upcoming investigations on microperfusion and MD. Secondly, StO_2 was evaluated without reference values of an accompanied vascular occlusion test on the upper arm due to potential disruption

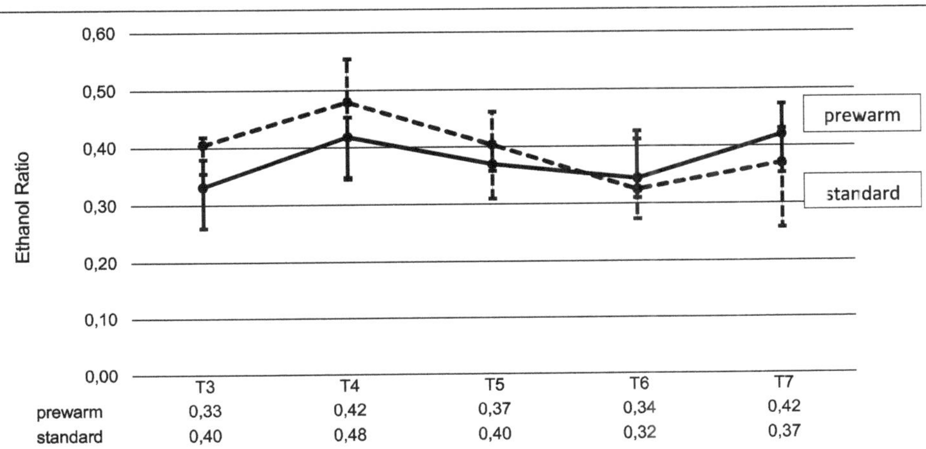

Fig. 6 Secondary endpoints: Ethanol ratio in MD before prewarming (T_1) and during operation ($T_4$to T_6) and at the end of surgery (T_7) [median and quartile (25%; 75%)]

and damage to the microdialysis catheter, which was inserted on the same side. Lastly, prewarming did not allow a blinding at all times. A concealed randomization was performed. Furthermore the anesthesiologist in charge of the patient was not involved in the collection of study related data. So the likelihood of bias was reduced.

Conclusion

In conclusion, forced-air prewarming at 43 °C during epidural catheter placement and induction of GA without interfering with the perioperative routine setting is effective to reduce the core temperature drop. Furthermore, prewarming maintains intraoperative normothermia until the end of surgery and up to two hours after ICU admission without any shivering or mechanically ventilation due to hypothermia postoperatively. A statistically significant impact of prewarming on microperfusion as measured by MD could not be detected by this study. However, reduced ethanol ratio and increased glucose concentration in the microdialysis as well as an increased tissue oxygenation may point to a better maintained microperfusion in prewarmed patients compared to those receiving standard treatment. The use of hemodynamic parameters, transfusion rates, StO_2, dCO_2 and MD parameters as surrogate parameters influencing microperfusion should be controlled in further randomized, controlled studies investigating the impact of temperature management in surgical patients.

Abbreviations

BCT: body core temperature; BCT_{drop}: drop in body core temperature; CO: cardiac output; CRF: case reporting form; dCO_2: carbon dioxide difference; ECRC: Experimental & Clinical Research Center; EDA: Epidural anesthesia; FFP: fresh frozen plasma; GA: General anesthesia; GFR: glomerular filtration rate; GINA: Global Initiative for Asthma; HR: heart rate; i.v.: intravenous; ICU: Intensive Care Unit; LV-EF: left ventricular ejection fraction; MAP: mean arterial pressure; MD: microdialysis; OR: operating room; PACU: post-anesthesia care unit; PCEA: patient-controlled epidural analgesia; PPV: pulse pressure variation; PW: prewarming; RBC: red blood cell concentrates; SD: standard deviation; SOP: standard operating procedures; StO_2: tissue oxygenation; SV: stroke volumen; SVV: stroke volume variation; T_1: Temperature at time before induction of anesthesia; T_2: Temperature after induction of anesthesia; T_3: Temperature after 15 min of induction of anesthesia; T_4: Temperature after 60 min of induction of anesthesia; T_5: Temperature after 120 min of induction of anesthesia; T_6: Temperature after 180 min of induction of anesthesia; T_7: Temperature at the end of operation; T_{ICU}: Temperature on admission to the ICU; T_{ICU2h}: Temperature until 2 h after ICU admission

Acknowledgements

Not applicable

Study presentation

This trial was presented in parts at the annual meetings of the American Society of Anesthesiologists 2017 and the European Society of Anesthesiology 2018.

Authors contribution

Substantial contributions to conception and design: LK, CvH, PN. Acquisition of data: PN, TB, SC, MB. Analysis and Interpretation of data: AB, JS, MB, CS, AH, CvH. Drafting the manuscript: LK, AB. Revision of the manuscript: PN, TB, SC, JS, MB, CS, AH, CvH. Final approval: LK, PN, TB, SC, JS, AB, MB, CS, AH, CvH. Agreement to be accountable for all aspects of the work: LK, PN, TB, SC, JS, AB, MB, CS, AH, CvH. All Authors meet the criteria for authorship according to the ICMJE guidelines.

Competing interests

PN, TB, SC, AB, JS, MB, AH have no conflict of interest. LK reports grants from 3 M during the conduct of the study; personal fees from HICC Deutschland GbR., Novo Nordisk, Sintetica, CSL Behring, outside the submitted work. CvH reports personal fees from Bayer AG, CSL Behring, Boehringer Ingelheim, Pfizer GmbH, Bristol Myers Squibb, Shire, Ferring GmbH, Sanofi Aventis, Mitsubishi Pharma, Novo Nordisk, HICC GbR, grants and personal fees from Daiichi Sankyo, outside the submitted work.
CS received funding from European Union funded seventh framework research program (FP7/2007–2013), under the grant agreement No. HEALTH-F2-2014-60246, Bio Cog, grants from Dr. Köhler Chemie GmbH, AppAdventure, J&P Medical Research Ltd., Pharmaceutical Research Associate GmbH, Delcath Systems Inc., INC Research UK Ltd., La Jolla Pharmaceutical Company, ARIDIS Pharmaceutical Inc., B. Braun Melsungen AG, Drägerwerk AG & CoKGaA, Grünenthal GmbH, Infectopharm GmbH, Sedana Medical Ltd., Arbeitsgemeinschaft industrieller Forschungsvereinigungen "Otto von Guericke" e.V. (AiF)/German Federation of Industrial Research Associations, Berufsverband deutscher Anästhesisten e.V. (BDA)/ Professional Associationof German Anaesthesiologists, Deutsche Forschungsgemeinschaft/ German Research Society, Deutsches Zentrum für Luft- und Raumfahrttechnik e.V. (DLR)/German Aerospace Center, Einstein Stiftung Berlin/Einstein Foundation Berlin, European Society of Anaesthesiology, Gemeinsamer Bundesausschuss/Federal Joint Commitee (G-BA), inneruniversitäre Forschungsförderung/Inner university grant, Projektträger im DLR/Project Management Agency, Stifterverband/Non-Profit Society Promoting Science and Education, WHOCC, Westfälische Wilhelms- Universität Münster/ DFG, AbbVie Deutschland GmbH & CoKG, Aguettant Deutschland GmbH, MAQUET Vertrieb und Service Deutschland GmbH, Orion Pharma GmbH, Philips Electronics Nederland B.V., Sintetica GmbH, Baxter Deutschland GmbH, Biotest AG, Cytosorbents Europe GmbH, Edwards Lifesciences Germany GmbH, Fresenius Medical Care, Masimo Europe Ltd., Medtronic GmbH, Pfizer Pharma PFE GmbH, European Commission, BMUB (Bundesministerium für Umwelt, Naturschutz und nukleare Sicherheit), personal fees from B. Braun Melsungen AG, Georg Thieme Verlag; outside the submitted work. CS has a patent 10 2014 215 211.9 pending, a patent application No. PCT/EP2015/067730 pending to Graft Gesellschaft von Architekten mbH and a patent application No. PCT/ EP2015/067731 pending to Graft Gesellschaft von Architekten mbH.
All authors report no conflict of interest relating to this work.

Author details

[1]Department of Anaesthesiology and Operative Intensive Care Medicine (CCM, CVK), Charité-Universitätsmedizin Berlin, Corporate Member of Freie Universität Berlin, Humboldt-Universität zu Berlin, and Berlin Institute of Health, Campus Virchow-Klinikum, Augustenburger Platz 1, 13353 Berlin, Germany. [2]Department of Anaesthesia, Intensive Care Medicine, Emergency Medicine and Pain Therapy, Vivantes Klinikum im Friedrichshain, Berlin, Germany. [3]Department of Gynaecology, Charité-Universitätsmedizin Berlin, Berlin, Germany. [4]Institut für Klinische Chemie und Pathobiochemie, Klinikum rechts der Isar der Technischen Universität München, Munich, Germany. [5]Experimental & Clinical Research Center, ECRC, Charité-Universitätsmedizin Berlin CCB, Berlin, Germany.

References

1. Forstot RM. The etiology and management of inadvertent perioperative hypothermia. J Clin Anesth. 1995;7(8):657–74.
2. Grote R, Wetz AJ, Bräuer A, Menzel M. Prewarming according to the AWMF S3 guidelines on preventinginadvertentt perioperative hypothermia 2014:: retrospective analysis of 7786 patients. Anaesthesist. 2018;67(1):27–33.
3. Sessler DI. Perioperative thermoregulation and heat balance. Lancet. 2016;387(10038):2655–64.
4. Sessler DI. Perianesthetic thermoregulation and heat balance in humans. FASEB J. 1993;7(8):638–44.
5. Fotopoulou C, Savvatis K, Steinhagen-Thiessen E, Bahra M, Lichtenegger W, Shouli J. Primary radical surgery in elderly patients with epithelial ovarian Cancer. Int J Gynecol Cancer. 2010;20:34–40.

6. Kurz A, Go JC, Sessler DI, Kaer K, Larson MD, Bjorksten AR. Alfentanil slightly increases the sweating threshold and markedly reduces the vasoconstriction and shivering thresholds. Anesthesiology. 1995;83(2):293–9.
7. Michelson AD, MacGregor H, Barnard MR, Kestin AS, Rohrer MJ, Valeri CR. Reversible inhibition of human platelet activation by hypothermia in vivo and in vitro. Thromb Haemost. 1994;71(5):633–40.
8. Schmied H, Reiter A, Kurz A, Sessler DI, Kozek S. Mild hypothermia increases blood loss and transfusion requirements during total hip arthroplasty. Lancet. 1996;347(8997):289–92.
9. Kurz A, Sessler DI, Lenhardt R. Perioperative normothermia to reduce the incidence of surgical-wound infection and shorten hospitalization. Study of wound infection and temperature group. N Engl J Med. 1996;334(19):1209–15.
10. Rosdahl H, Ungerstedt U, Jorfeldt L, Henriksson J. Interstitial glucose and lactate balance in human skeletal muscle and adipose tissue studied by microdialysis. J Physiol. 1993;471(1):637–57.
11. Horn E-P, Bein B, Böhm R, Steinfath M, Sahili N, Höcker J. The effect of short time periods of pre-operative warming in the prevention of perioperative hypothermia: pre-operative warming in the prevention of perioperative hypothermia. Anesthesia. 2012;67(6):612–7.
12. Horn EP, Bein B, Broch O, Iden T, Böhm R, Latz S-K, et al. Warming before and after epidural block before general anesthesia for major abdominal surgery prevents perioperative hypothermia: A randomized controlled trial. Eur J Anaesthesiol. 2016;33(5):334–40.
13. Vanni SMD, Braz JRC, Módolo NSP, Amorim RB, Rodrigues GR. Preoperative combined with intraoperative skin-surface warming avoids hypothermia caused by general anesthesia and surgery. J Clin Anesth. 2003;15(2):119–25.
14. Andrzejowski J, Hoyle J, Eapen G, Turnbull D. Effect of prewarming on post-induction core temperature and the incidence of inadvertent perioperative hypothermia in patients undergoing general anesthesia. Br J Anaesth. 2008;101(5):627–31.
15. Wong PF, Kumar S, Bohra A, Whetter D, Leaper DJ. Randomized clinical trial of perioperative systemic warming in major elective abdominal surgery. Br J Surg. 2007;94(4):421–6.
16. Torossian A, Bein B, Bräuer A. German S3 Guideline „Vermeidung von perioperativer Hypothermie". AWMF Register. 2014;001–018.
17. Camus Y, Delva E, Sessler DI, Lienhart A. Pre-induction skin-surface warming minimizes intraoperative core hypothermia. J Clin Anesth. 1995;7(5):384–8.
18. Melling AC, Ali B, Scott EM, Leaper DJ. Effects of preoperative warming on the incidence of wound infection after clean surgery: a randomized controlled trial. Lancet. 2001;358(9285):876–80.
19. Mäkinen MT, Pesonen A, Jousela I, Päivärinta J, Poikajävi S, Albäck A, et al. Novel zero-heat-flux deep body temperature measurement in lower extremity vascular and cardiac surgery. J Cardiothorac Vasc Anesth. 2016;30: 973–8.
20. Spies C, Kerner T, Kastrup M, Melzer-Gartzke C, Zielke H. SOPs in Anästhesiologie und Schmerztherapie. Stuttgart: Thieme Verlag 2013. ISBN: 9783131694317.
21. Futier E, Robin E, Jabaudon M, Guerin R, Petit A, Bazin J-E, Constantin J-M, Vallet B. Central venous O2 saturation and venous-to-arterial CO2 difference as complementary tools for goal-directed therapy during high-risk surgery. Crit Care. 2010;14(5):R193.
22. Lau A, Lowlaavar N, Cooke EM, West N, German A, Morse DJ, et al. Effect of preoperative warming on intraoperative hypothermia: a randomized controlled trial. Can J Anesth/J Can Anesth. 2018;65:1029.
23. Cho YJ, Lee SY, Kim TK, Hong DM, Jeon Y. Effect of Prewarming during induction of anesthesia on microvascular reactivity in patients undergoing off-pump coronary artery bypass surgery: a randomized clinical trial. PLoS One. 2016;11(7):e0159772.
24. Bahlmann L, Wagner K, Heringlake M, Wirtz C, Fütterer T, Schmucker P, et al. Subcutaneous microdialysis for metabolic monitoring in abdominal aortic surgery. J Clin Monit Comput. 2002;17(5):309–12.

10

Effects of anesthetic method on inflammatory response in patients with Parkinson's disease

Won Jung Hwang, Min A. Joo and Jin Joo*

Abstract

Background: The pathogenesis of Parkinson's disease (PD) involves degeneration of dopaminergic neurons, which is influenced by innate and adaptive immunity. IL-17 is a characteristic cytokine secreted by Th17 cells, which acts as a powerful stimulator of neutrophil migration and infiltration and promotes the secretion of inflammatory cytokines. General anesthesia and surgical stress induce immune and inflammatory responses that activate the immunosuppressive mechanism in the perioperative period. The present study investigated changes in levels of inflammatory cytokines, such as IL-17, IL-1β, and TNF-α, in patients with PD undergoing general anesthesia with inhalational anesthetics or TIVA.

Methods: Adult patients, aged 40–75 years, scheduled for cerebral stimulator implantation were enrolled. Upon arrival at the operating theater, patients were allocated to the inhalational (I) or TIVA (T) group using block randomization. In group I, anesthesia was induced by tracheal intubation 1–2 min after intravenous administration of propofol (1–2 mg/kg) and rocuronium (0.6–1 mg/kg). Thereafter, anesthesia was maintained with 1–2 vol% sevoflurane, 0.01–0.2 μg/kg/min remifentanil, and O_2/air (FiO_2 0.4). In group T, propofol (3–6 μg/mL), remifentanil (2–6 ng/mL), and rocuronium (0.6–1 mg/kg) were administered using target controlled infusion (TCI) for induction of anesthesia. Blood samples were obtained preoperatively (T0), 2 h after induction of anesthesia (T1), and 24 h after surgery (T2). IL-17, IL-1β, and TNF-α levels were evaluated by ELISA.

Results: Serum levels of IL-17 were elevated at T2 in group I compared to group T but the difference was not statistically significant. IL-1β tended to be greater in group I compared to group T, but the differences were not significant. TNF-α was slightly higher at all time points in group T and showed a tendency to increase at T2 in both groups, but this was not statistically significant.

Conclusions: TIVA may be useful for inhibiting neuroinflammation by inhibiting the increase in serum levels of IL-17 24 h after implantation surgery. Serum IL-17 level may be used as a biomarker for PD progression.

Keywords: Parkinson's disease, Inhalational anesthetic, Total intravenous anesthesia (TIVA), Inflammatory response

* Correspondence: jiyo1004@catholic.ac.kr
Department of Anesthesiology and Pain Medicine, Seoul St. Mary's Hospital, College of Medicine, The Catholic University of Korea, 222 Banpodaero, Seocho-gu, Seoul 06591, South Korea

Background

Parkinson's disease (PD) is a progressive central nervous system (CNS) movement disorder, and is the second most common inflammatory neurodegenerative disorder after Alzheimer's disease [1]. About 2–3% of elderly people above 65 years old have PD [2]. The earliest symptoms are bradykinesia, resting tremor, rigidity, and impairment of balance. These motor symptoms are caused by a decrease in levels of the neurotransmitter dopamine, due to death of dopaminergic neurons in the substantia nigra [3]. This degeneration of dopaminergic neurons is accompanied by inflammatory changes in microglia (innate immunity) and infiltration of T lymphocytes (adaptive immunity) [4].

There have been a number of studies of the relations between PD and immunity, and Th17 cells play an important role in neurodegeneration in experimental models of PD [5]. In patients with PD, Th17 cell effector molecules are upregulated and the immune pathways of Th17 cells are activated. Th17 cells produce cytokines, such as IL-17, IL-21, IL-1β, and TNF-α, resulting in neuronal apoptosis [5, 6]. IL-17 is a characteristic cytokine secreted by Th17 cells that acts as a powerful stimulator of neutrophil migration and infiltration. It promotes the secretion of other inflammatory cytokines, such as IL-1, TNF-α, and IL-6, by microglial cells [7]. These cytokines lead to neuronal cell death, resulting in neurodegeneration.

General anesthesia and surgical stress induce immune and inflammatory responses that activate the immunosuppressive mechanism in the perioperative period [8]. Unlike inhalation anesthetics, propofol shows antioxidant activity that protects cells and tissues from toxic free radicals [9, 10]. There has been a great deal of research on the relations between general anesthesia and immunity. Inhalational anesthetics have a greater immunosuppressive effect than total intravenous anesthesia (TIVA) using propofol. With the aging of the population, increasing numbers of elderly patients with PD are undergoing various types of surgery under general anesthesia [11]. However, there have been no studies on the effects of anesthetic method on inflammatory responses in patients with PD. The present study investigated changes in levels of inflammatory cytokines, such as IL-17, IL-1β, and TNF-α, in patients with PD undergoing general anesthesia with inhalational anesthetics or TIVA.

Methods

The protocol of this study adheres to CONSORT guidelines.

Study population and ethical approval

The study protocol was approved by the Institutional Review Board of Seoul St. Mary's Hospital, The Catholic University of Korea (approval no. KC17RESI0365) and has been registered with the Clinical Research Information Service of Korea National Institute of Health (CRIS, identification number: KCT0002061). Each patient provided written and oral informed consent. Adult patients, aged 40–75 years who were scheduled for deep brain stimulation (DBS) surgery to control symptoms between June 2018 and December 2019 were enrolled in this randomized, prospective study. Patients who had no medical histories and who had hypertension and diabetes without any complications were included. Patients with myocardial infarction or coronary artery disease, patients with lung diseases, such as asthma or chronic obstructive pulmonary disease (COPD), with AST/ALT greater than normal, and with a medical history of hypersensitivity to inhalation anesthetics or propofol were excluded.

Anesthetic management

Patients were not allowed to eat and drink 8 h before surgery in consideration of slowed gastric emptying time in PD patients [12], except for the sips of water when they had to take their routine PD medication. Upon arrival at the operating theater, patients were allocated to the inhalational (I) or TIVA (T) group using block randomization. Basic monitoring, including ECG, noninvasive blood pressure (NIBP), pulse oximetry, and bispectral index (BIS), was used. Blood was drawn from peripheral blood vessels before induction of general anesthesia (T0). In group I, anesthesia was induced by tracheal intubation 1–2 min after intravenous administration of propofol (1–2 mg/kg), rocuronium (0.6–1 mg/kg) and remifentanil (0.01–0.2 μg/kg/min). Thereafter, anesthesia was maintained with 1–2 vol% sevoflurane, 0.01–0.2 μg/kg/min remifentanil, and O_2/air (FiO_2 0.4). In group T, propofol (3–6 μg/mL), remifentanil (2–6 ng/mL) using target controlled infusion (TCI), and rocuronium (0.6–1 mg/kg) were administered for induction of anesthesia. After tracheal intubation, anesthesia was maintained with propofol (2–4 μg/mL), remifentanil (2–4 ng/mL), O_2/air (FiO_2 0.4). In both groups, the depth of anesthesia was adjusted to the anesthetic dose with a BIS of 40–50. Blood pressure and pulse were maintained at around 20% of the respective baseline. At the end of surgery, anesthetics were discontinued and sugammadex was used to reverse the muscle relaxant effect. At this time, blood was taken from the peripheral blood vessels (T1). Extubation was carried out when the patient's breathing had returned sufficiently, and then the patient was moved to the recovery room. Blood was taken from peripheral blood vessels 24 h after surgery (T2). Patients discharged from hospital at postoperative 2 day.

Cytokine analyses

Blood samples were centrifuged at 1500 rpm for 10 min at room temperature. Serum was removed and stored in 200 μL aliquots at − 80 °C until assays were performed. Serum was dispensed onto coated ELISA plates. Levels of cytokines in the serum samples were determined by ELISA using the following kits in accordance with the manufacturer's instructions: IL-1β, sensitivity: 6.5 pg/mL (ab46052; Abcam, Cambridge, MA); TNF-α, sensitivity: 4.32 pg/mL (181,421; Abcam); IL-17, sensitivity: < 10 pg/mL (100,556; Abcam). ELISA plates were analyzed using a microtiter plate reader (BioTek Instruments, Inc., Winooski, VT) at 450 nm after stopping the reaction.

Data collection and statistical analyses

For sample size calculation, IL-17 levels described in a previous animal study were used [12]. With a 10 pg/dL difference in mean value between groups and a standard deviation of 8, the sample size required at a significance level of 5% (two-sided $\alpha = 0.05$) and a power of 80% ($1 - \beta = 0.8$) was 15 patients per group, taking a 10% dropout rate into consideration. All data were analyzed using SPSS (ver. 18.0; SPSS, Inc., Chicago, IL). Demographic data were compared using the $\chi 2$ test and t test as appropriate. Repeated-measures ANOVA was performed to compare the cytokines between the groups, with group and time point as independent variables, after confirming the normality of the distribution with the Shapiro–Wilk test ($p > 0.05$). The interaction term was calculated with Bonferroni's correction for repeated measures. In all analyses, $p < 0.05$ was taken to indicate statistical significance.

Results

A total of 30 patients were recruited for the study; two were excluded from data analyses (one in each group) due to low blood pressure maintained during surgery and loss to follow-up (Fig. 1). Demographic data and perioperative data are shown in Table 1.

There were no significant differences in preoperative baseline (T0) IL-17 level between groups I and T (675.6 ± 398.4 vs. 705.7 ± 312.7 pg/mL, respectively; $p > 0.05$). IL-17 did not show any increase at T1 (799.21 ± 423.8 vs. 694.2 ± 395.6 pg/mL, respectively; $p > 0.05$) in either group; it tended to increase at T2 in group I compared to group T (843 ± 384.1 vs. 695.5 ± 391.2 pg/mL, respectively; $p > 0.05$), but the difference was not statistically significant (Fig. 2).

There were no significant differences in preoperative baseline (T0) IL-1β level between groups I and T (11.76 ± 9.5 vs. 19.5 ± 11.5 pg/mL, respectively; $p > 0.05$). IL-1β tended to increase in group I compared to group T (15.1 ± 13.0 vs. 16.4 ± 15.1 pg/mL in T1, and 21.2 ± 20.0 vs. 13.2 ± 10.8 pg/mL in T2, respectively; $p > 0.05$), but the differences were not significant (Fig. 3). There were no significant differences in preoperative baseline (T0) TNF-α level between groups I and T (9.9 ± 6.2 vs. 11.9 ± 6.0 pg/mL, respectively; $p > 0.05$). TNF-α showed a tendency to increase at T2 in both groups (9.6 ± 3.8 vs. 11.3 ± 6.4 in T1, and 10.5 ± 4.4 vs. 12.4 ± 8.4 pg/mL in T2, respectively; $p > 0.05$), but this was not statistically significant (Fig. 4).

Discussion

Various studies have demonstrated that the pathogenesis of PD involves neuroinflammation, which is affected by both innate and adaptive immunity. They have shown that the levels of proinflammatory cytokines are elevated in PD patients [5, 13–16]. Th17 cells are among the most important lymphocytes involved in degeneration of dopaminergic neurons in PD [5]. Th17 cells secrete the proinflammatory cytokine IL-17, which is commonly associated with allergic responses. IL-17 promotes the secretion of other cytokines, such as IL-1β and TNF-α, and plays a pivotal role in the early stages of inflammation. These cytokines bind to receptors on dopaminergic neurons, resulting in apoptosis [4, 6, 17].

To the best of our knowledge, this is the first study to investigate the effects of anesthetic method on inflammatory response in patients with PD. IL-17 at 24 h after surgery tended to increase under inhalational anesthesia, while it was maintained at the preoperative baseline level under TIVA. IL-1β and TNF-α also tended to increase at 24 h after surgery under inhalational anesthesia, but the effect was not significant. Surgical stress and anesthesia induce inflammatory responses by disturbing the balance between pro- and anti- inflammatory cytokines [8], which may result in aggravation of the neuroinflammatory response in PD patients. Previous studies have indicated that TIVA has superior effects in inhibiting inflammatory responses to inhalational anesthetics [9, 18–20]. The influence of different inhalational anesthetics on inflammatory response are still controversial [21–24]. We chose to use sevoflurane, one of the commonly used inhalational anesthetics, because it helps rapid induction and recovery. Shan et al. [25] reported that sevoflurane aggravated the prognosis of PD in a Drosophila model. We attributed the lack of statistical significance in this study to the relatively short duration of DBS surgery and the follow-up due to short hospitalization period. These may not have been sufficient to reveal cytokine changes. A decline of immunity due to surgery and anesthesia is known to occur from roughly 2 h after induction of anesthesia, and the peak of immunosuppression occurs 3 days after surgery [8]. We obtained blood samples 2 h after induction of anesthesia when changes in the immune responses had just begun and 24 h after surgery when changes had not yet reached their peak. Another reason for lack of the statistical significance may be attributed to relatively long period of fasting. Preoperative fasting is one of the stress inducing factors during perioperative periods [26]. Prolonged fasting time may have resulted in the

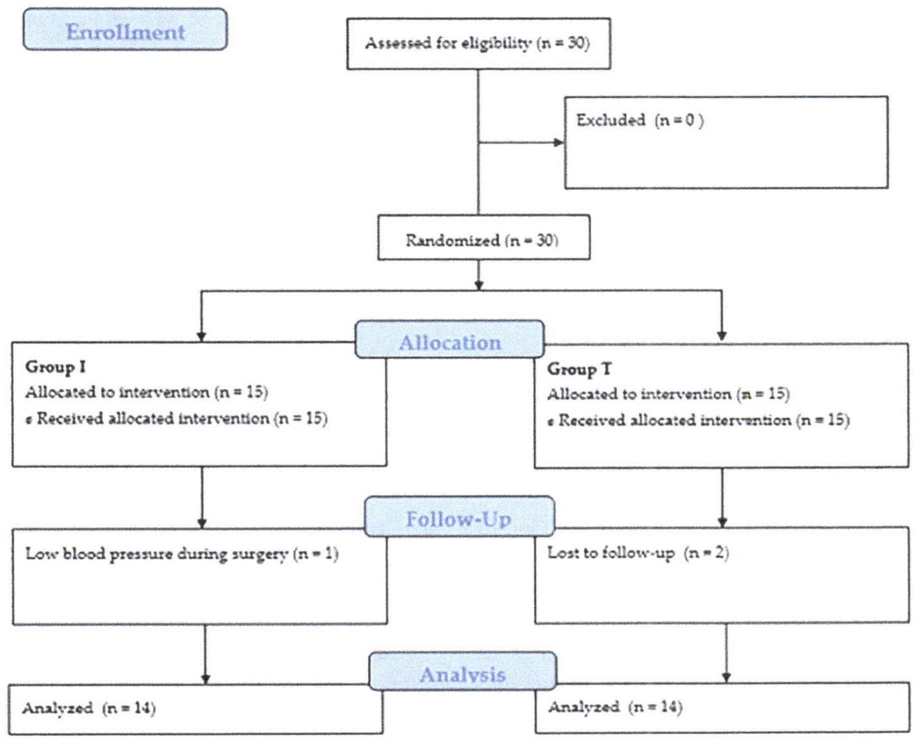

Fig. 1 Consort flow diagram

increases in the cytokines in both groups, masking the effect of the different anesthetics on inflammatory response. Guidelines for preoperative fasting period have recently been changed. Meanwhile, gastric emptying time is known to be prolonged in PD patients [12]. Given this, we did not allow the patients to eat and drink from 8 h before surgery, except for the time when they had to take the routine PD medications. However, these results demonstrate the possibility that TIVA have advantages with regard to inhibition of neuroinflammation after surgery in PD patients despite its lack of statistical significance since all the cytokines showed tendency of increase at 24 h after surgery.

The baseline IL-17 level in this study was about 700 pg/mL. Sommer et al. [27] reported that IL-17 levels in PD patients were about 350 pg/mL, while they were below 50 pg/mL in controls. Resting tremor, rigidity, bradykinesia, and impairment of balance are characteristic motor symptoms of PD. Shan et al. [21] reported that impairment of locomotor abilities is aggravated with exposure to sevoflurane in a Drosophila PD model. Tuon et al. [13] reported that IL-17 levels decrease after

Table 1 Patient data

	Group I	Group T	*p*-value
Age (yrs)	71.2 ± 6.4	72.0 ± 6.8	0.987
Sex (M/F)	8 / 6	7 / 7	0.705
Height (cm)	160.6 ± 10.5	161.5 ± 6.7	0.784
Weight (kg)	60.5 ± 12.0	63.4 ± 13.5	0.541
Years after diagnosis of Parkinson's disease	10.4 ± 6.8	9.5 ± 5.2	0.688
Blood loss (ml)	25.4 ± 16.9	27.3 ± 15.8	0.819
Crystalloid infused (ml)	544.3 ± 305.7	507.9 ± 206.7	0.715
Surgery time (min)	167.5 ± 77.0	177.6 ± 47.5	0.363
Anesthesia time (min)	190.9 ± 34.5	195.0 ± 35.5	0.678

Categorical variables are shown as numbers and other variables are shown as means ± standard deviation

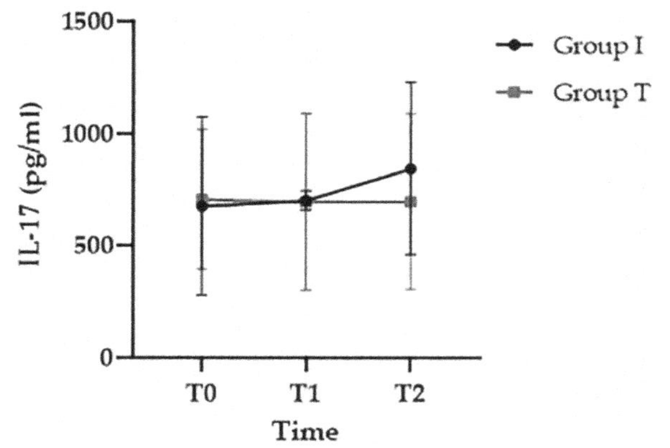

Fig. 2 Changes in IL-17. T0, preoperative baseline; T1, 2 h after induction of anesthesia; T2, 24 h after surgery

physical training in an experimental mouse model of PD. Williams-Gray et al. [2] showed that serum levels of cytokines, such as IL-1β, TNF-α, and IL-10, are higher in PD patients than in age-matched non-PD controls; higher TNF-α levels are associated with faster rates of motor decline and higher IL-1β levels are associated with a faster rate of cognitive decline. These studies suggest that IL-17 and TNF-α are closely related to the motor symptoms of PD. Our cohort consisted of patients who had been diagnosed with PD for about 10 years and required DBS surgery to manage motor symptoms that were not controlled by medications. These observations suggest that serum levels of IL-17 increase with the progression of PD. That is, neuroinflammation induced by Th-17 cells causing neuronal cell apoptosis may be an important factor in the progression of PD symptoms. Thus, serum IL-17 may be used as a biomarker for PD progression.

One of the limitations of this study is that we used the results from an experimental animal study for sample size calculation [13] because no similar clinical studies have been reported in the literature. In that study, the authors analyzed the levels of IL-17 in the brain tissue of a mouse model of PD 24 h after the intervention. However, the baseline IL-17 level is different between mice and humans, especially PD patients. Nevertheless, we believe that this study was worthwhile as a cornerstone in that it determined the baseline serum level of IL-17 for use in future human clinical studies on PD. In addition, we did not examine the motor symptoms before and after surgery in relation with cytokine changes. We selected PD patients undergoing brain stimulator implantation, and it would have been difficult to evaluate the motor symptoms before surgery due to the severity of PD and after surgery due to the stimulation. We intend to compare changes in short- and long-term motor symptoms in relation to cytokine changes in a future study.

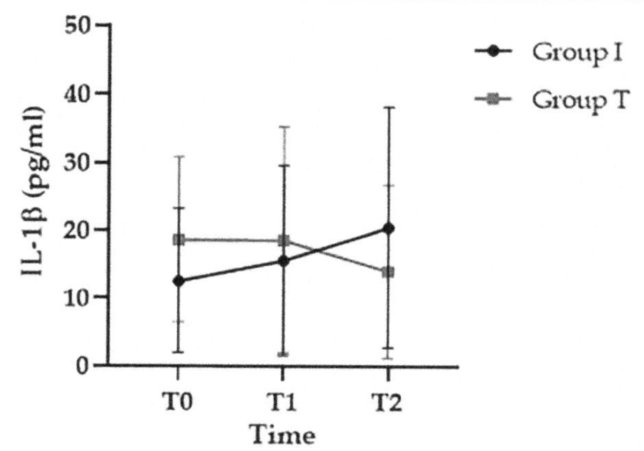

Fig. 3 Changes in IL-1β. T0, preoperative baseline; T1, 2 h after induction of anesthesia; T2, 24 h after surgery

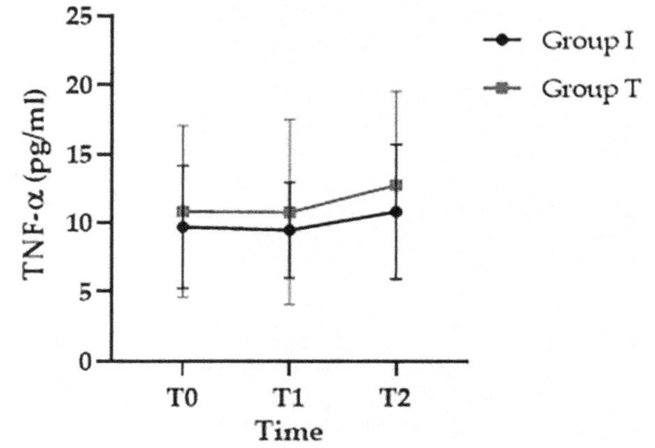

Fig. 4 Changes in TNF-α. T0, preoperative baseline; T1, 2 h after induction of anesthesia; T2, 24 h after surgery

In conclusion, this study did not demonstrate the superiority of TIVA to sevoflurane in inhibiting neuroinflammation 24 h after DBS surgery in PD patients. However, the larger increase of IL-17 at 24 h after DBS surgery under inhalation study reveals the possibility that TIVA have advantages with regard to inhibition of neuroinflammation after surgery. Serum IL-17 level may be used as a biomarker for PD progression since it was much higher in PD patients with severe motor symptoms. Further clinical trials to investigate the relationships between changes in cytokine levels and motor symptoms are needed.

Abbreviations

PD: Parkinson's disease; CNS: Central nervous system; TIVA: Total intravenous anesthesia; BIS: Bispectral index; DBS: Deep brain stimulation

Acknowledgements

Not applicable.

Authors' contributions

WJH and JJ contributed study design. WJH, MAJ and JJ collected and analyzed data. WJH and JJ drafted the manuscript. WJH, MAJ and JJ made critical revisions of the manuscript. All authors read and approved the final analysis of the manuscript.

Authors' information

Department of Anesthesiology and Pain Medicine, Seoul St. Mary's Hospital, College of Medicine, The Catholic University of Korea, Seoul, Korea.

References

1. Delenclos M, Jones DR, McLean PJ, Uitti RJ. Biomarkers in Parkinson's disease: advances and strategies. Parkinsonism Relat Disord. 2016;22(Suppl 1):S106–10.
2. Williams-Gray CH, Wijeyekoon R, Yarnall AJ, Lawson RA, Breen DP, Evans JR, et al. Serum immune markers and disease progression in an incident Parkinson's disease cohort (ICICLE-PD). Mov Disord. 2016;31(7):995–1003.
3. Schlachetzki JC, Winkler J. The innate immune system in Parkinson's disease: a novel target promoting endogenous neuroregeneration. Neural Regen Res. 2015;10(5):704–6.
4. Appel SH. CD4+ T cells mediate cytotoxicity in neurodegenerative diseases. J Clin Invest. 2009;119(1):13–5.
5. Reynolds AD, Stone DK, Hutter JA, Benner EJ, Mosley RL, Gendelman HE. Regulatory T cells attenuate Th17 cell-mediated nigrostriatal dopaminergic neurodegeneration in a model of Parkinson's disease. J Immunol. 2010; 184(5):2261–71.
6. Appel SH, Beers DR, Henkel JS. T cell-microglial dialogue in Parkinson's disease and amyotrophic lateral sclerosis: are we listening? Trends Immunol. 2010;31(1):7–17.
7. Lock C, Hermans G, Pedotti R, Brendolan A, Schadt E, Garren H, et al. Gene-microarray analysis of multiple sclerosis lesions yields new targets validated in autoimmune encephalomyelitis. Nat Med. 2002;8(5):500–8.
8. Coffey JC, Wang JH, Smith MJ, Bouchier-Hayes D, Cotter TG, Redmond HP. Excisional surgery for cancer cure: therapy at a cost. Lancet Oncol. 2003; 4(12):760–8.
9. Schneemilch CE, Ittenson A, Ansorge S, Hachenberg T, Bank U. Effect of 2 anesthetic techniques on the postoperative proinflammatory and anti-inflammatory cytokine response and cellular immune function to minor surgery. J Clin Anesth. 2005;17(7):517–27.
10. Mathy-Hartert M, Mouithys-Mickalad A, Kohnen S, Deby-Dupont G, Lamy M, Hans P. Effects of propofol on endothelial cells subjected to a peroxynitrite donor (SIN-1). Anaesthesia. 2000;55(11):1066–71.
11. Garcia-Perez L, Linertova R, Lorenzo-Riera A, Vazquez-Diaz JR, Duque-Gonzalez B, Sarria-Santamera A. Risk factors for hospital readmissions in elderly patients: a systematic review. QJM. 2011;104(8):639–51.
12. Knudsen K, Szwebs M, Hansen AK, Borghammer P. Gastric emptying in Parkinson's disease - a mini-review. Parkinsonism Relat Disord. 2018;55:18–25.
13. Tuon T, Souza PS, Santos MF, Pereira FT, Pedroso GS, Luciano TF, et al. Physical training regulates mitochondrial parameters and Neuroinflammatory mechanisms in an experimental model of Parkinson's disease. Oxidative Med Cell Longev. 2015;2015:261809.
14. Brodacki B, Staszewski J, Toczylowska B, Kozlowska E, Drela N, Chalimoniuk M, et al. Serum interleukin (IL-2, IL-10, IL-6, IL-4), TNFalpha, and INFgamma concentrations are elevated in patients with atypical and idiopathic parkinsonism. Neurosci Lett. 2008;441(2):158–62.
15. Garcia-Esparcia P, Llorens F, Carmona M, Ferrer I. Complex deregulation and expression of cytokines and mediators of the immune response in Parkinson's disease brain is region dependent. Brain Pathol. 2014;24(6):584–98.
16. Lane EL, Soulet D, Vercammen L, Cenci MA, Brundin P. Neuroinflammation in the generation of post-transplantation dyskinesia in Parkinson's disease. Neurobiol Dis. 2008;32(2):220–8.
17. Tzartos JS, Craner MJ, Friese MA, Jakobsen KB, Newcombe J, Esiri MM, et al. IL-21 and IL-21 receptor expression in lymphocytes and neurons in multiple sclerosis brain. Am J Pathol. 2011;178(2):794–802.
18. Kushida A, Inada T, Shingu K. Enhancement of antitumor immunity after propofol treatment in mice. Immunopharmacol Immunotoxicol. 2007;29(3–4):477–86.
19. Ren XF, Li WZ, Meng FY, Lin CF. Differential effects of propofol and isoflurane on the activation of T-helper cells in lung cancer patients. Anaesthesia. 2010;65(5):478–82.
20. Mitsuhata H, Shimizu R, Yokoyama MM. Suppressive effects of volatile anesthetics on cytokine release in human peripheral blood mononuclear cells. Int J Immunopharmacol. 1995;17(6):529–34.
21. Pirbudak Cocelli L, Ugur MG, Karadasli H. Comparison of effects of low-flow Sevoflurane and Desflurane anesthesia on neutrophil and T-cell populations. Curr Ther Res Clin Exp. 2012;73(1–2):41–51.
22. Jiao B, Yang C, Huang NN, Yang N, Wei L, Xu H. Relationship between volatile anesthetics and tumor progression: unveiling the mystery. Curr Med Sci. 2018;38(6):962–7.
23. Marana E, Russo A, Colicci S, Polidori L, Bevilacqua F, Viviani D, et al. Desflurane versus Sevoflurane: a comparison on stress response. Minerva Anestesiol. 2013;79(1):7–14.
24. Allaouchiche B, Debon R, Goudable J, Chassard D, Duflo F. Oxidative stress status during exposure to Propofol, Sevoflurane and Desflurane. Anesth Analg. 2001;93(4):981–5.
25. Shan Z, Cai S, Zhang T, Kuang L, Wang Q, Xiu H, et al. Effects of sevoflurane on leucine-rich repeat kinase 2-associated Drosophila model of Parkinson's disease. Mol Med Rep. 2015;11(3):2062–70.26.
26. Ljungqvist O. Modulating postoperative insulin resistance by preoperative carbohydrate loading. Best Pract Res Clin Anaesthesiol. 2009;23(4):401–9.
27. Sommer A, Marxreiter F, Krach F, Fadler T, Grosch J, Maroni M, et al. Th17 lymphocytes induce neuronal cell death in a human iPSC-based model of Parkinson's disease. Cell Stem Cell. 2019;24(6):1006.

11

Patients' perception of the practice of anaesthesia in a teaching hospital in Northern Jordan

Adel M. Bataineh[1,2*], Ibraheem Y. Qudaisat[3], Khaled El-Radaideh[1], Rawand A. Alzoubi[1] and Mohammad I. Abu-Shehab[1]

Abstract

Background and aim: Despite big leaps of progress in its scope, the practice of anesthesia is still suffering from poor public image, especially in developing countries. Little research investigated the public awareness of anesthesia in the Middle East. This study aimed to examine the perception of the practice of anaesthesia among Jordanian patients.

Methods: A standard questionnaire with 29 questions was administered through personal interview to consenting patients. Questions tested patients' correct knowledge of the identity of anesthetists, their roles and scope of their practice. Awareness was measured using the frequency of correct answers to each survey question. A total awareness score was calculated as the percentage ratio of the number of correct answers to the total number of questions. We classified this score into: Poor< 50%. Moderate 50–75%, and Good > 75% to reflect patient's overall perception of anesthetists and their roles. Effects of demographic variables on results were also investigated. Appropriate statistical tests were used to summarize and compare results. A total of 513 patients admitted for elective surgery were sequentially approached for enrolment.

Results: Five hundred and five patients were enrolled. Most patients identified anesthesia as a separate practice from surgery (86%). The anaesthetist was identified as a physician by only 37% of patients. Equal importance to both anaesthetists and surgeons was assumed by 71.5% of patents. Only 15% of patients showed good level of total knowledge of anaesthetist roles, while 51% scored poorly. Highest awareness was of anaesthetist's preoperative roles (65.1%). Age was the only demographic factor affecting studied awareness ($P = 0.009$).

Conclusion: Although the importance of anesthetist is well perceived among Jordanian patients, there is still some ignorance in their knowledge of the details of anesthesia practice. Active communication efforts and patient education by anesthetists are needed to improve the public status of the specialty.

Keywords: Anaesthesia, Anaesthetist roles, Perception, Jordan

* Correspondence: ambataineh3@just.edu.jo
[1]Department of Anesthesia and Recovery, Faculty of Medicine, Jordan University of Science and Technology, Irbid, Jordan
[2]Department of Anaesthesia and Recovery, King AbduLLAH-I University Hospital, Irbid, Jordan

Background

Since its early beginnings in the nineteenth century, the practice of anesthesia had been in a state of continuous evolution [1]. This evolution culminated in the announcement of anesthesia as a specialty in 1939 during the New York World Fair [2]. Its scope of medical care had extended beyond the perioperative period to include more and more medical services. In addition to the perioperative anesthetic care, the practice now covers acute and chronic pain management, intensive care units, and resuscitation care services. This is in addition to the well-established role of anaesthetists in undergraduate medical education [3]. Consequently, the role of the anaesthetist, as a medical care giver, has grown tremendously and extended beyond the boundaries of operating theatres.

Unfortunately, the status of anesthesia is still underestimated within medical specialties, and its role misunderstood among lay communities who are not trained, qualified or experienced in medical field [4]. Even in the developed world, the progress of this understanding was slow and is still incomplete, except for few countries like Switzerland [4, 5]. The perception of anesthesia and role of anaesthetist in the developing countries is still lagging behind that in the developed world [6].

Anesthetic care in Jordan is currently provided by a qualified anesthesia specialist doctor assisted by an anesthesia technician who is a graduate from a two-year study program from a community college. The aim of our study was to investigate the state of perception of anaesthesia and role of anaesthetist among Jordanian patients admitted for elective surgery in a teaching hospital in the north of Jordan.

Methods

Study design, settings and participants

A cross-sectional questionnaire-based opinion survey was carried out through personal interviews at King Abdullah University Hospital, Al Ramtha-Jordan, in the period between March and June 2019. After obtaining approval from the research committee of the faculty of medicine at Jordan University of Science and Technology, and hospital's IRB committee, 18-year-old and above patients, admitted for elective surgery the next day in different surgical specialties, were approached in their wards for participation in the survey. Exclusion criteria included patients who were mentally incapacitated, physically or emotionally unstable, patient with pain score ≥ 4 on the visual analogue scale, and those receiving any medications that can alter their decision making. The study was performed following the guidelines of the Declaration of Helsinki [7].

Questionnaire

After a review of previous similar literature, a questionnaire with a total of 29 questions was developed and structured by the first two authors to cover the intended study objectives. It was then reviewed by the other three researchers. It consisted of three parts: the first part was of demographic data including previous surgery, the second part contained questions about patients' perception of anaesthetists in terms of their qualifications (i.e. fulfilling the official requirements for a specific practice in the medical field), and importance (how much their role counts in maintaining the wellbeing of the patient in the perioperative period), and the last part examined patients' awareness of the roles of anaesthetist both inside and outside theatre, (Additional file 1). The survey questionnaire was administered through personal interviews in the commonly spoken (colloquial), non-formal Arabic language. It was first piloted to 10 patients, and necessary modifications in questions were made before embarking on the survey proper. Responses from each patient were recorded on a separate form, given a serial number, and the patient's identity was kept anonymous. After completion each interview, the data was entered into an Excel database file for future processing and analysis.

Study outcomes

The primary outcome of this study was to determine patients' knowledge and perceptions of anesthesia and anaesthetists. In order to achieve that, we used the frequencies of correct responses to the different relative questions. Also, we calculated a knowledge percentage score of anaesthetist roles as the percentage of correct answers out of responses to all 19 questions. A similar score was also calculated for each stage of perioperative management and for the roles of anaesthetist outside the operating theatre. We classified the knowledge percentage score scale into poor, moderate, and good as follows: Poor< 50%. Moderate 50–75%, and Good > 75%. The secondary outcome was to assess the effect of demographic factors on this perception and knowledge.

Statistics

Statistical Analysis was carried out using SPSS version 22 software (IBM, Chicago, IL, USA). Descriptive statistics were used to summarize data using frequencies for nominal data and mean (±SD) for continuous variables. For secondary study outcomes, chi-square test and independent samples t-test were used as appropriate for comparisons between demographic subgroups.

Results

Five hundred and thirteen patients were sequentially approached for participation in the survey. Eight patients declined participation, and 505 patients agreed to be enrolled, giving a response rate of 98%. The mean age of participants was 43.5 (14.9±) years, and 276 (55%) were females. Most patients (92%) were city dwellers, and (44%) had education higher than high school. Two hundred and sixty-three patients (52%) had previous surgeries, 39% of them were in teaching hospitals. All enrolled patients completed the survey without withdrawals. Table 1 summarizes the details of demographic variables.

Only 37% of patients were aware that the one who administers anesthesia is a fully qualified physician, compared to 41% who believed that a technician does the job. However, 17% did not know what to answer, with negligible percentages of patients assuming the job done by other professions, Fig. 1. Most of our patients (83%), identified the anaesthetist as a separate practitioner from the surgical team, and 86% knew that he does not leave the theatre during surgery. About 71.5% of patients in our study considered the roles of both anesthetists and surgeons equally important in maintaining patients' well-being in the perioperative period, Fig. 2.

Table 2 summarizes the frequencies of patients' correct perception of the perioperative roles of the anaesthetist. Preoperative evaluation of patients including ordering investigations and asking for necessary consultations was recognized as an anaesthetist role by about half of the participants. Two-thirds of patients were aware that the decisions on fitness for surgery under anesthesia and the required fasting time were also roles of the anaesthetist. A higher proportion of about three-quarters of patients were aware of the role of anaesthetist in obtaining informed consent from each patient before anesthesia.

Patients' awareness of anaesthetist's intraoperative roles was not uniform. It was most apparent for putting patients to sleep (75%), monitoring them throughout surgery (73%), and waking them up at the end (72%). Recognition

Table 1 Demographic data of study participants

Variable			*n*	%
GENDER		Male	229	45.3
		Female	276	54.7
AGE GROUP		< 60 yr	426	84.4
		> = 60 yr	79	15.6
EDUCATION		up to High school	281	55.6
		Higher education	224	44.4
RESIDENCE		City	332	65.7
		other	173	34.3
PREVIOUS SURGERY	Yes	Teaching hospital	197	39
		other hospital	166	32.9
		Total	363	71.9
	No		142	28.1

of other roles was only observed in about one-third of patients for the administration of analgesic drugs, other medications, and fluid needs. Blood transfusion was believed to be an anaesthetist role by only 22% of patients.

Escorting patients to the post-anesthesia care unit (PACU), and following them up there, were believed to be roles of the anaesthetist by a little more than half of patients. Surprisingly, only 32% of our patients considered the management of postoperative medical complications in PACU an anaesthetist job.

Most patients were not aware of the roles of anaesthetists outside the operating theatres. Awareness was highest for cardiopulmonary resuscitation (40%), followed by the management of acute and chronic pain (28%). Awareness of the role of looking after intensive care patients was observed only in 25% of responses.

Almost half of our patients (51%) showed poor level of knowledge of anaesthetists' roles. Good level of knowledge was shown by only 15% and moderate level by the remaining 34% of participants. Age was the only demographic finding that had significant effect on the level of awareness among patients of the roles of anaesthetists Table 3. Older patients (> 60 yr) were significantly more aware of the roles of anaesthetists compared to younger ones ($P = 0.009$). The genders had almost the same level of awareness while higher education, city-dwelling, previous surgery, and teaching hospital surgical experience had a minimal positive effect that did not reach statistical significance.

On the other hand, when we calculated the average score for each stage of perioperative care separately, the preoperative roles of the anaesthetist turned out to be enjoying the highest level of awareness among patients (65%). Nonetheless, this score was still in the moderate level of knowledge. The level of awareness of anaesthetists' roles in other stages of patients' care were unfortunately poor, Table 4.

Discussion

The results of this survey of Jordanian patients admitted for elective surgery in a teaching hospital about their perception of anaesthetists and their roles, showed a mixture of appreciation and misconception. Patients were aware of the standalone nature of anesthetic practice from the surgical team and were also informed that the anaesthetist is committed to his patient in the operating theatre. Furthermore, the importance assumed by most of our patients to the role of anaesthetists was equal to that of surgeon by 71.5% of them. However, only 37% of them recognized the anaesthetist as a specialized doctor. Furthermore, the anaesthetist was thought to be a technician by an even higher percentage of patients (41%). This misconception may be because anesthetic services in Jordan used to be provided mainly

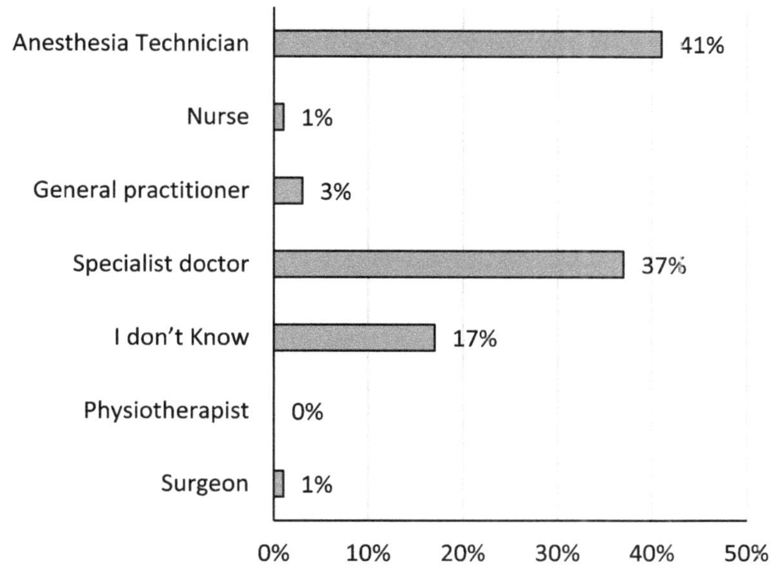

Fig. 1 Frequencies of patients' perception of anaesthetist qualification

by anesthesia technicians in the past. The scarcity of anaesthetists in the country mandated this level of qualifications until the mid-eighties of the last century. At that time, regulations were set by the ministry of health, which limited the provision of anesthetic care to physician anaesthetists. Unfortunately, there are no previous national baseline values to compare our results with. However, it is apparent, after about three and half decades, that the rise in the public awareness of the professional identity of the anaesthetist is slow. This slow progress of awareness about anaesthetists was observed even in developed countries at some point and reflected deficient perioperative teaching and communication on the side of anaesthetists about their practice [4].

Our patients' awareness of the different roles of the anaesthetist is consistent with their perception of his qualifications. This consistency was most apparent in the awareness results of the intraoperative roles of the anaesthetist, Table 2. Here, patients voted most for the roles that are mainly concerned with the sleep process, while more medical roles, like fluid management, blood transfusion, and administration of other necessary drugs, were perceived only poorly. On the other hand, the medical roles of preoperative patient assessment and postoperative management of complications were also considered least by patients to be roles of anaesthetists. Our results about the physician status of anaesthetists are close to those reported in previous studies from different countries in the developing world [8–11].

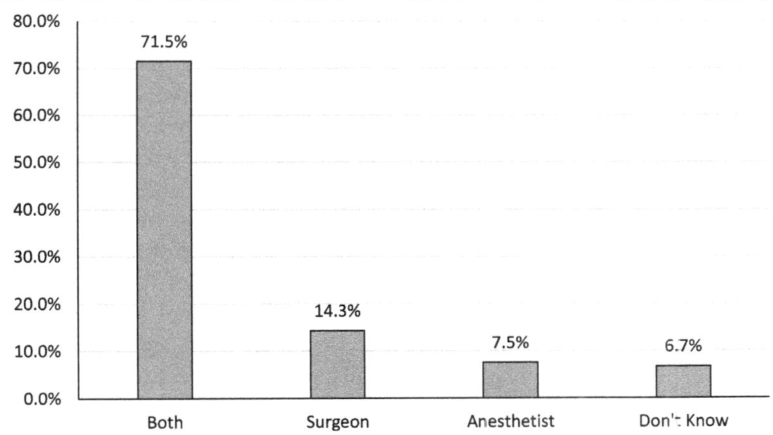

Fig. 2 Patients' perception of the more important doctor in the operating theatre

Table 2 Frequencies of patients' correct answers to knowledge questions about the roles of anaesthetists

Role		Correct answer	
		No.	%
Pre-operative Roles	Preoperative assessment of patients	266	52.7
	Asking for investigations and consultations	279	55.2
	Deciding on patient fitness to undergo surgery	332	65.7
	Dermining required fasting duration	305	60.4
	Expalining anesthetic details before operation	388	76.8
	Answering all patient questions about anesthesia	402	79.6
Intra-operative Roles	Giving patient the required hypnotic drugs	380	75.2
	Giving patients the required analgesic drugs	186	36.8
	Administering any medications that the patient may need in OR	153	30.3
	Continuously monitoring the patient without leaving the OR	368	72.9
	looking after patients needs of fluids	156	30.9
	Estimating blood loss and carrying out necessary blood TX	112	22.2
	Waking patient up in the operting room at the end of surgery	363	71.9
Postoperative Roles	Escorting patient to the recovery room	268	53.1
	Superising patient in the recovery room	279	55.2
	Treating any complications in the recovery room	161	31.9
Roles outside operating theater	Managing patients in the intensive care unit	128	25.3
	Doing cardiopulmonary resuscitation	202	40.0
	Chronic and acute pain management	143	28.3

Compared to other perioperative and outside-theatre roles, the preoperative duties of anaesthetists were the most recognized duties by our patients, with a knowledge score of 65.1%, Table 3. A possible explanation could be that the patient's knowledge about the roles of anaesthetists was likely obtained by witnessing rather than education. The total loss of consciousness during general anesthesia and the residual effects of anesthetic drugs in the recovery room will deprive patients of this resource of learning.

Age was the only demographic factor significantly affecting our patients' level of awareness of the roles of anaesthetists, Table 4. This finding is intriguing as older patients are more familiar with the older system of anaesthetist qualifications and roles. However, once again, if the practice of anesthesia was not brought to patient's awareness through ongoing education and proper role modelling, patients will end up with the implicit type of learning through exposure to the different sources of information like friends, media, and observation during previous surgical experiences. This implicit type of learning is believed to be preserved with healthy aging, and older patients will have the privilege of higher exposure to information through this type of learning [12]. The active role of educating patients about this specialty seems to be deficient so far among anaesthetists in our country and unfortunately even in teaching hospitals.

Table 3 Patients' knowledge score of the anaesthetist's roles at different points of care

Knowledge Score	Mean
All roles	50.8 (23.1)
Preoperative roles	65.1 (28.7)
Intraoperative roles	48.6 (25.5)
Postoperative roles	46.7 (37.9)
Roles outside operating theaters	31.2 (34.6)

Regardless of their level of education, there is always a desire amongst patients to know more about their management, and efforts in this regard are mandatory to increase awareness of the specialty [13, 14]. The benefits of educating patients about anesthesia and what to expect from their anaesthetists are multiple. Patients' fear from the loss of control over their own bodies during anesthesia can negatively affect their perioperative course of management to the extent that they may choose to cancel their surgeries. Enlightening patients with the details of their perioperative anesthetic care in terms of personnel and practice, will alleviate much of their anxiety and make them feel better in control over this part of their hospital experience [15, 16]. On the other hand, anaesthetists will be able to build rapport with their patients during their preoperative physician-patient encounters [4, 17]. This rapport fosters the trust

Table 4 Effects of demographic factors on level of patients' knowledge of anaesthetists' roles

Demographic variable	Subgroup	n.	Knowledge percentage Score (%)	*P value*
Gender	M	229	50.77 (23.1)	0.977
	F	276	50.76 (23.2)	
Age group	< 60 yr	426	49.6 (23.1)	0.006
	> = 60	79	57.3 (22.2)	
Education group	school	363	49.7 (22.2)	0.325
	> school	142	51.9 (23.7)	
Residence	City	332	52.0 (23.2)	0.093
	other	173	48.4 (22.8)	
Previous surgery	Yes	363	51.4 (23.0)	0.304
	No	142	49.1 (23.5)	
Previous surgery Hospital	Teaching	197	49.8 (25.8)	0.353
	non-teaching	166	47.3 (24.8)	

and confidence of patients in their anaesthetists and will help improve the poor public image of the practice of anesthesia and even reduce incidence of malpractice litigations [4, 18]. The patients' perception and knowledge of the practice of anesthesia was shown to be improved by active patient education endeavors [15]. This education can take multiple forms which include: preoperative assessment clinics, informative preoperative visits, use of educational videos, use of public media, educating other health professionals about anesthesia, and getting anaesthetists involved in administrative hospital committees [4, 19–21].

Our data collection and analysis were completed before the start of the Coronavirus pandemic. However, in their justification for the country's lockdown, the national Coronavirus committee raised the concern that the health system may be overwhelmed by the probable large numbers of critical Covid-19 victims. Media discussions about the adequacy of the country's repository of beds, ventilators, and staff followed. These events shed a good light on the importance of anesthetists. So, if our study was to be repeated nowadays, we expect that it will reveal positive changes in the results especially those of anesthetist identity and the critical care part of the practice. Results about anesthetist's perioperative roles are expected to minimally change.

Our survey was carried out in the northern part of Jordan, and our results may have changed had the data been collected from other country regions too. Another limitation was the unfortunate lack of external peer-reviewing of our study questionnaire, which could have increased confidence in its effectiveness.

Our study results gave an idea about the current state of patients' perception of anesthesia and anaesthetists in Jordan. We believe that results represent an addition to the medical literature from this part of the world in this field and can be used as a reference for any future studies in this regard.

Conclusion

Our study showed that, although patients in Jordan are aware of the importance of anesthetists in maintaining their well-being during perioperative care, there is still ignorance in their knowledge about the details of their practice. Efforts to educate patients about anesthesia in terms of practice and personnel are needed to improve the current state of perception to meet international standards.

The leading role of intensive care practitioners, including anesthetists during the recent pandemic of the Coronavirus, may have played a role in improving the public's perception of this particular role of anesthetists.

Abbreviation

PACU: Post-Anaesthesia Care Unit

Acknowledgements

None.

Authors' contributions

AB and IQ: Coming up with rresearch idea, doing literature review and study design. Training data collection team did data analysis and preparation of manuscript. KE: reviewing research idea, sharing literature review and reviewing study design and manuscript body. RAA; MIA: shared literature review, did data collection, review of manuscript. All authors have read and approved the manuscript.

Authors' information

Nothing of necessity for the study.

Author details

[1]Department of Anesthesia and Recovery, Faculty of Medicine, Jordan University of Science and Technology, Irbid, Jordan. [2]Department of Anaesthesia and Recovery, King AbduLLAH-I University Hospital, Irbid, Jordan. [3]Department of Anesthesia and Intensive Care, School of Medicine, University of Jordan, Amman, Jordan.

References

1. Robinson DH, Toledo AH. Historical development of modern anesthesia. J Investig Surg. 2012;25(3):141–9.
2. Bacon DR, Lema MJ, Yearley CK. For all the world to see: anesthesia at the 1939 New York World's fair. J Clin Anesth. 1993;5(3):252–8.
3. Brull R, Bradley JW. The role of anesthesiologists in Canadian undergraduate medical education. Can J Anesth Can Anesth. 2001;48(2):147–52.
4. Klafta JM, Roizen MF. Current understanding of patients' attitudes toward and preparation for anesthesia. Anesth Analg. 1996;83(6):1314–21.
5. Kindler CH, Harms C, Alber C. Das Berufsbild des Anästhesisten. Anaesthesist. 2002;51(11):890–6.
6. Mooruth V. Knowledge and perceptions of patients regarding anaesthetists and anaesthesia. Johannesburg: University of the Witwatersrand, 2015. available from: https://pdfs.semanticscholar.org/734a/ab4119dc3b1e2ff38d6103b8256974754de6.pdf. Accessed 2 May 2020.
7. World Medical Association Declaration of Helsinki. JAMA [Internet]. 2013 27; 310(20):2191. Available from: http://jama.jamanetwork.com/article.aspx?doi=10.1001/jama.2013.281053; Accessed 1 May 2020.
8. Jathar D, Shinde V, Patel R, Naik L. A study of patients ' perception about knowledge of Anaesthesia & Anaesthesiologist. Indian J Anaesth. 2002;46(1): 26–30.
9. Baaj J, Takrouri MS, Hussein BM, Al AH. Saudi patients' knowledge and attitude toward anesthesia and anesthesiologists--a prospective cross-sectional interview questionnaire. Middle East J Anaesthesiol. 2006;18(4): 679–91.
10. Bhattarai B, Kandel S, Adhikari N. Perception about the role of anesthesia and anesthesiologist among the paramedical staffs: perspective from a medical college in Nepal. Kathmandu Univ Med J (KUMJ). 2012;10(38):51–4. https://doi.org/10.3126/kumj.v10i2.7344.
11. Hariharan S. Knowledge and attitudes of patients towards anesthesia and anesthesiologists. A review. Anest México. 2009;21((3)):174–8.
12. Ward E V., Berry CJ, Shanks DR. Age effects on explicit and implicit memory. Front Psychol. 2013;4.
13. Naithani U, Purohit D, Bajaj P. Public awareness about anaesthesia and anaesthesiologists: a survey. Indian J Anaesth. 2007;51:420–6.
14. Lonsdale M, Hutchison GL. Patients' desire for information about anaesthesia Scottish and Canadian attitudes. Anaesthesia. 1991;46(5):410–2.
15. Imran M, Khan F. Change In Patient's Perception And Knowledge Regarding Anaesthetic Practice After A Preoperative Anaesthesia Clinic Visit. Internet J Anesthesiol. 2012;30(3).
16. Anderson EA. Preoperative preparation for cardiac surgery facilitates recovery, reduces psychological distress, and reduces the incidence of acute postoperative hypertension. J Consult Clin Psychol. 1987;55(4):513–20.
17. Deledda G, Moretti F, Rimondini M, Zimmermann C. How patients want their doctor to communicate. A literature review on primary care patients' perspective. Patient Educ Couns. 2013;90(3):297–306.
18. Usha Gurunathan RJ. The public's perception of anaesthesiologists - Indian attitudes. Indian J Anaesth. 2004;48:456–60.
19. Markus MacGill. What do anesthesiologists do?. Medical News Today 2017. Available from: https://www.medicalnewstoday.com/articles/287857#what-does-an-anesthesiologist-do? Accessed 5 May 2020.
20. Baskett PJK, Armitage EN. The public image of the speciality. Anaesthesia. 1978;33(1):64–5.
21. American Society of Anesthesiologists. Anesthesia as Career. Available from: https://www.asahq.org/education-and-career/careerresources/anesthesia-as-a-career. Accessed 13 May 2020.

12

Comparison of spinal anesthesia and general anesthesia in inguinal hernia repair in adult

Lin Li[†], Yi Pang[†], Yongchao Wang, Qi Li and Xiangchao Meng[*]

Abstract

Background: Inguinal hernia repair is one of the most commonly performed surgical procedures. To date, there is no consensus on which anesthesia should be used. The objective of this meta-analysis was to assess the efficacy of spinal anesthesia (SA) vs. general anesthesia (GA) in inguinal hernia repair in adults.

Methods: Eligible studies were identified before January 2020 from PubMed, Embase, ScienceDirect, Cochrane Library, Scopus database as well as reference lists. Outcomes included surgery time, the time in the operation room, the length of hospital stay, pain scores, patient satisfaction, and postoperative complications. Subgroup analysis based on surgical approaches was conducted.

Results: Six randomized controlled trials (RCT) and five cohort studies were included. A total of 2593 patients were analyzed. Compared to GA, SA was associated with a longer surgery time (weighted mean difference [WMD]: − 3.28, 95%confident interval [CI]: − 5.76, − 0.81), particularly in laparoscopic repair. Postoperative pain at 4 h and 12 h were in favor of SA following either open or laparoscopic repairs (standard mean difference [SMD]: 1.58; 95%CI: 0.55, 2.61, SMD: 0.99, 95%CI: 0.37, 1.60, respectively); and considering borderline significance, patients receiving SA might be more satisfied with the anesthesia they used for herniorrhaphy (SMD: -0.32, 95%CI: − 0.70, 0.06). Some major complications of scrotal edema, seroma, wound infection, recurrence, shoulder pain were comparable between the two groups. However, patients receiving SA had an increased risk of postoperative urinary retention and headache when compared with GA (relative ratio [RR]: 0.44, 95% CI: 0.23, 0.86, RR: 0.33, 95% CI: 0.12, 0.92, respectively). There was a tendency that the incidence of postoperative nausea and vomiting was lower in SA than GA (RR: 2.12, 95%CI: 0.95, 4.73), especially in open herniorrhaphy.

Conclusions: SA can be another good choice for pain relief no matter in open or laparoscopic hernia repairs, but it can't be confirmed that SA is better than GA.

Keywords: Inguinal hernia repair, Spinal anesthesia, General anesthesia, Meta-analysis

* Correspondence: XiangchaoMeng@yeah.net
[†]Lin Li and Yi Pang contributed equally to this work.
Department of Thyroid, Breast, Hernia Surgery, Tianjin the third Central Hospital, NO.83, Jintang Road, Tianjin 300170, China

Background

Inguinal hernia repair is one of the most commonly performed surgical procedures every year [1]. Patients always expect to undergo this operation with little anesthetic risk, minimal discomfort, and early recovery and discharge home. To date, there is no consensus on which anesthesia should be used. The choice of anesthetic techniques ranges from local infiltration to regional block to general endotracheal. Local anesthesia (LA) is more frequently used in specialist hernia centers, however, infiltration is painful and 85% of patients experience pain intraoperatively [2]. The most commonly used regional anesthesia technique is spinal anesthetic (SA), which has the advantage of avoiding paralytic agents and endotracheal intubation [3]. General anesthesia (GA) is most preferred by patients because of anxiety and fear of surgery, with a frequency of 60–70% [4]. Many studies have attempted to explore the benefits among the three anesthetic techniques for inguinal hernia repair. However, to date, no pooled analyses of the results focusing on the comparison between SA and GA in adults have surfaced. The purpose of this meta-analysis was to assess the efficacy of SA vs. GA in inguinal hernia repair in adults, in terms of surgery time, the time in operation room, hospital stay, pain scores, patient satisfaction, and major postoperative complications.

Methods

This meta-analysis was carried out according to the guidelines of the Preferred Reporting Items for Systematic Reviews and Meta-Analysis statement [5].

Search strategy

The primary search of electronic databases was conducted in PubMed, Embase, ScienceDirect, Cochrane Library, and Scopus database before January 2020. Supplemental identification was conducted by cross-checking of reference lists. Combinations of search terms 'spinal anesthesia', 'general anesthesia', and 'inguinal hernia' were used. Two reviewers independently checked the titles and abstracts of potentially relevant studies. Studies were excluded due to duplication, non-related topics and other article types (review, case report, etc.). Differences between reviewers were resolved by discussion until agreement was reached.

Study inclusion criteria

Only randomized controlled trails (RCTs) or cohort studies that compared spinal anesthesia with general anesthesia used in inguinal hernia repair in adults could be included. The language reported on need to be English, but region and publication date were free from limitation. Study results should cover intraoperative or

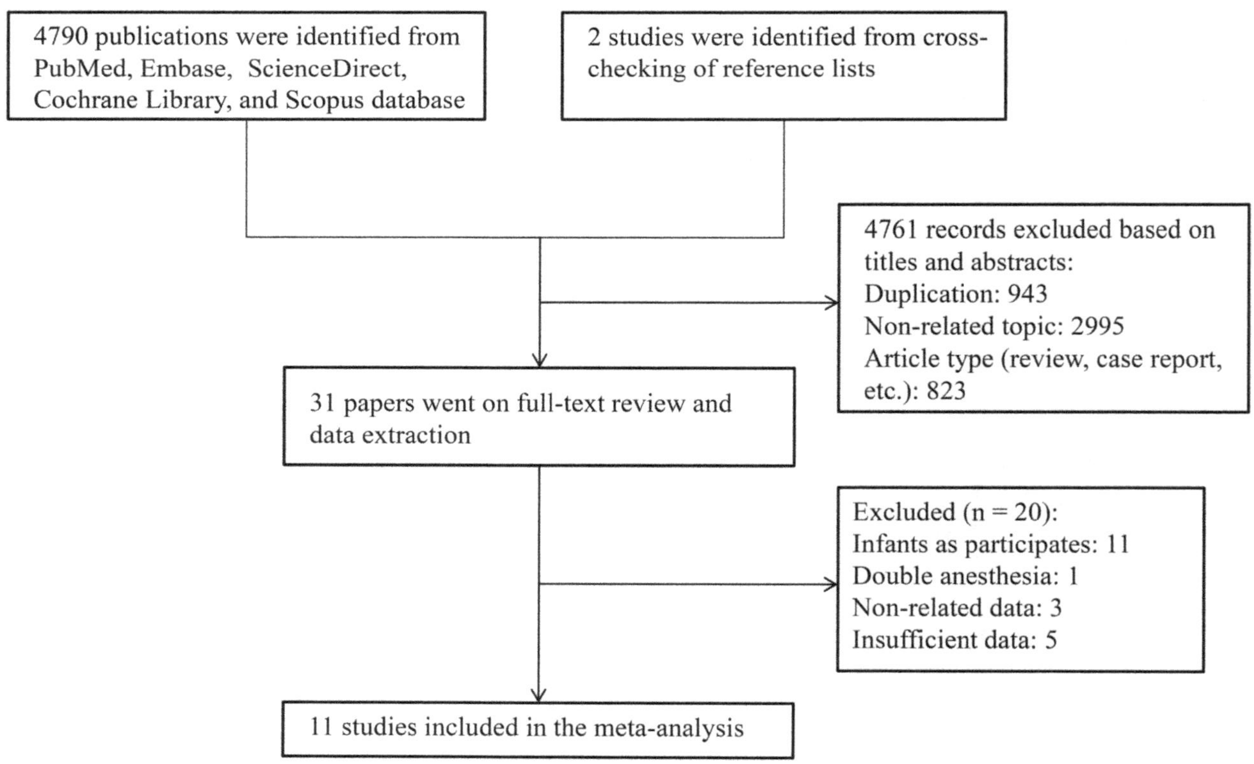

Fig. 1 Flow diagram describing the article search and inclusion in meta-analysis

Table 1 Study characteristics

Study	Design	Group	Total N	Age	N	Inclusion	Exclusion	Repair used
Burney RE 2004 [4]	RCT	SA	33	≥18 years	15	Unilateral hernia	Recurrent or bilateral hernia	Open inguinal repair
		GA		≥ 18 years	18			
Donmez T 2016 [8]	RCT	SA	50	37.16 ± 10.85	25	Uncomplicated hernia	Complicated inguinal hernia (irreducible, obstructed, or strangulated); Recurrent hernias	TEP
		GA		35.36 ± 11.40	25			
Ismail M 2009 [10]	Cohort study	SA	652	46.1 ± 14.1	636	Reducible inguinal hernia	Obstructed and strangulated hernias, pediatric hernias, and other hernias, such as ventral hernias	TEP
		GA		43.3 ± 15.6	16			
Ozgün H 2002 [15]	RCT	SA	50	51.4 ± 15.1	25	Unilateral, reducible, direct or indirecthernia; types II and III according to the Nyhus classication	Scrotal, sliding, recurrent hernias	Open inguinal repair
		GA		46.9 ± 19.8	25			
Pere 2016 [16]	RCT	SA	100	51 ± 15	49	Unilateral	Not reported	Open inguinal repair
		GA		54 ± 15	51			
Sarakatsianou C 2017 [11]	RCT	SA	70	58.85 ± 13.54	34	Non-high risk; primary, unilateralinguinal hernia	Non-reducible/obstructed hernias, bilateral hernias, big scrotal hernias	TAPP
		GA		57.64 ± 15.77	36			
Sinha R 2008 [9]	Cohort study	SA	529	32.2	480	Unilateral or bilateral, direct or indirect, recurrent inguinal hernia	Obstructed and strangulatedinguinal hernia	TEP
		GA		33.7	49			
Sunamak 2018 (1) [12]	Cohort study	SA	207	31.8 ± 10.9	96	Unilateral hernia	Recurrent hernias, strangulated, incarcerated, or bilateral hernia	TEP
		GA		39.9 ± 16.2	111			
Sunamak 2018 (2) [12]	Cohort study	SA	233	38.1 ± 16.8	116	Unilateral hernia	Recurrent hernias, strangulated, incarcerated, or bilateral hernia	Open inguinal repair
		GA		39.1 ± 16.5	117			
Symeonidis 2013	Cohort study	SA	75	56.04 ± 13.44	50	Unilateral	Scrotal, recurrent, bilateral, strangulated, or incarcerated hernias	Open inguinal repair
		GA		61.28 ± 11.42	25			
Urbach 1964 [13]	RCT	SA	514	48 (17–71)	236	Unilateral or bilateral inguinal hernia	Not reported	Open inguinal repair
		GA		43 (18–75)	278			
Yildirim D 2017 [14]	Cohort study	SA	80	35.0 ± 11.3	40	Direct or indirect hernia	Strangled, bilateral, hernia, recurrent hernia	TEP
		GA		36.4 ± 10.0	40			

RCT Randomized controlled trail, *SA* Spinal anesthesia, *GA* General anesthesia, *TEP* Laparoscopic total extraperitoneal hernia repair, *TAPP* Laparoscopic transabdominal preperitoneal inguinal hernia repair

Table 2 Quality assessment for each included cohort study

Item	Ismail M 2009 [10]	Sinha R 2008 [9]	Sunamak 2018 [12]	Symeonidis 2013	Yildirim D 2017 [14]
Item 1: The selection of the study groups					
Representativeness of the exposed cohort	☆	☆	☆	☆	☆
Selection of the non exposed cohort	☆	☆	☆	☆	☆
Ascertainment of exposure	☆	☆	☆	☆	☆
Demonstration that outcome of interest was not present at start of study	☆	☆	☆	☆	☆
Item 2: The comparability of the groups	☆☆	☆☆	☆☆	☆☆	☆☆
Item 3: The ascertainment of either the exposure or outcome of interest for cohort studies					
Assessment of outcome	☆	☆	☆	☆	☆
follow-up long enough for outcomes to occur	☆	☆	☆	☆	☆
Adequacy of follow up of cohorts	☆		☆	☆	☆

☆: one ☆ means one score; each domain of Item 1 and 3 worth one ☆, Item 2 worth two ☆

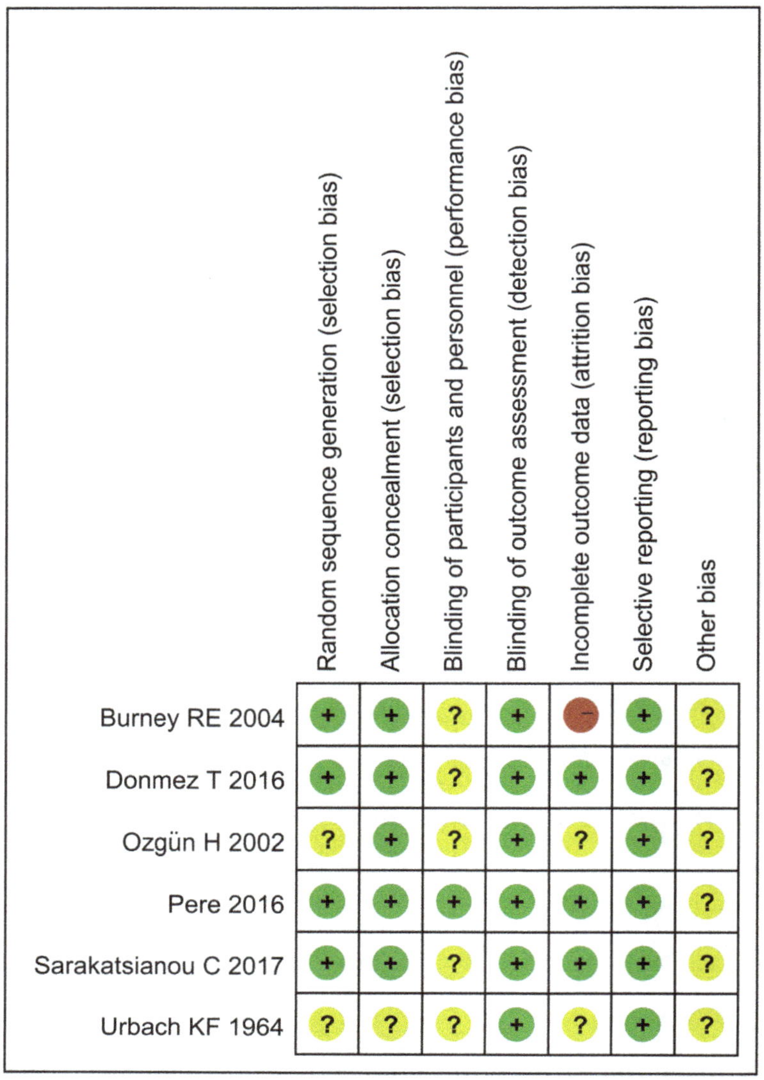

Fig. 2 Risk of bias summary of five included RCTs

postoperative outcome measures. However, studies that included a double anesthetic procedure to the same group of patients were eliminated from this analysis.

Data extraction

Data from eligible records were reviewed and extracted into an Excel spreadsheet. Our measurements encompass surgery time, the time in the operation room, the length of hospital stay, pain score, patient satisfaction, and postoperative complications. Outcomes of complications assessed in at least three papers were considered for meta-analysis. For the study of Sunamak et al. assessing open and laparoscopic total extraperitoneal repairs under GA and SA, we extracted two sets of data for meta-analysis, namely data for open repair and data for laparoscopic repair.

We defined the surgery time as the duration between beginning of the skin incision and skin closure; the time in the operating room as the period from the beginning of anesthesia to discharge from the operating room. Complications include scrotal edema, seroma, wound infection, recurrence, shoulder pain, urinary retention, headache, and postoperative nausea and vomiting (PONV).

Quality assessment

Quality of each included RCT was evaluated using the Cochrane Collaboration tool for assessing the risk of bias [6]. The method contains seven domains, namely, random sequence generation, allocation concealment, blinding of participants and personnel, blinding of outcome assessment, incomplete outcome data, selective reporting, and other bias. For each domain, RCTs were assessed to be high (red), unclear (yellow), or low (green) in risk of bias. As to the quality assessment of cohort studies, the Newcastle-Ottawa Scale was used [7]. The tool includes three domains: the selection of the study groups; the comparability of the groups; and the ascertainment of either the exposure or outcome of interest for cohort studies. For each evaluation, a 'star system' was applied to score from 0 star to 9 stars.

Data analysis

We conducted all statistical analysis using Stata software version 15.0 (Stata Corporation, College Station, TX, USA) software. Pooled relative ratios (RRs) and 95% confidence intervals (CIs) were calculated for postoperative

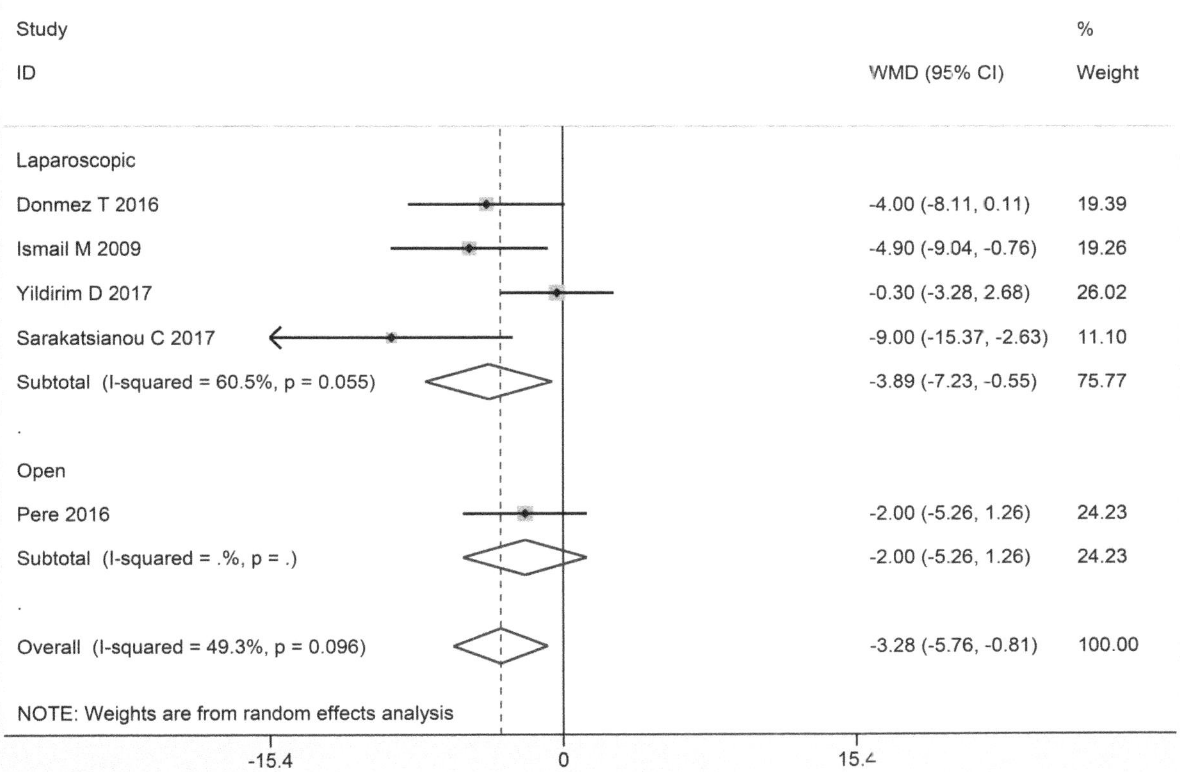

Fig. 3 The surgery time when GA and SA compared

complications. Weighted mean differences (WMDs) and 95% CIs were calculated for surgery time, operation time, and the length of hospital stay; standard mean differences (SMDs) and 95% CIs were calculated for pain scores and patient satisfaction. Heterogeneity across the studies was estimated by the I^2 statistics. $I^2 > 50\%$ was defined as significant heterogeneity. In case of $I^2 > 50\%$, a random effects model was used, otherwise, a fixed effects model was preferred. Sensitivity analysis was performed when significant heterogeneity was found. Sensitivity analysis was conducted by removing one study at a time to disclose if one particular study could affect the overall result. Subgroup analyses of laparoscopic and open techniques were also conducted. Pooled outcomes were presented in forest plots and considered as statistically significant if *P* value < 0.05.

Results

Study screening

The initial search of electronic databases produced 4790 studies. Two supplemental records were identified through checking the references of above mentioned studies. Further screening removed 4761 articles due to duplication, non-related topics and other article types (reviews, case reports, etc). Thirty one potentially eligible studies remained and went on a full-text review. We finally included 11 studies that matched the aforementioned criteria for this meta-analysis. The flow diagram describing the article search was shown in Fig. 1.

Study characteristics

Six RCTs and five cohort studies were included [3, 8–17]. A total of 2593 patients were recruited into this analysis. The patient age was comparable in each selected study, and the inguinal hernia included in all studies were uncomplicated hernia. Open inguinal hernia repair was performed in six studies, and laparoscopic surgical techniques were used in six. Study characteristics were summarized in Table 1.

Study quality

The evaluation for quality of each study was shown in Table 2 and Fig. 2. Both randomization and the method of sequence generation were mentioned in three RCTs

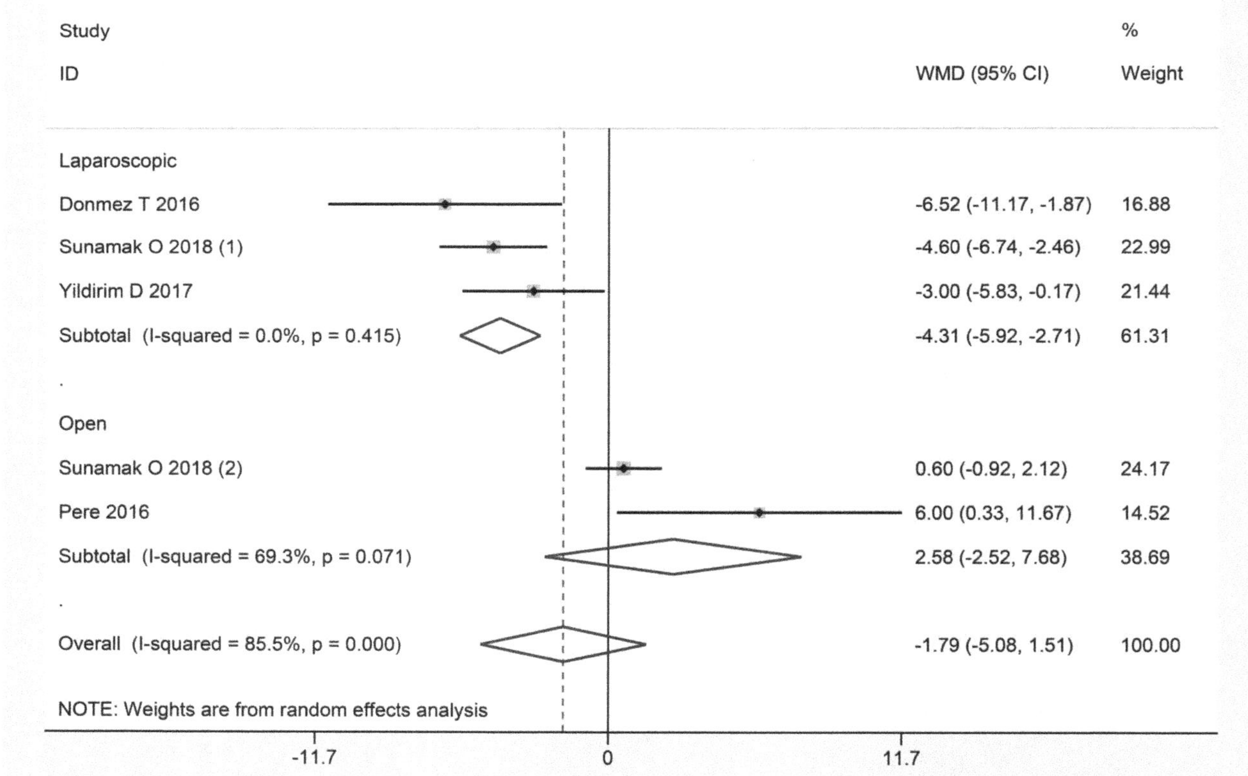

Fig. 4 The time in operation room when GA and SA compared

[3, 8, 11], whilst allocation concealment was described in four RCTs [3, 8, 11, 15]. All the five RCTs failed to provide adequate information of blinding, so they might involve an unclear risk of bias. And all the RCTs analyzed were judged to have low or unclear risk of incomplete outcome data, selective outcome reporting and other potential source of bias. On the other hand, four cohort studies satisfied all criteria and scored 9 stars [10, 12, 14]. Only one cohort study scored 8 stars owing to inadequacy of follow up [9].

Outcomes

Five studies evaluated the surgery time and the pooled WMD was − 3.28 (95%CI: − 5.76, − 0.81; $I^2 = 49.3\%$) in favor of GA ($P = 0.01$); however, subgroup analysis suggested the statistical significance to only remain in laparoscopic repair group (WMD: -3.89, 95%CI: − 7.23, − 0.55, $P = 0.02$) (Fig. 3).

Data synthesis of operating time from five cohorts generated a WMD of − 1.79 (95%CI: − 5.08, 1.51; $I^2 = 85.5\%$), indicating the time in the operating room was comparable between SA and GA groups ($P = 0.29$). Sensitivity analysis did not change the result or heterogeneity. Interestingly, by subgroup analysis we found SA group had significantly longer operation time than GA group following laparoscopic repair (WMD: -4.31, 95%CI: − 5.92, − 2.71, $P < 0.01$) (Fig. 4).

There was no significant difference in the length of hospital stay between patients under SA and GA (WMD: -0.04, 95%CI: − 1.04, 0.96, $I^2 = 56.5\%$, $P = 0.94$). This comparable results remained in both subgroups of laparoscopic and open repairs (Fig. 5).

We assessed pain scores at 4 h and 12 h after operation. The overall results showed that pain scores were significantly higher in patients under GA compared to SA at these two time points (SMD: 1.58, 95%CI: 0.55, 2.61, $I^2 = 96.0\%$, $P < 0.01$; SMD: 0.99, 95%CI: 0.37, 1.60, $I^2 = 91.8\%$, $P < 0.01$, respectively) (Fig. 6). In the subgroup of laparoscopic repair, statistical significance remained between the two groups. In the subgroup of open repair, there were also trends that patients with GA had higher pain scores than those with SA at these two time points, though there were no statistical significances (Table 3).

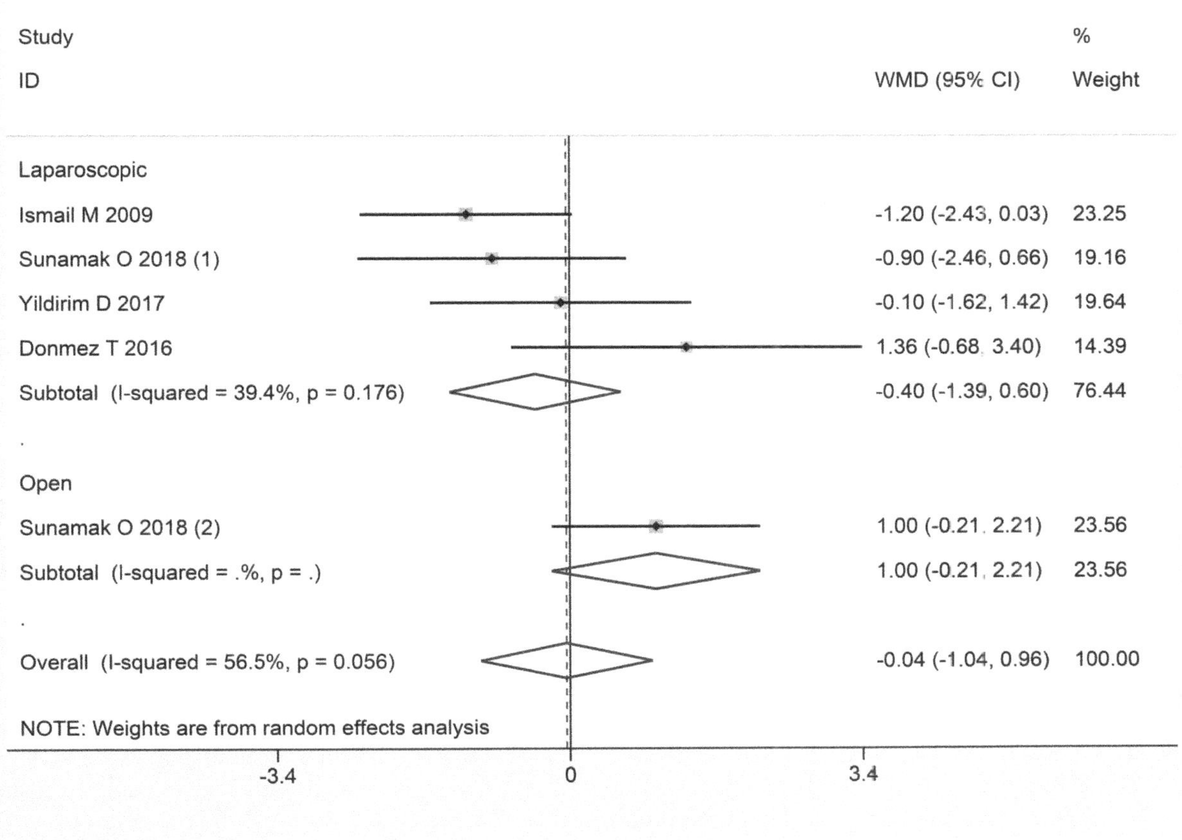

Fig. 5 The hospital stay when GA and SA compared

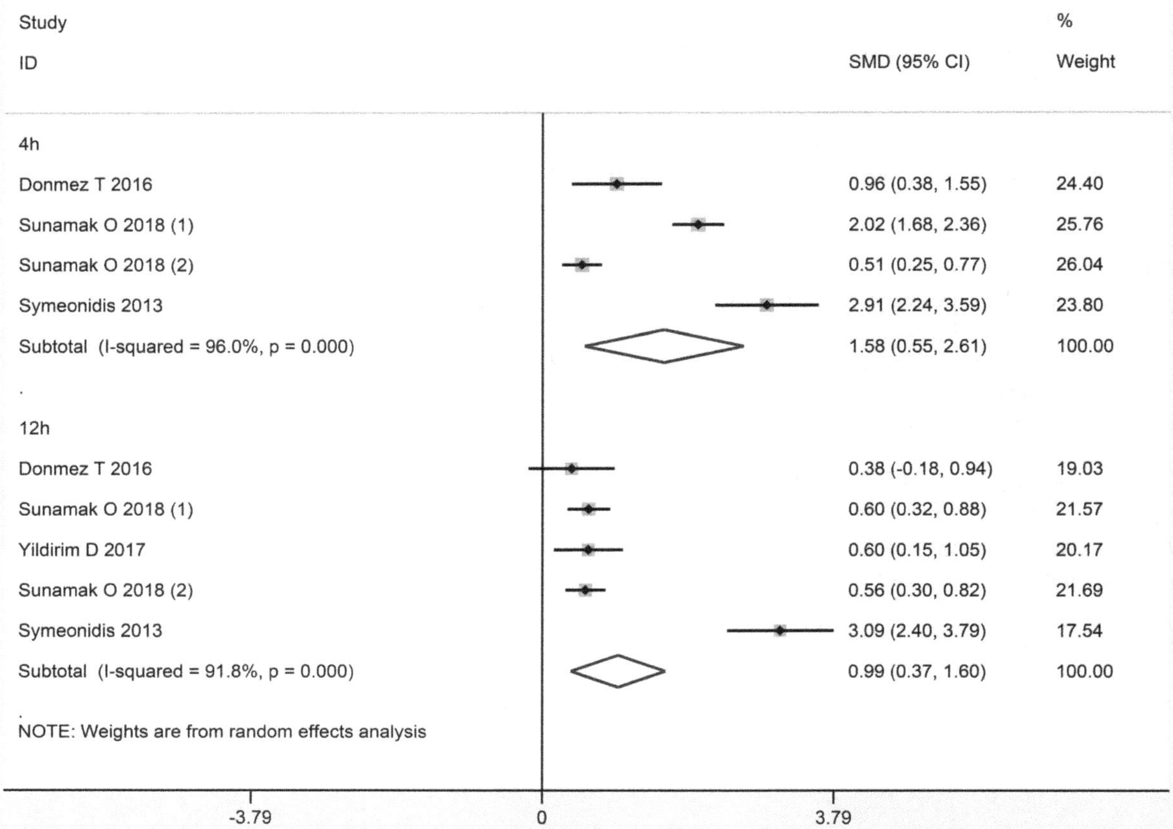

Fig. 6 The pain scores at 4 h and 12 h after operation when GA and SA compared

Only four cohorts reported patient satisfaction and the pooled SMD was − 0.32 (95%CI: − 0.70, 0.06, $I^2 = 77.5\%$, $P = 0.10$), indicating a trend that patients receiving SA were more satisfied with the anesthesia they used for herniorrhaphy as compared to GA (Fig. 7). Subgroup analysis further revealed that the difference between the two groups regarding satisfaction was significant in favor of SA in the laparoscopic group.

Meta-analysis of postoperative complications was shown in Fig. 8. We found the incidences of scrotal edema, seroma, wound infection, recurrence, and shoulder pain were comparable between the two groups irrespective of laparoscopic or open repairs. However, the incidences of urinary retention and headache were significantly higher in SA group than GA group (RR: 0.44, 95%CI: 0.23, 0.86, $I^2 = 48.1\%$, $P = 0.02$; RR: 0.33, 95%CI: 0.12, 0.92, $I^2 = 91.8\%$, $P = 0.03$, respectively); but we found in subgroup analysis that the significance only remained in laparoscopic repair group. For the incidence of PONV, borderline significance suggested that there was a tendency for patients under GA to suffer more PONV (RR: 2.12, 95%CI: 0.95, 4.73, $I^2 = 75.2\%$, $P = 0.07$); and the difference between SA and GA was noticeable in the subgroup of open repair (Table 3).

Discussion

Inguinal hernia repair is one of the most common surgeries in the world [1]. But it's still undetermined that which anesthesia should be used. In order to improve the safety and effect of the repair, many previous studies or reviews attempted to compare local anesthesia and regional anesthesia and general anesthesia, and to disclose the advantages and disadvantages among these anesthesia. Our meta-analysis of eleven studies comparing SA and GA showed that patients receiving SA might have less pain intensity post operatively and it seems that SA was associated with higher patient satisfaction than GA, which suggests that SA can be an effective option for pain relief in hernia repair compared to the gold standard GA. However, It can not be confirmed that SA

Table 3 Summary of subgroup analysis comparing pain scores and complications between SA and GA

Outcomes	Subgroups	SMD (95% CI)	RR (95% CI)	I^2 value	*P* value*
Pain scores					
4 h	Laparoscopic	1.52 (0.49, 2.55)	–	89.3%	< 0.01
	open	1.69 (−0.66, 4.05)	–	97.6%	0.16
12 h	Laparoscopic	0.57 (0.35, 0.78)	–	0.0%	< 0.01
	open	1.81 (−0.68, 4.29)	–	97.8%	0.15
Complications					
Scrotal edema	Laparoscopic	–	0.64 (0.34, 1.21)	0.0%	0.17
	open	–	1.26 (0.48, 3.26)	–	0.64
Seroma	Laparoscopic	–	0.72 (0.36, 1.44)	0.0%	0.35
	open	–	1.36 (0.61, 3.02)	0.0%	0.45
Wound infection	Laparoscopic	–	0.93 (0.40, 2.17)	0.0%	0.87
	open	–	1.17 (0.49, 2.76)	0.0%	0.73
Recurrence	Laparoscopic	–	1.57 (0.44, 5.62)	0.0%	0.49
	open	–	1.21 (0.37, 3.99)	20.9%	0.75
Shoulder pain	Laparoscopic	–	1.02 (0.52, 1.98)	0.0%	0.95
	open	–	–	–	–
Urinary retention	Laparoscopic	–	0.38 (0.15, 0.95)	0.0%	0.04
	open	–	0.47 (0.18, 1.22)	71.7%	0.12
Headache	Laparoscopic	–	0.20 (0.06, 0.68)	0.0%	0.01
	open	–	0.48 (0.09, 2.47)	78.7%	0.38
PONV	Laparoscopic	–	2.15 (0.50, 9.26)	84.1%	0.31
	open	–	1.76 (1.10, 2.80)	0.0%	0.02

*: comparisons of outcomes between SA and GA; *CI* Confidence interval, *PONV* Postoperative nausea and vomiting, *RR* Relative ratio, *SMD* Standard mean difference

is better than GA as reported by previous studies, because surgery time in the SA group was longer and patients receiving SA might have an increased risk of postoperative headache and urinary retention, especially following laparoscopic repair.

Surgery duration and operating time in SA group for laparoscopic inguinal hernia repair were longer as compared to GA group, which was in line with most previous studies; while we found comparable results between the two groups for open hernia repair. However, significant heterogeneity precluded us to draw a conclusive conclusion, and further limitations on these results might be small sample size and operator variability. More robust evidence therefore is needed to verify our findings. Moreover, the hospital stay period is an important parameter to explore the effectiveness of the techniques. By data synthesis, we concluded that patients treated by either SA or GA had a similar hospitalization.

Pain in the early postoperative period, after inguinal hernia operations, is the most common patient complaint. Our meta-analysis showed that pain scores at 4 h and 12 h post operatively were lower in SA group than GA group, no matter following laparoscopic or open repairs. That is, compared with GA, SA shows an advantage in term of early postoperative pain as demonstrated by many studies [18, 19]. Furthermore, we found the superiority of SA over GA in early postoperative pain was more significant in laparoscopic repair than open repair. Less early pain in the SA group can help patients to breathe easier and get mobilized earlier, and reduces the need for additional analgesia. Likewise, patient satisfaction increases in the SA group attributed to less pain during the first postoperative hours and the similar length of hospital stay [20]. All the eleven studies analyzed concluded that the patients under SA techniques had slightly or significantly better satisfaction when compared with GA, following either open hernia repair or laparoscopic hernia repair. Besides, through our meta-analysis of four cohorts we found patients seem to be more satisfied with SA for inguinal hernia repair, especially in laparoscopic method. This means patients were happy and would probably recommend SA to his friends. However, given the fact that the sample size in the open repair group was relatively small, the outcomes need to be interpreted with caution and similar studies

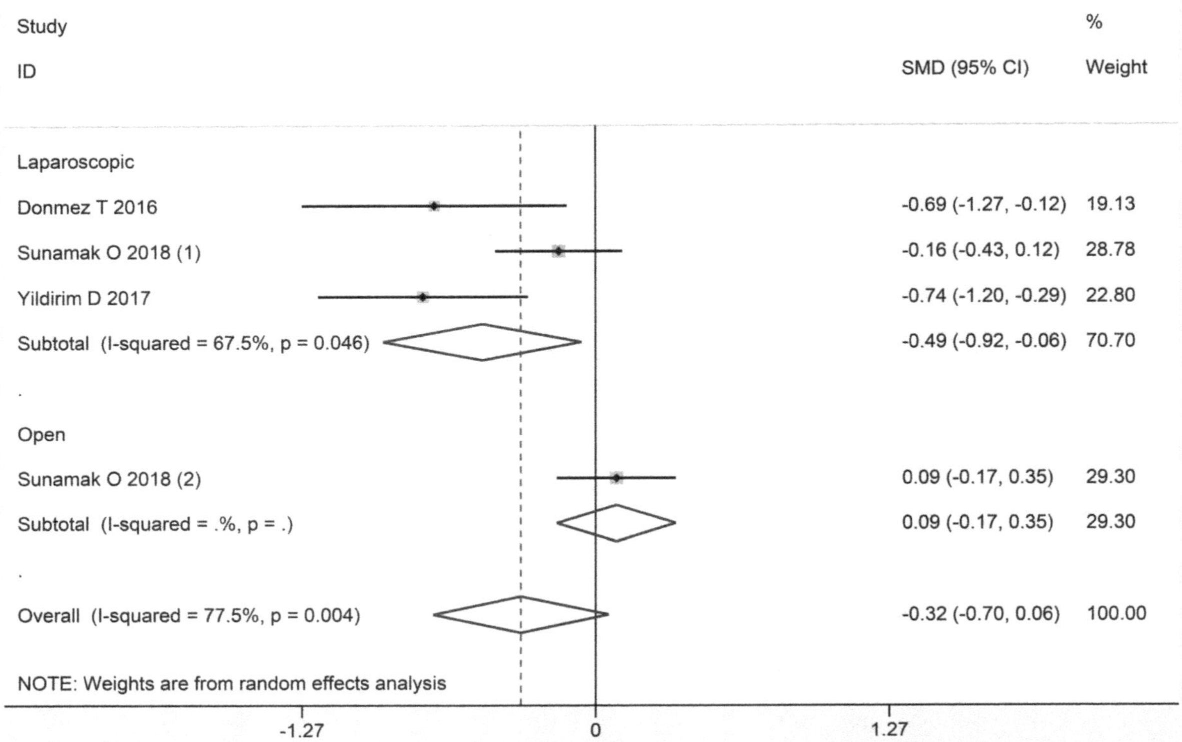

Fig. 7 The patients satisfaction when GA and SA compared

based on surgical approaches under SA and GA are warranted.

General complications, as one of the most determinant outcome measures, were reported comparable between groups in our results, including scrotal edema, seroma, wound infection, recurrence, shoulder pain. Urinary retention was one of the most frequent postoperative complications. Contradiction regarding urinary retention always exists. A higher frequency of urinary retention was often reported in previous studies. By meta-analysis, we found it was a tendency for patients under SA to experience more urinary retention than GA, in agreement with the most recent guidelines concluding that urinary retention might be more frequent following regional anesthesia [21]. Moreover, Reiner and his colleagues found that the age of the patients with urinary retention was significantly higher than patients without urinary retention, and suggested that urinary retention is seen more often in elderly patients [22]. Another study demonstrated that using short-acting agent, lidocaine, for SA virtually eliminates problems with urinary retention that occurs with long-acting SA agents [3]. Therefore, a deeper search into the incidence of urinary retention among specific groups with large sample size and adequate data is needed.

To our knowledge, headache is a very common complication following SA that always draws our attention. Our analysis showed that the incidence of headache was indeed higher in patients under SA than GA, but this difference was not significant in open herniorrhaphy. It's hypothesized that varying use of anesthetic may have an influence on this outcome in the open repair group; and insufficient data for subgroup analysis may be responsible for the inconsistency. PONV is another important postoperative adverse effect that discomforts patients [23]. From the pooled analysis, we detected a trend that PONV created a higher morbidity in the GA group, which reached agreement with most studies. PONV is highest after GA, especially when nitrous or opiates or reversal agents are utilized and has been reported in up to 60–70% of patients [24]. The incidence is as high as 30% even with the newer agents like propofol and isoflurane [25]. It seems that the type of anesthetic agents used in the surgery influence the frequency of PONV among patients under GA. But to our

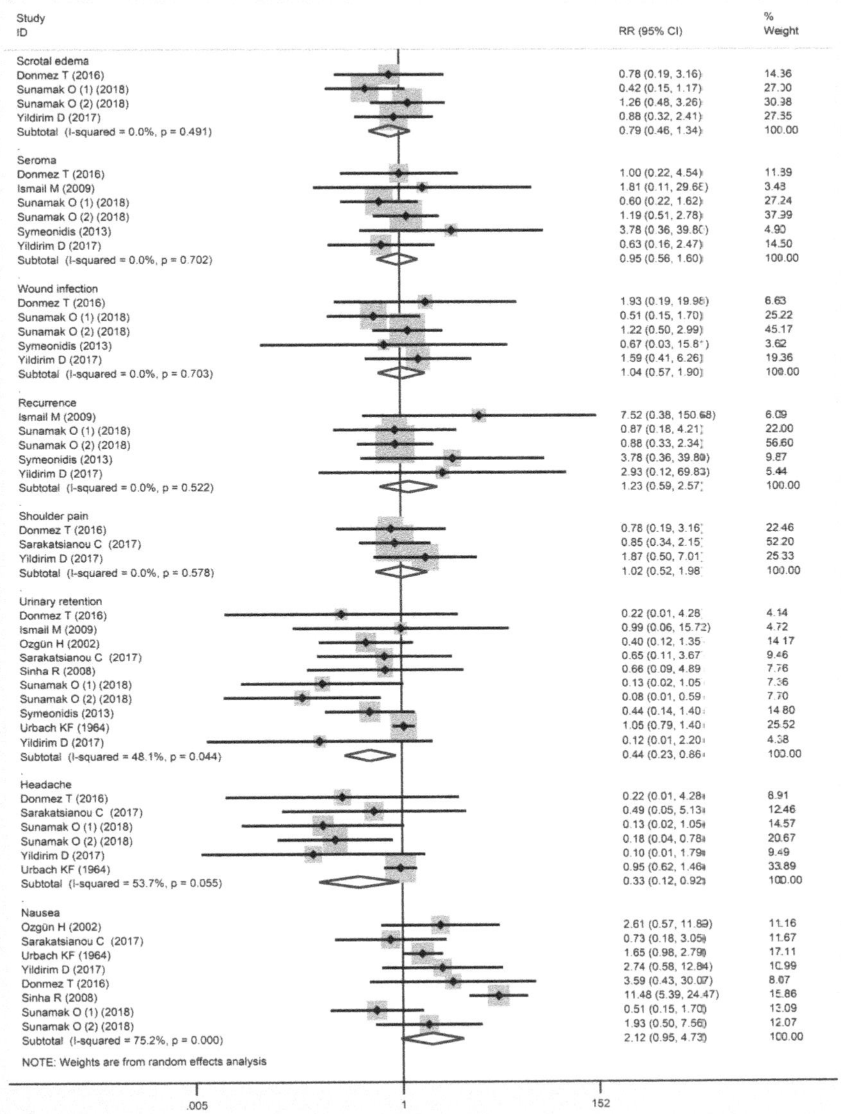

Fig. 8 The postoperative complications when GA and SA compared

knowledge, in most cases, SA has an advantage over GA in terms of the incidence of PONV due to the freedom from endotracheal intubation.

Several limitations should be acknowledged. The major limitations were significant heterogeneity and small study sample size that will greatly weaken our conclusion. Moreover, it's reported by a Danish study with a very large sample that the risk of complications after herniorrhaphy increased with increasing age [26]; patient age can be a critical factor affecting our results of complications, but subgroup analysis based on age did not work in our meta-analysis for the lack of information. Therefore, clinical application of our assessment regarding complications should be cautious. Another limitation of the analysis was the outcome measures failed to cover some other commonly concerned aspects due to inadequate data, such as minor complications, conversion to GA during repair, and return to work and normal activity. Furthermore, the combined analysis of RCTs and cohort studies produces less powerful evidence than the studies only recruiting RCTs. To improve the future comparison of inguinal hernia repair studies, a consensus should be reached regarding study designs and outcome measures.

Conclusion

In conclusion, SA is a feasible and effective method for inguinal hernia repair in adults comparable to the gold standard GA as far as postoperative pain and patient satisfaction are concerned. However, patients receiving SA need a longer surgery time and may experience more urinary retention and headache postoperatively, especially following laparoscopic repair. Therefore, SA can be another good choice for pain relief in inguinal repair, but it can't be confirmed that SA is better than GA. Further studies are still warranted to validate our conclusions.

Abbreviations

CI: Confidence intervals; GA: General anesthesia; PONV: Postoperative nausea and vomiting; RCT: Randomized controlled trails; RR: Relative ratios; SA: Spinal anesthesia; SMD: Standardized mean difference; WMD: Weighted mean difference

Acknowledgements

Not applicable.

Authors' contributions

LL and YP made contribution to the conception of the study and draft the manuscript and revision. YW and QL were responsible for study search and data collection and statistical analyses. XM made contribution to final result and figures using data processing software, and was the corresponding author. All authors have read and approved the final manuscript.

References

1. Kulacoglu H, Alptekin A. Current options in local anesthesia for groin hernia repairs. Acta Chir Iugosl. 2011;58(3):25–35.
2. Teasdale C, Mccrum A, Williams N, Horton R. A randomised controlled trial to compare local with general anaesthesia for short-stay inguinal hernia repair. Ann R Coll Surg Engl. 1982;64(4):238–42.
3. Burney R, Prabhu M, Greenfield M, Amy S, Michael O. Comparison of spinal vs general anesthesia via laryngeal mask airway in inguinal hernia repair. Arch Surg. 2004;139(2):183–7.
4. Nordin P, Staffan H, Willem V, Erik N. Choice of anesthesia and risk of reoperation for recurrence in groin hernia repair. Ann Surg. 2004;240(1):187–92.
5. Moher D, Liberati A, Tetzlaff J, Altman DG, PRISMA Group, et al. PLoS Med. 2009;6(7):e1000097.
6. Higgins JPT, Green S. Cochrane Handbook for Systematic Reviews of Interventions Version 5.1.0 [updated March 2011]: The Cochrane Collaboration; 2011. Available from http://www.cochrane-handbook.org.
7. Wells G, Shea B, O'Connell D. The newcastle-ottawa scale (nos) for assessing the quality of non-randomized studies in meta-analysis. Appl Eng Agric. 2012;18:727–34.
8. Donmez T, Erdem V, Sunamak O, Erdem D, Avaroglu H. Laparoscopic total extraperitoneal repair under spinal anesthesia versus general anesthesia: a randomized prospective study. Ther Clin Risk Manag. 2016;12:1599–608.
9. Sinha R, Gurwara A, Gupta S. Laparoscopic total extraperitoneal inguinal hernia repair under spinal anesthesia: a study of 480 patients. J Laparoendosc Adv Surg Tech A. 2008;18(5):673.
10. Ismail M, Garg P. Laparoscopic inguinal total extraperitoneal hernia repair under spinal anesthesia without mesh fixation in 1,220 hernia repairs. Hernia. 2009;13(2):115–9.
11. Sarakatsianou C, Georgopoulou S, Baloyiannis I, Chatzimichail M, Vretzakis G, Zacharoulis D, et al. Spinal versus general anesthesia for transabdominal preperitoneal (TAPP) repair of inguinal hernia: interim analysis of a controlled randomized trial. Ther Clin Risk Manag. 2017;214(2):239–45.
12. Sunamak O, Donmez T, Yildirim D, Hut A, Erdem VM, Erdem DA, et al. Open mesh and laparoscopic total extraperitoneal inguinal hernia repair under spinal and general anesthesia. Ther Clin Risk Manag. 2018;14:1839–45.
13. Urbach K, Lee W, Sheely L, Lang F, Sharp R. Spinal or general anesthesia for inguinal hernia repair? A comparison of certain complications in a controlled series. J Am Med Assoc. 1964;190(1):25–9.
14. Yildirim D, Hut A, Uzman S, Kocakusak A, Demiryas S, Cakir M, et al. Spinal anesthesia is safe in laparoscopic total extraperitoneal inguinal hernia repair. A retrospective clinical trial. Wideochir Inne Tech Maloinwazyjne. 2017;12(4):417–27.
15. Ozgun H, Meryem N, Ibrahim K, Mehmet H. Comparison of local, spinal, and general anesthesia for inguinal herniorrhaphy. Eur J Surg. 2002;168:455–9.
16. Pere P, Harju J, Kairaluoma P, Remes V, Turunen P, Rosenberg P. Randomized comparison of the feasibility of three anesthetic techniques for day-case open inguinal hernia repair. J Clin Anesth. 2016;34:166–75.
17. Symeonidis D, Baloyiannis I, Koukoulis G, Pratsas K, Georgopoulou S, Efthymiou M, et al. Prospective non-randomized comparison of open versus laparoscopic transabdominal preperitoneal (TAPP) inguinal hernia repair under different anesthetic methods. Surg Today. 2014;44(5):906–13.
18. Behnia R, Hashemi F, Stryker S, Ujiki G, Poticha S. A comparison of general versus local anesthesia during inguinal herniorrhaphy. Surg Gynecol Obstet. 1992;174(4):277–80.
19. Roberge C, Mcewen M. The effects of local anesthetics on postoperative pain. AORN J. 1998;68(6):1003–12.
20. Asuri K, Misra M, Virinder Kumar B, Subodh K, Rajeshwari S, Anjolie C. Laparoscopic inguinal hernia repair: transabdominal preperitoneal (TAPP) versus totally extraperitoneal (TEP) approach: a prospective randomized controlled trial. Surg Endosc. 2012;26(3):639–49.
21. Hernia Surge Group. International guidelines for groin hernia management. Hernia. 2018;22(1):1–165.
22. Reiner M, Bresnahan E. Laparoscopic total extraperitoneal hernia repair outcomes. JSLS. 2016;20(3):e2016.00043.
23. Myles P, Williams D, Hendrata M, Anderson H, Weeks A. Patient satisfaction after anaesthesia and surgery: results of a prospective survey of 10,811 patients. Br J Anaesth. 2000;84(1):6–10.
24. Sood J, Kumra V. Anesthesia for laparoscopic surgery. IJS. 2003;65:232–40.
25. Malins A, Field J, Nesling P, Cooper G. Nausea and vomiting after gynaecological laparoscopy: comparison of premedication with oral ondansetron, metoclopramide and placebo. Br J Anaesth. 1994;72(2):231–3.
26. Bay-Nielsen M, Kehlet H. Anaesthesia and post-operative morbidity after elective groin hernia repair: a nation-wide study. Acta Anaesthesiol Scand. 2008;52(2):169–74.

13

Effect of ancillary drugs on sevoflurane related emergence agitation in children undergoing ophthalmic surgery

Dan Tan[1*], Haifa Xia[2], Shujun Sun[2] and Fuquan Wang[2]

Abstract

Background: The comparative efficacy of ancillary drugs on sevoflurane related emergence agitation (EA) in children undergoing ophthalmic surgery remains controversial.

Methods: The databases were retrieved in an orderly manner from the dates of their establishment to October, 2018, including PubMed, The Cochrane Library and Web of Science, to collect randomized controlled trials (RCT) of different anesthetic drugs combined with sevoflurane for ophthalmic surgery. Then a network meta-analysis was conducted using R and Stata 12.0 softwares.

Results: The meta-analysis showed that, in reducing sevoflurane related EA, dexmedetomidine, ketamine, propofol, fentanyl, midazolam, sufentanil, remifentanil and clonidine were superior to placebo ($P < 0.05$). The network meta-analysis showed that the effects of ancillary drugs combine with sevoflurane in reducing risk of EA in children undergoing ophthalmic surgery was superior to placebo: dexmedetomidine (OR = 0.17, 95% CrI 0.12–0.22), ketamine (OR = 0.30, 95% CrI 0.11–0.49), propofol (OR = 0.24, 95% CrI 0.09–0.63), fentanyl (OR = 0.16, 95% CrI 0.08–0.56), midazolam (OR = 0.20, 95% CrI 0.09–0.40), sufentanil (OR = 0.27, 95% CrI 0.14–0.41), remifentanil (OR = 0.18, 95% CrI 0.08–0.54) and clonidine (OR = 0.14, 95% CrI 0.07–0.41). The SUCRA of placebo, dexmedetomidine, ketamine, propofol, fentanyl, midazolam, sufentanil, remifentanil, clonidine were respectively 0.26, 77.93, 27.71, 42.8, 69.43, 52.89, 59.83, 57.62 and 61.53%.

Conclusions: The effects of dexmedetomidine combine with sevoflurane in reducing risk of emergence agitation in children undergoing ophthalmic surgery was superior to other drugs.

Keywords: Ophthalmic surgery, Emergence agitation, Anesthetic drugs, Network meta-analysis, Randomized control trial

Background

Ophthalmic surgery is one of the common operations in children [1]. In ophthalmic surgery, especially in children's ophthalmology, the operation time is short, and the patient's self-control ability is weak, so the quality of anesthesia is required to be high [2]. It is a necessary condition for the operation to effectively inhibit the stress response and oculocardiac reflex caused by the operation under the anesthesia. Moreover, children may experience severe adverse events during the course of anesthesia, for instance, cardiac arrest, bronchial hyper-reactivity, upper respiratory tract infection, and obstructive sleep apnea. Therefore, the selection of appropriate anesthetic inducing drugs is of great significance for the implementation of the operation [3, 4].

Sevoflurane is the most commonly used inhalation anesthetic in pediatric anesthesia [5]. It has the characteristics of fast induction, rapid clearance, rapid awakening and easy adjustment of anesthesia depth. In addition, the drug has little effect on heart rate, airway stimulation is also very small, can achieve the role of relaxation of

* Correspondence: tandan_dta@163.com
[1]Editorial Office, Journal of New Medicine, Zhongnan Hospital of Wuhan University, No.169 Donghu Road, Wuchang District, Wuhan 430071, Hubei Province, China

smooth muscle [6]. However, when it is used as the only anesthetic, it is associated with a high incidence of emergence agitation (EA) and may be harmful to patients [7–9]. Anesthetic adjuvants such as metomidine, ketamine, propofol, fentanyl, midazolam, sufentanil, remifentanil, clonidine and other drugs have been effectively used to prevent EA. However, these drugs may increase the sedative effect after anesthesia, leading to slow awakening and, in some cases, adverse side effects, such as nausea and vomiting [10, 11]. Studies have shown that the combination of anesthetic adjuvant and sevoflurane can produce synergistic effect, not only maintain good anesthetic effect, rapid recovery after operation, but also do not cause respiratory inhibition. It can maintain the analgesic effect for a long time after operation, and effectively reduce the EA, crying and other adverse reactions in children [12].

In this study, we tried to investigate eight adjuvant drugs in combination with sevoflurane in children undergoing ophthalmic surgery. We use a Bayesian network to determine which adjuvant drugs combine with sevoflurane can affect the incidence of EA in children undergoing ophthalmic surgery.

Methods and analysis

Eligibility criteria

Eligibility criteria will be designed according to the PICOS (Participant-Intervention-Comparator-Outcome-Study design) framework.

Selection of studies

We will include studies assessing the effect of different anesthetic drugs combined with sevoflurane for ophthalmic surgery.

Study design

We only include randomized controlled trials.

Participants

We will include patients with undergoing ophthalmic surgery and those receiving sevoflurane under 0 and 18 years.

Interventions

The control group was given an anesthetic adjuvant or placebo, and the experimental group was given an anesthetic adjuvant.

Outcome measurements

Contains the main outcome indicator is number of patients with EA. EA is known as emergence delirium which is often accompanied with revival after pediatric anesthesia.

Search strategy

By using the combination of subject words and free words, the databases were retrieved in an orderly manner from the dates of their establishment to October, 2018, including PubMed, The Cochrane Library and Web of Science, with keywords including "Ophthalmic

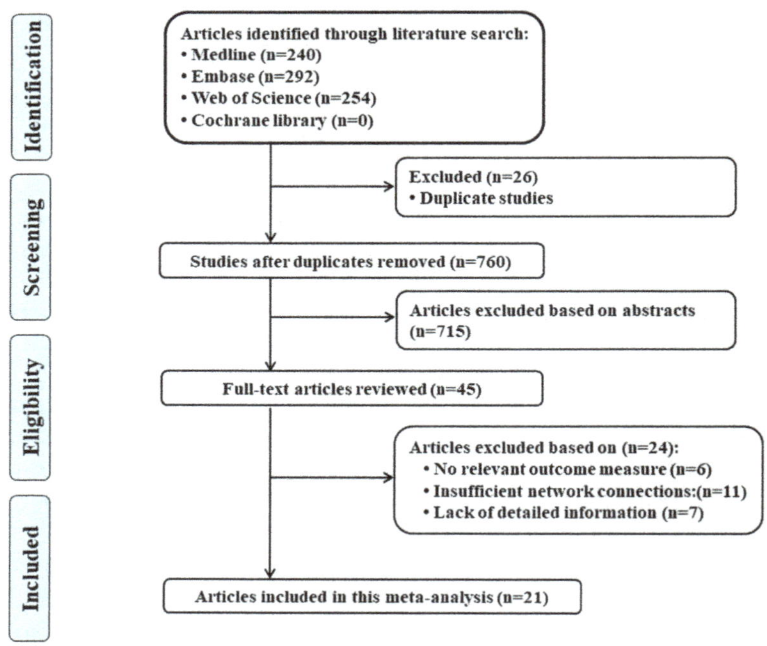

Fig. 1 Flow diagram of the study selection process

surgery" [MeSH] OR "Eye surgery" [MeSH] AND "Anesthetic Drugs" [MeSH] OR "Anesthetic Agents" [MeSH] OR "Anesthetic Effect" [MeSH] OR "Dexmedetomidine" [MeSH] OR "Ketamine" [MeSH] OR "Propofol" [MeSH] OR "Fentanyl" [MeSH] OR "Midazolam" [MeSH] OR "Sufentanil" [MeSH] OR "Remifentanil" [MeSH] OR "Clonidine" [MeSH] AND "sevoflurane" [MeSH] AND "Randomized Controlled Trial" [MeSH] OR "RCT" [MeSH].

Data extraction

According to the inclusion criteria, the titles and abstracts of the literature were screened by two researchers independently of each other, and the unrelated literature was eliminated. Then through reading the full text, exclude the literature that does not accord with this research scheme, and record the reasons and quantity of exclusion. Finally, the selected literature was cross-checked by two researchers. Using Excel 2013 Software design data extraction table to extract the key information in the literature after the inclusion of the literature.

Risk of bias assessment

The quality of included literature was evaluated by Cochrane collaboration network evaluation risk tool. The quality of literature was evaluated according to random method, distribution concealment, blind method, incomplete outcome data, selective outcome report and other biased sources.

Statistical analysis

Stata 12.0 software was used for statistical analysis. χ^2 test was used to analyze the heterogeneity among the studies, and I^2 was used for quantitative analysis. If $I^2 < 50\%$, it indicated that there was homogeneity among the studies, which could be directly combined and analyzed by fixed effect model. If $I^2 \geq 50\%$, the heterogeneity of each study is indicated, and the random effect model is used for statistical analysis [13]. The biggest difference between the network meta analysis and the traditional Meta analysis is that it can compare multiple intervention measures at the same time. The two interventions which do not have direct comparison are indirectly compared and quantitatively analyzed through the mesh relationship, and the best scheme is obtained according to the advantages and disadvantages of the outcome index. Bayesian network model based on Markov chain Monte Carlo operation for analyzing the therapeutic effects of drugs in two groups and multiple groups. All the included drugs were sorted using the surface under the cumulative ranking (SUCRA) to determine the pros and cons of the drug treatment on sevoflurane related EA in children undergoing ophthalmic surgery. The larger the

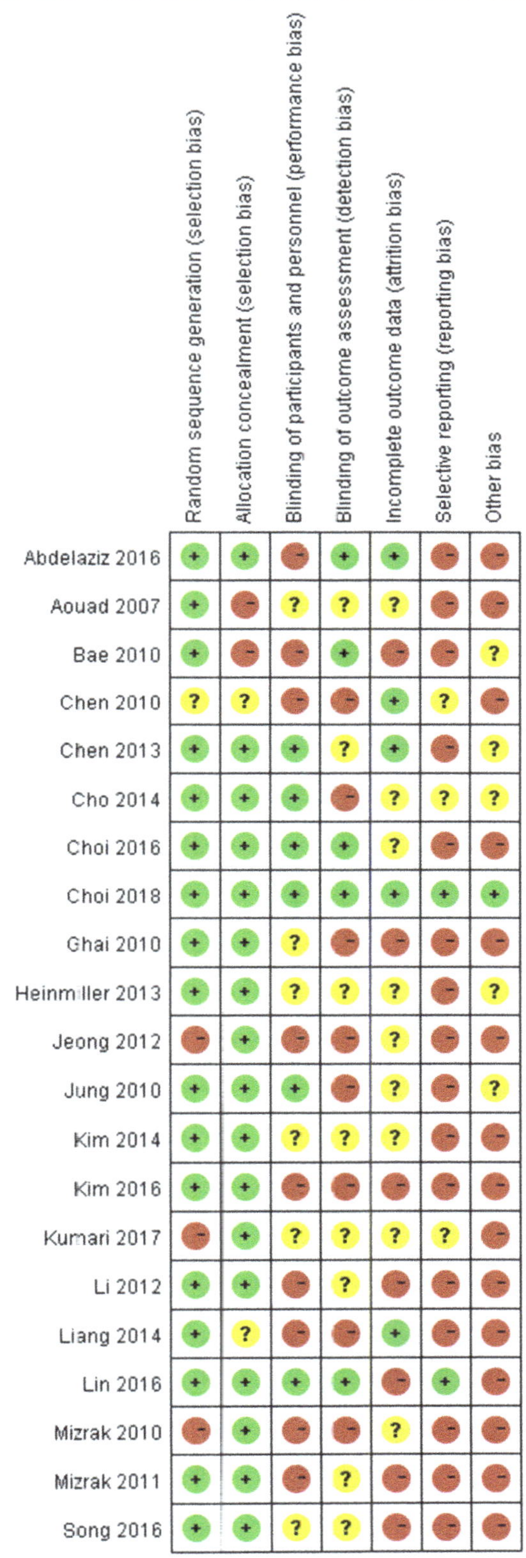

Fig. 2 Risk of bias of the included RCTs (Review authors' judgments about each risk of bias item for each included study. +, low risk; –, high risk;?, unclear risk)

Table 1 Characteristics of included studies

Author	Year	Treatments											
		Treatments 1	Age (year)	Male (%)	Cases /n	Treatments 2	Age (year)	Male (%)	Cases /n	Treatments 3	Age (year)	Male (%)	Cases /n
Aouad et al	2007	Propofol	4.2 ± 1.4	46	8/41	Placebo	4.3 ± 1.3	58	17/36				
Bae et al	2010	Midazolam	4.9 ± 1.6	53	2/15	Placebo	4.1 ± 1.4	47	19/45				
Chen et al	2010	Midazolam	3.6 ± 1.9	–	5/40	Propofol	3.7 ± 1.7	–	8/40	Ketamine	3.8 ± 2.0	–	15/40
Chen et al	2013	Dexmedetomidine	4.1 ± 1.3	63	3/28	Ketamine	4.2 ± 1.2	67	6/28	Placebo	4.3 ± 1.1	62	11/28
Cho et al	2014	Midazolam	8.0 ± 2.1	33	10/60	Placebo	8.0 ± 2.1	30	13/30				
Choi et al	2018	Remifentanil	6.0 ± 1.1	44	2/39	Placebo	5.6 ± 1.1	49	14/41				
Choi et al	2016	Placebo	6.1 ± 2.3	48	21/33	Remifentanil	6.2 ± 2.0	50	11/34				
Jeong et al	2012	Placebo	4.8 ± 0.4	55	15/20	Ketamine	5.0 ± 0.4	50	10/40				
Jung et al	2010	Ketamine	5.4 ± 1.9	48	4/23	Fentanyl	7.5 ± 2.0	33	0/24				
Kim et al	2014	Dexmedetomidine	4.3 ± 1.4	38	7/47	Placebo	4.3 ± 1.0	55	33/47				
Kim et al	2016	Midazolam	4.1 ± 1.4	47	15/34	Ketamine	4.2 ± 1.3	48	11/33				
Liang et al	2014	Sufentanil	5.1 ± 1.3	57	9/30	Fentanyl	4.8 ± 1.3	47	11/30	Placebo	5.5 ± 1.4	43	19/30
Li et al	2012	Dexmedetomidine	5.0 ± 2.0	53	3/30	Placebo	4.0 ± 1.0	57	13/30				
Lin et al	2016	Dexmedetomidine	4.7 ± 1.9	60	10/60	Placebo	4.1 ± 1.6	50	24/30				
Mizrak et al	2010	Ketamine	7.7 ± 3.1	37	5/30	Propofol	6.9 ± 3.0	40	5/30				
Mizrak et al	2011	Dexmedetomidine	8.5 ± 2.6	50	6/30	Placebo	8.6 ± 2.8	43	16/30				
Song et al	2016	Dexmedetomidine	4.3 ± 1.7	50	6/28	Placebo	3.8 ± 1.5	50	17/28				
Abdelaziz et al	2016	Dexmedetomidine	2.7 ± 1.5	52	4/35	Midazolam	2.5 ± 1.2	52	7/35	Placebo	2.8 ± 1.7	56	15/35
Kumari et al	2017	Dexmedetomidine	7.9 ± 3.2	57	3/30	Clonidine	7.5 ± 2.9	63	1/30	Midazolam	6.6 ± 2.8	60	0/30
Heinmiller et al	2013	Clonidine	4.3 ± 1.5	40	6/25	Placebo	4.1 ± 1.3	48	15/25				
Ghai et al	2010	Clonidine	3.4 ± 1.5	62	3/39	Placebo	3.0 ± 1.4	60	16/40				

SUCRA, the better the effect. Bayesian network analysis using R software.

Results

Literature search results

A total of 240 studies from Medline, 292 studies from Embase and 254 studies from Web of Science. After removing duplicates study, 760 studies were identifed. After reviewing their titles and abstracts, 715 citations were excluded. The remaining 45 citations were assessed in more detail for eligibility by reading the full text. Among them, 6 studies were excluded due to no relevant outcome measure; 11 studies were excluded due to insufficient network connections; 7 study was excluded due to lack of detailed information. Finally, 21 studies were used for the final data synthesis [14–34]. The flow chart of literature searching was presented in Fig. 1. Figure 2 showed the risk of bias of 21 studies included in this meta-analysis. The characteristics of the included studies are shown in the Table 1. Figure 3 showed the pattern of evidence within the network is displayed.

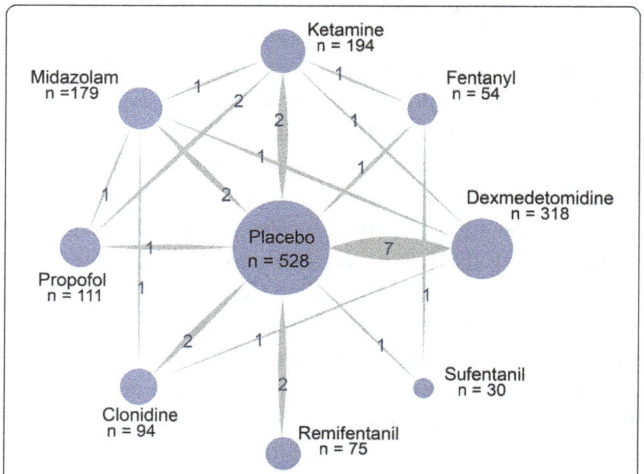

Fig. 3 Network of randomized controlled trials comparing different adjuvant therapies for EA in ophthalmic surgery. The thickness of the connecting lines represents the number of trials between each comparator, and the size of each node corresponds to the number of subjects who received the same pharmacological agent (sample size)

Results of pairwise meta-analysis

Table 2 displayed the results produced by pairwise meta-analysis. The effects of ancillary drugs combine with sevoflurane in reducing risk of EA in children undergoing ophthalmic surgery was superior to placebo: dexmedetomidine(OR = 0.26, 95% CrI 0.17–0.39), ketamine (OR = 0.41, 95% CrI 0.20–0.86), propofol (OR = 0.39, 95% CrI 0.18–0.83), fentanyl (OR = 0.56, 95% CrI 0.29–0.89), midazolam (OR = 0.40, 95% CrI 0.21–0.75), sufentanil (OR = 0.47, 95% CrI 0.38–0.58), remifentanil (OR = 0.35, 95% CrI 0.17–0.73) and clonidine (OR = 0.29, 95% CrI 0.13–0.66).

Network meta-analysis

Table 3 displayed the results produced by network meta-analysis. The effects of ancillary drugs combine with sevoflurane in reducing risk of EA in children undergoing ophthalmic surgery was superior to placebo: dexmedetomidine(OR = 0.17, 95% CrI 0.12–0.22), ketamine (OR = 0.30, 95% CrI 0.11–0.49), propofol (OR = 0.24, 95% CrI 0.09–0.63), fentanyl (OR = 0.16, 95% CrI 0.08–0.56), midazolam (OR = 0.20, 95% CrI 0.09–0.40), sufentanil (OR = 0.27, 95% CrI 0.14–0.41), remifentanil (OR = 0.18, 95% CrI 0.08–0.54) and clonidine (OR = 0.14, 95% CrI 0.07–0.41)(Fig. 4).

The corresponding results of SUCRA values are presented in Fig. 5. The SUCRA of placebo, dexmedetomidine, ketamine, propofol, fentanyl, midazolam, sufentanil, remifentanil, clonidine were respectively 0.26, 77.93, 27.71, 42.8, 69.43, 52.89, 59.83, 57.62 and 61.53%. The effects of dexmedetomidine combine with sevoflurane in reducing risk of emergence agitation in children undergoing ophthalmic surgery was superior to other drugs.

Consistency, publication bias of included studies

One of the main assumptions of the network meta-analysis is the consistency between direct evidence and indirect evidence. The degree of indirect evidence is consistent with direct evidence by the node splitting method. The evidence in the network seems to be consistent with most comparisons ($P > 0.05$)(Fig. 6). All data points are evenly distributed on both sides of the inverted funnel plot, suggesting that there is less likelihood of publication bias (Fig. 7).

Discussion

The anesthetics used in pediatric ophthalmic surgery can meet the requirements of fast effect, stable effect, quick awakening, easy adjustment, small stimulation and low incidence of complications [35, 36]. Although sevoflurane is the most commonly used inhaled anesthetic in pediatric anesthesia and it has incomparable advantages over other anesthetic in the induction period of pediatric surgical anesthesia, sevoflurane alone can lead to high risk of EA. EA during awakening refers to a state of mind in which consciousness and behavior are separated from the awakening of general anesthesia, manifested as inability to appease and irritability. The incidence of EA

Table 2 Summary odds ratios of emergence agitation and heterogeneity for each direct comparison

Comparison	OR (95% CI)	P-heterogeneity	I-squared	Tau-squared
Dexmedetomidine vs. Placebo	*0.26 (0.17, 0.39)*	0.697	0.0%	< 0.001
Ketamine vs. Placebo	*0.41 (0.20, 0.86)*	0.514	0.0%	0.018
Propofol vs. Placebo	*0.39 (0.18, 0.83)*	–	–	< 0.001
Fentanyl vs. Placebo	*0.56 (0.29, 0.89)*	–	–	< 0.001
Midazolam vs. Placebo	*0.40 (0.21, 0.75)*	0.912	0.0%	0.004
Sufentanil vs. Placebo	*0.47 (0.38, 0.58)*	–	–	< 0.001
Remifentanil vs. Placebo	*0.35 (0.17, 0.73)*	0.173	46.1%	0.005
Clonidine vs. Placebo	*0.29 (0.13, 0.66)*	0.399	0.0%	0.003
Ketamine vs. Dexmedetomidine	2.00 (0.46, 8.80)	–	–	0.359
Midazolam vs. Dexmedetomidine	0.97 (0.33, 2.83)	0.126	47.3%	0.851
Clonidine vs. Dexmedetomidine	0.33 (0.03, 3.39)	–	–	0.353
Propofol vs. Ketamine	0.66 (0.30, 1.43)	0.455	0.0%	0.292
Fentanyl vs. Ketamine	0.11 (0.05, 2.09)	–	–	0.140
Midazolam vs. Ketamine	0.73 (0.37, 1.43)	0.159	46.3%	0.360
Midazolam vs. Propofol	0.63 (0.19, 2.07)	–	–	0.443
Sufentanil vs. Fentanyl	0.82 (0.30, 2.26)	–	–	0.699
Clonidine vs. Midazolam	0.96 (0.17, 5.60)	–	–	0.506

P value less than 0.05 is considered as significance with italic fonts

Table 3 Network meta-analysis comparisons

	Placebo	Dexmedetomidine	Ketamine	Propofol	Fentanyl	Midazolam	Sufentanil	Remifentanil	Clonidine
Placebo	1	*5.89 (4.55, 8.33)*	*3.33 (2.04, 9.10)*	*4.20 (1.60, 11.0)*	*6.00 (1.70, 13.0)*	*5.00 (2.50, 11.0)*	*3.70 (2.43, 7.14)*	*5.60 (1.90, 13.0)*	*6.90 (2.50, 14.0)*
Dexmedetomidine	*0.17 (0.12, 0.22)*	1	0.43 (0.18, 1.10)	0.55 (0.18, 1.70)	0.77 (0.20, 4.00)	0.64 (0.28, 1.60)	0.77 (0.17, 4.50)	*0.37 (0.23, 0.53)*	0.88 (0.29, 3.10)
Ketamine	*0.30 (0.11, 0.49)*	2.30 (0.94, 5.80)	1	1.30 (0.50, 3.30)	1.80 (0.49, 9.00)	1.50 (0.70, 3.60)	1.80 (0.38, 11.0)	1.70 (0.45, 7.10)	2.10 (0.61, 8.10)
Propofol	*0.24 (0.09, 0.63)*	1.80 (0.59, 5.30)	0.78 (0.30, 2.20)	1	1.40 (0.31, 8.00)	1.20 (0.45, 3.40)	1.40 (0.26, 9.20)	1.30 (0.31, 6.20)	1.70 (0.42, 7.20)
Fentanyl	*0.16 (0.08, 0.56)*	1.30 (0.24, 4.90)	0.56 (0.11, 2.10)	0.69 (0.11, 3.10)	1	0.79 (0.16, 3.30)	0.98 (0.20, 4.30)	0.92 (0.14, 5.10)	1.10 (0.19, 5.80)
Midazolam	*0.20 (0.09, 0.40)*	1.60 (0.61, 3.50)	0.66 (0.28, 1.40)	0.84 (0.28, 2.30)	1.20 (0.30, 5.80)	1	1.20 (0.24, 6.70)	1.10 (0.29, 4.40)	1.40 (0.41, 4.90)
Sufentanil	*0.27 (0.14, 0.41)*	1.30 (0.23, 5.80)	0.56 (0.10, 2.70)	0.71 (0.10, 3.90)	1.00 (0.25, 4.90)	0.82 (0.15, 4.10)	1	0.95 (0.14, 6.10)	1.20 (0.18, 7.00)
Remifentanil	*0.18 (0.08, 0.54)*	*2.70 (1.20, 4.40)*	0.59 (0.14, 2.20)	0.76 (0.16, 3.30)	1.10 (0.20, 6.80)	0.89 (0.22, 3.40)	1.10 (0.17, 7.40)	1	1.20 (0.25, 5.80)
Clonidine	*0.14 (0.07, 0.41)*	1.10 (0.31, 3.40)	0.46 (0.12, 1.60)	0.61 (0.14, 2.40)	0.85 (0.17, 5.20)	0.70 (0.20, 2.40)	0.86 (0.14, 5.70)	0.80 (0.17, 3.80)	1

***P* value less than 0.05 is considered as significance with italic fonts**

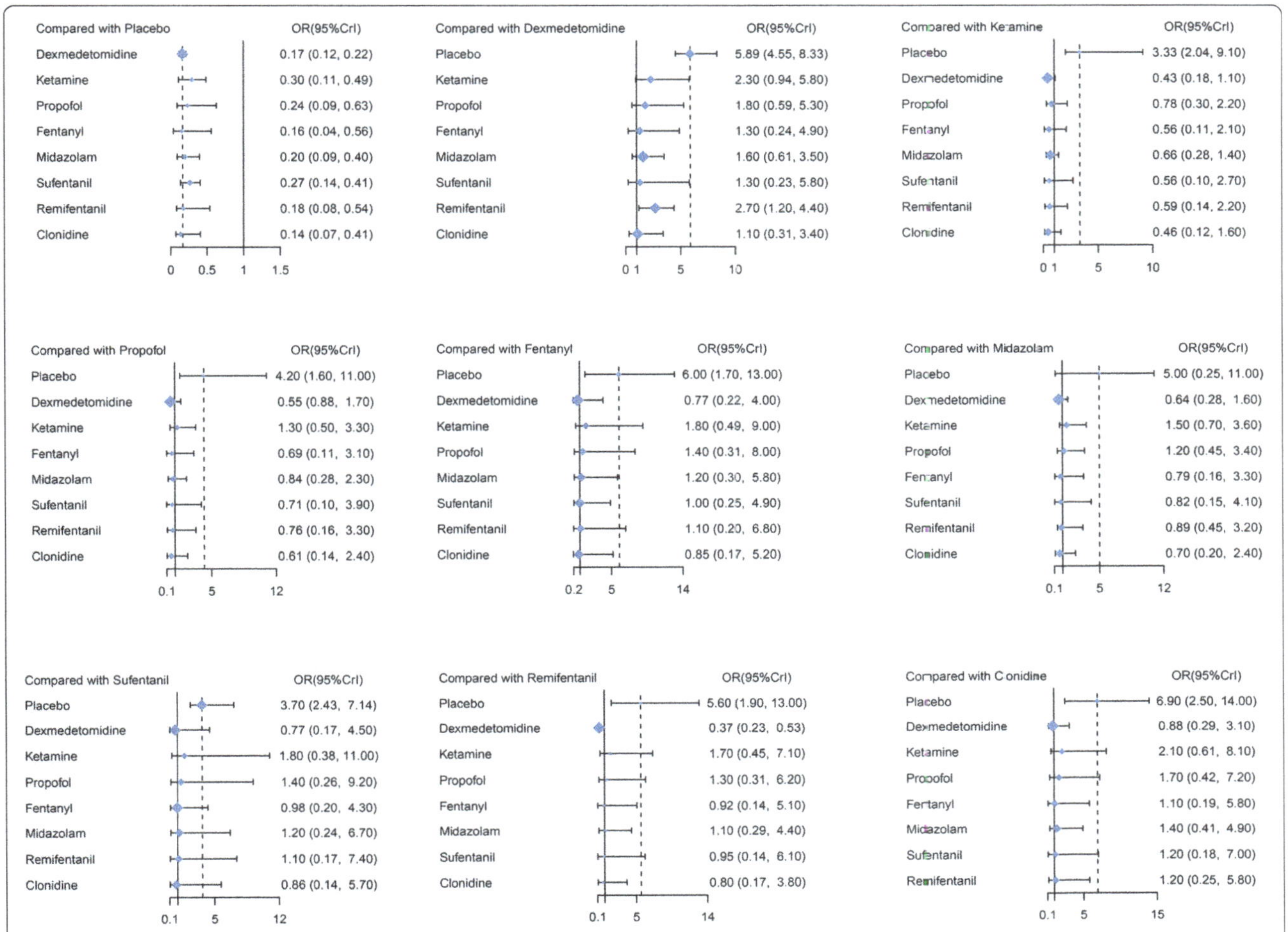

Fig. 4 Forest plots of odds ratios (95% creditable intervals) produced by network meta-analysis

in children undergoing ophthalmic surgery under anesthesia is high [37]. In clinical practice, other anesthetic adjuvants can be combined with sevoflurane to prevent EA. However, the results are contradictory.

This network meta-analysis attempted to explain the effectiveness of ancillary drugs employed in sevoflurane related emergence agitation in children undergoing ophthalmic surgery treatment. Our analysis suggests that the effects of dexmedetomidine on sevoflurane related emergence agitation in children undergoing ophthalmic surgery were superior to other drugs, and fentanyl was close behind. Dexmetomidine is a novel, highly selective α2 adrenergic receptor agonist, which acts on α2 adrenergic receptor and inhibits sympathetic nerve activity [38]. It can produce sedative and analgesic effects, reduce the dose of anesthetics, maintain hemodynamic stability, no respiratory inhibition, postoperative amnesia, anti-vomiting and diuretic effects [39]. Dexmedetomidine has been widely used and recognized in ICU sedation and general anesthesia because of its fast absorption, fast effect, complete metabolism [40, 41]. As a highly selective central α2 adrenergic receptor agonist, dexmedetomidine was sedative and analgesic effects and can produce synergistic effects with anesthetics and analgesics.

Dexmetomidine is a new choice of anesthetic auxiliary drugs, which provides effective sedation for ophthalmic surgery anesthesia patients, and can provide a certain degree of analgesic effect. At the same time, it has the effect of compliance amnesia, especially in sober sedation, it has no respiratory inhibition and less side effect which makes it show its unique superiority and application value in clinical anesthesia practice. Existing studies have confirmed that the sedative, hypnotic and anti-anxiety effects of dexmetomidine are dose-dependent [42]. Therefore, the application of dexmetomidine in ophthalmic anesthesia surgery has the following advantages: 1) to provide patients with satisfactory and comfortable sedation without reducing the degree of cooperation of intraoperative patients; 2) it can increase the tolerance

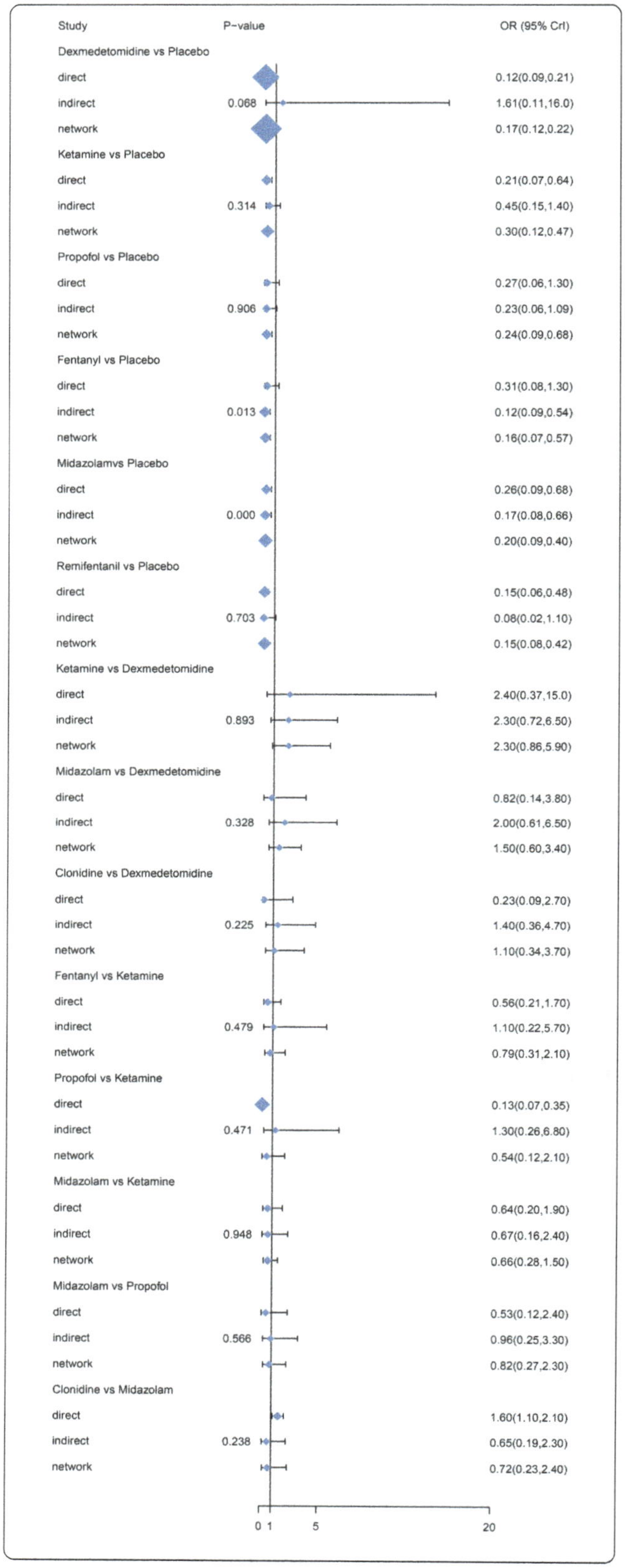

Fig. 5 Surface under the Cumulative Ranking Curve (SUCRA), expressed as percentages, ranking the therapeutic effects and safety of treatments for EA in ophthalmic surgery. For efcacy and safety assessment, the pharmacological agent with the highest SUCRA value would be the most efcacious and safe treatment

of ophthalmic anesthesia patients to pain; 3) can maintain the stability of hemodynamics and reduce the degree of stress in intraoperative patients; 4) can eliminate the bad memory of ophthalmic local anesthesia patients with anesthesia and surgical operation, etc. It has a certain anterograde amnesia effect; 5) no increase in the incidence of postoperative adverse reactions.

Fentanyl is a classical opioid anesthetic with strong fat solubility, which can maintain the drug effect near 30 min after a single administration, and the blood concentration can show the second peak at 20~90 min [43]. Fentanyl can maintain analgesic effect for a long time after operation. These characteristics meet the clinical anesthesia needs of short operation time, no savings and rapid recovery after ophthalmic surgery in children. Studies have shown that the combination of fentanyl and sevoflurane in the anesthesia induction stage can produce synergistic effect and effectively improve the analgesic and sedative effect [44]. Therefore, the application of fentanyl in the induction stage of anesthesia combined with sevoflurane to maintain intraoperative anesthesia can give full play to the advantages of the two drugs, not only to maintain a good anesthetic effect, but also to recover quickly after operation. The drug has less savings in the body, and the use of fentanyl to induce a single low dose of the drug will not cause respiratory inhibition, and can maintain a longer postoperative analgesic effect, in order to alleviate the pain caused by the regression of sevoflurane during the recovery period [45]. It can effectively reduce the restlessness, crying and other adverse reactions in children. In this sudy, we found fentanyl combine with sevoflurane also can effectively reduce risk of emergence agitation in children undergoing ophthalmic surgery [46].

There are some limitations in this study. First of all, different doses included in the literature, different administration schemes, and different age of the patients resulted in clinical heterogeneity. Secondly, we only evaluated the incidence of EA, while the incidence of postoperative nausea and vomiting and other adverse reactions (such as dizziness, chills) could not be analyzed due to the lack of relevant data. Finally, the quality and quantity of the literature included are on the low side, which leads to the decrease of the test efficiency of the results of this study, the small sample size of the interventions included in the study, and the possible shortage of statistical efficiency may be insufficient. Based on the shortcomings of the existing research, clinicians should

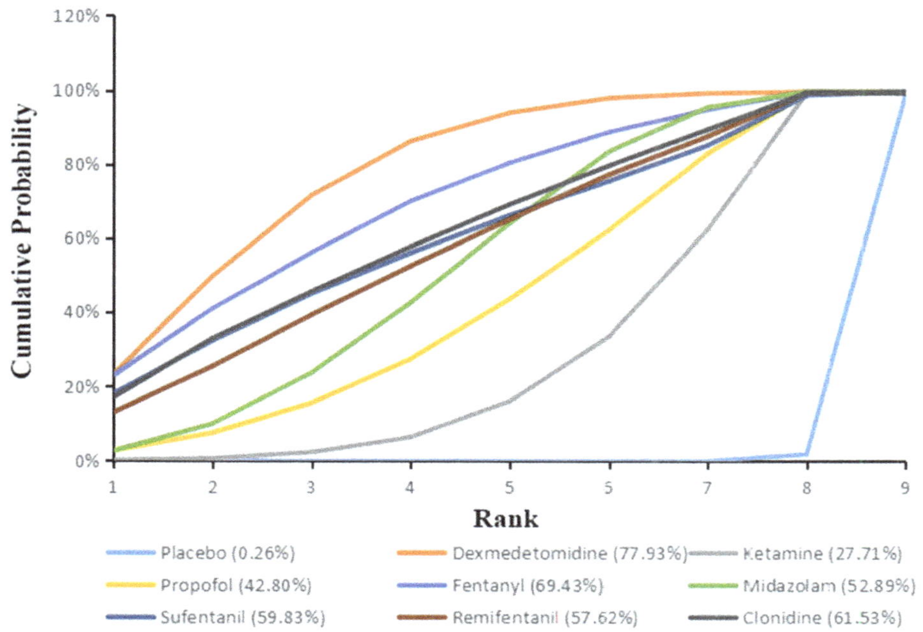

Fig. 6 Node splitting results for each comparison

consider the influence of the above factors and choose carefully when applying the conclusions of this study.

Conclusion

In summary, based on this study, the results of network meta analysis showed that dexmedetomidine, ketamine, propofol, fentanyl, midazolam, sufentanil, remifentanil or clonidine combine with sevoflurane also can effectively reduce risk of emergence agitation in children undergoing ophthalmic surgery compare wirh placebo. The effects of dexmedetomidine combine with sevoflurane in reducing risk of emergence agitation in children undergoing ophthalmic surgery was superior to other drugs.

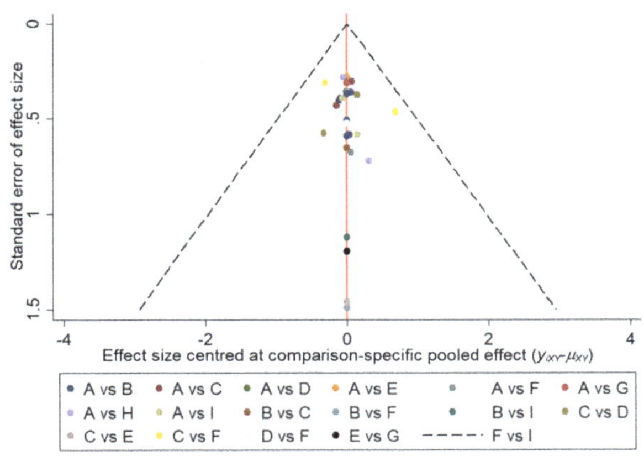

Fig. 7 Comparison-adjusted funnel plot for the network meta-analysis. The red line suggests the null hypothesis that the study-specifc effect sizes do not differ from the respective comparison-specifc pooled effect estimates. Different colors represent different comparisons

Abbreviations

EA: Emergence agitation; RCT: Randomized controlled trials; SUCRA: Surface under the cumulative ranking

Acknowledgements

Not applicable

Authors' contributions

Substantial contributions to conception and design: DT. Data acquisition, data analysis and interpretation: HX, SS. Drafting the article or critically revising it for important intellectual content: DT, FW. Final approval of the version to be published: All authors. Agreement to be accountable for all aspects of the work in ensuring that questions related to the accuracy or integrity of the work are appropriately investigated and resolved: All authors.

Author details

[1]Editorial Office, Journal of New Medicine, Zhongnan Hospital of Wuhan University, No.169 Donghu Road, Wuchang District, Wuhan 430071, Hubei Province, China. [2]Department of Anesthesiology, Institute of Anesthesia and Critical Care, Union Hospital, Tongji Medical College, Huazhong University of Science and Technology, Wuhan, China.

References

1. de Sa L, Hoyt CS, Good WV. Complications of pediatric ophthalmic surgery. Int Ophthalmol Clin. 1992;32(4):31–9.
2. Daoud YJ, Hutchinson A, Wallace DK, Song J, Kim T. Refractive surgery in children: treatment options, outcomes, and controversies. Am J Ophthalmol. 2009;147(4):573–582.e572.

3. Khanna P, Ray BR, Govindrajan SR, Sinha R, Chandralekha TP. Anesthetic management of pediatric patients with Sturge-Weber syndrome: our experience and a review of the literature. J Anesth. 2015;29(6):857–61.
4. Gayer S, Tutiven J. Anesthesia for pediatric ocular surgery. Ophthalmol Clin N Am. 2006;19(2):269–78.
5. Sakai EM, Connolly LA, Klauck JA. Inhalation anesthesiology and volatile liquid anesthetics: focus on isoflurane, desflurane, and sevoflurane. Pharmacotherapy. 2005;25(12):1773–88.
6. Cravero J, Surgenor S, Whalen K. Emergence agitation in paediatric patients after sevoflurane anaesthesia and no surgery: a comparison with halothane. Paediatr Anaesth. 2000;10(4):419–24.
7. Dahmani S, Stany I, Brasher C, Lejeune C, Bruneau B, Wood C, Nivoche Y, Constant I, Murat IJBJA. Pharmacological prevention of sevoflurane- and desflurane-related emergence agitation in children: a meta-analysis of published. studies. 2010;104(2):216–23.
8. Kulka P, Bressem M, Tryba MJAA: Clonidine prevents sevoflurane-induced agitation in children. 2001, 93(2):335–338, 332nd contents page.
9. Park JH, Lim BG, Kim HZ, Kong MH, Lim SH, Kim NS, Lee IO. Comparison of emergence agitation between sevoflurane/nitrous oxide administration and sevoflurane administration alone in children undergoing adenotonsillectomy with preemptive ketorolac. Korean J Anesthesiol. 2014; 66(1):34–8.
10. Lodes U. Total intravenous anesthesia (TIVA) and balanced anesthesia with short-acting anesthetics for ENT surgery in children. Anaesthesiol Reanim. 1999;24(1):13–8.
11. Maze M, Tranquilli W. Alpha-2 adrenoceptor agonists: defining the role in clinical anesthesia. Anesthesiology. 1991;74(3):581–605.
12. Lysakowski C, Dumont L, Pellegrini M, Clergue F, Tassonyi E. Effects of fentanyl, alfentanil, remifentanil and sufentanil on loss of consciousness and bispectral index during propofol induction of anaesthesia. Br J Anaesth. 2001;86(4):523–7.
13. Higgins JP, Thompson SG, Deeks JJ, Altman DG. Measuring inconsistency in meta-analyses. Bmj. 2003;327(7414):557–60.
14. Ghai B, Ram J, Chauhan S, Wig J. Effects of clonidine on recovery after sevoflurane anaesthesia in children undergoing cataract surgery. Anaesth Intensive Care. 2010;38(3):530–7.
15. Aouad MT, Yazbeck-Karam VG, Nasr VG, El-Khatib MF, Kanazi GE, Bleik JH. A single dose of propofol at the end of surgery for the prevention of emergence agitation in children undergoing strabismus surgery during sevoflurane anesthesia. Anesthesiology. 2007;107(5):733–8.
16. Bae JH, Koo BW, Kim SJ, Lee DH, Lee ET, Kang CJ. The effects of midazolam administered postoperatively on emergence agitation in pediatric strabismus surgery. Korean J Anesthesiol. 2010;58(1):45–9.
17. Chen J, Li W, Hu X, Wang D. Emergence agitation after cataract surgery in children: a comparison of midazolam, propofol and ketamine. Paediatr Anaesth. 2010;20(9):873–9.
18. Chen JY, Jia JE, Liu TJ, Qin MJ, Li WX. Comparison of the effects of dexmedetomidine, ketamine, and placebo on emergence agitation after strabismus surgery in children. Can J Anaesth. 2013;60(4):385–92.
19. Cho EJ, Yoon SZ, Cho JE, Lee HW. Comparison of the effects of 0.03 and 0. 05 mg/kg midazolam with placebo on prevention of emergence agitation in children having strabismus surgery. Anesthesiology. 2014;120(6):1354–61.
20. Choi EK, Lee S, Kim WJ, Park SJ. Effects of remifentanil maintenance during recovery on emergence delirium in children with sevoflurane anesthesia. Paediatr Anaesth. 2018;28(8):739–44.
21. Choi YH, Kim KM, Lee SK, Kim YS, Kim SJ, Hwang WS, Chung JH. Effects of remifentanil and remifentanil-alfentanil administration on emergence agitation after brief ophthalmic surgery in children. BMC Anesthesiol. 2016;16(1):50.
22. Jeong WJ, Kim WY, Moon MG, Min DJ, Lee YS, Kim JH, Park YC. The effect of ketamine on the separation anxiety and emergence agitation in children undergoing brief ophthalmic surgery under desflurane general anesthesia. Korean J Anesthesiol. 2012;63(3):203–8.
23. Jung HJ, Kim JB, Im KS, Oh SH, Lee JM. Effect of ketamine versus thiopental sodium anesthetic induction and a small dose of fentanyl on emergence agitation after sevoflurane anesthesia in children undergoing brief ophthalmic surgery. Korean J Anesthesiol. 2010;58(2):148–52.
24. Kim J, Kim SY, Lee JH, Kang YR, Koo BN. Low-dose dexmedetomidine reduces emergence agitation after desflurane anaesthesia in children undergoing strabismus surgery. Yonsei Med J. 2014;55(2):508–16.
25. Kim KM, Lee KH, Kim YH, Ko MJ, Jung JW, Kang E. Comparison of effects of intravenous midazolam and ketamine on emergence agitation in children: randomized controlled trial. J Int Med Res. 2016;44(2):258–66.
26. Kumari S, Agrawal N, Usha G, Talwar V, Gupta P. Comparison of Oral clonidine, Oral Dexmedetomidine, and Oral midazolam for premedication in pediatric patients undergoing elective surgery. Anesth Essays Res. 2017; 11(1):185–91.
27. Liang P, Zhou C, Ni J, Luo Z, Liu B. Single-dose sufentanil or fentanyl reduces agitation after sevoflurane anesthesia in children undergoing ophthalmology surgery. Pak J Med Sci. 2014;30(5):1059–63.
28. Lili X, Jianjun S, Haiyan Z. The application of dexmedetomidine in children undergoing vitreoretinal surgery. J Anesth. 2012;26(4):556–61.
29. Lin Y, Chen Y, Huang J, Chen H, Shen W, Guo W, Chen Q, Ling H, Gan X. Efficacy of premedication with intranasal dexmedetomidine on inhalational induction and postoperative emergence agitation in pediatric undergoing cataract surgery with sevoflurane. J Clin Anesth. 2016;33:289–95.
30. Mizrak A, Erbagci I, Arici T, Ozcan I, Ganidagli S, Tatar G, Oner U. Ketamine versus propofol for strabismus surgery in children. Clin Ophthalmol. 2010;4:673–9.
31. Mizrak A, Erbagci I, Arici T, Avci N, Ganidagli S, Oner U. Dexmedetomidine use during strabismus surgery in agitated children. Med Princ Pract. 2011; 20(5):427–32.
32. Song IA, Seo KS, Oh AY, Baik JS, Kim JH, Hwang JW, Jeon YT. Dexmedetomidine injection during strabismus surgery reduces emergence agitation without increasing the Oculocardiac reflex in children: a randomized controlled trial. PLoS One. 2016;11(9):e0162785.
33. Jain S, Sethi S, Ghai B, Ram J. Effect of dexmedetomidine on emergence agitation using desflurane in pediatric cataract surgery. Saudi J Anaesth. 2018;12(1):28–34.
34. Heinmiller LJ, Nelson LB, Goldberg MB, Thode AR. Clonidine premedication versus placebo: effects on postoperative agitation and recovery time in children undergoing strabismus surgery. J Pediatr Ophthalmol Strabismus. 2013;50(3):150–4.
35. Khokhar SK, Pillay G, Dhull C, Agarwal E, Mahabir M, Aggarwal P. Pediatric cataract. Indian J Ophthalmol. 2017;65(12):1340–9.
36. Ducloyer JB, Couret C, Magne C, Lejus-Bourdeau C, Weber M, Le Meur G, Lebranchu P. Prospective evaluation of anesthetic protocols during pediatric ophthalmic surgery. Eur J Ophthalmol. 2018; 1120672118804798.
37. Kanaya A. Emergence agitation in children: risk factors, prevention, and treatment. J Anesth. 2016;30(2):261–7.
38. Weerink MAS, Struys M, Hannivoort LN, Barends CRM, Absalom AR, Colin P. Clinical pharmacokinetics and pharmacodynamics of Dexmedetomidine. Clin Pharmacokinet. 2017;56(8):893–913.
39. Mahmoud M, Mason KP. Dexmedetomidine: review, update, and future considerations of paediatric perioperative and periprocedural applications and limitations. Br J Anaesth. 2015;115(2):171–82.
40. Keating GM. Dexmedetomidine: a review of its use for sedation in the intensive care setting. Drugs. 2015;75(10):1119–30.
41. Plambech MZ, Afshari A. Dexmedetomidine in the pediatric population: a review. Minerva Anestesiol. 2015;81(3):320–32.
42. Devasya A, Sarpangala M. Dexmedetomidine: a review of a newer sedative in dentistry. J Clin Pediatr Dent. 2015;39(5):401–9.
43. Suzuki J, El-Haddad S. A review: fentanyl and non-pharmaceutical fentanyls. Drug Alcohol Depend. 2017;171:107–16.
44. Schug SA, Ting S. Fentanyl formulations in the Management of Pain: an update. Drugs. 2017;77(7):747–63.
45. Thomson IR, Harding G, Hudson RJ. A comparison of fentanyl and sufentanil in patients undergoing coronary artery bypass graft surgery. J Cardiothorac Vasc Anesth. 2000;14(6):652–6.
46. Adelgais KM, Brent A, Wathen J, Tong S, Massanari D, Deakyne S, Sills MR. Intranasal fentanyl and quality of pediatric acute care. J Emerg Med. 2017; 53(5):607–615.e602.

14

Age-based prediction of uncuffed tracheal tube size in children to prevent inappropriately large tube selection

Hiroshi Hanamoto*, Hiroharu Maegawa, Mika Inoue, Aiko Oyamaguchi, Chiho Kudo and Hitoshi Niwa

Abstract

Background: This study aims to validate our previously reported prediction technique for uncuffed tracheal tube (TT) sizes in children younger than 2 years of age based on a calculated outer diameter (OD_{Cal}, mm) in each patient according to the regression equation $OD_{Cal} = 0.00223 \times$ age (day) + 4.88 and to investigate a better method to select initial TT sizes to decrease re-intubation frequency, especially since large tubes can damage the trachea.

Methods: We included patients younger than 2 years of age who underwent oral surgery under general anesthesia with tracheal intubation between July 2011 and December 2016 at the Osaka University Dental Hospital. The OD of the actual TT and the age in days were extracted from anesthesia records. Agreement rates, estimated numbers of required tubes, and size reduction frequencies were compared to obtain recommended OD (OD_{Rec}) values in 2 selection groups: "average selection" in the range "nearest to the OD_{Cal} value (OD_{Cal} - 0.35 < $OD_{Rec} \leq OD_{Cal}$ + 0.35)" and "safe selection" in the range "nearest to the value below OD_{Cal} (OD_{Cal} - 0.7 < $OD_{Rec} \leq OD_{Cal}$)".

Results: The agreement rates for an OD_{Rec} in the average selection and safe selection groups were 60.8 and 55.1%, respectively ($P = 0.001$). The estimated number of required tubes per patient were 1.40 ± 0.51 and 1.47 ± 0.55 ($P <$ 0.001), respectively. The estimated frequencies of size reductions were 13.3 and 4.0% ($P < 0.001$), respectively.

Conclusions: Because the size reduction frequency is lower despite a slightly higher number of required TTs, selecting an OD_{Rec} based on "safe selection" parameters is desirable to avoid complications due to intubation with larger TTs.

Keywords: Anesthesia, Intubation, Oral surgery, Pediatric surgery, Trachea

Background

In traditional pediatric airway management, uncuffed tracheal tubes (TTs) have been the gold standard for intubation in children under 8 years of age [1]. However, cuffed TTs are also used in pediatric practice [2]. Although cuffed TTs reduce the TT exchange rate, they do not affect the risk of complications compared with uncuffed TTs [3, 4]. Moreover, because ultrathin polyurethane Microcuff Pediatric Tracheal Tubes™ are expensive, uncuffed TTs are still regularly used in younger children in some hospitals.

Although age, height, and weight have been considered as accurate predictors of TT size, [5] the standard metric for determining it in pediatric patients younger than 2 years is controversial. Ultrasonography- [6–8] and radiography- [9] based predictions of TT sizes have been investigated in recent studies. Although these methods might well predict the actual TT size, using ultrasonography is cumbersome in some cases. Furthermore, chest radiography is not always successful because of an infant's movements, and the risk/benefit ratio of exposing children to X-rays should be considered. Therefore, even though the current age-based prediction method might be inferior to ultrasonography or radiography correlations, it might still be the most common method in

* Correspondence: hanamoto@dent.osaka-u.ac.jp
Department of Dental Anesthesiology, Osaka University Graduate School of Dentistry, 1-8 Yamada-Oka, Suita, Osaka 565-0871, Japan

clinical practice. We previously focused on uncuffed TT size in pediatric patients younger than 2 because Cole's formula [internal diameter (mm) = 0.25 × (age in years) + 4], which is commonly used, cannot be applied in such cases that require TT smaller than 4.0 mm. Therefore, we previously reported a regression formula for the outer diameter (OD) based on age in days [calculated OD (OD_{Cal}) = 0.00223 × age (days) + 4.88, $R^2 = 0.511$] based on data from 1035 general anesthesia cases between February 2003 and June 2011 in patients younger than 2 years [10].

Although commercially available TTs are made with an inner diameter of 0.5 mm, the OD differs depending on the type and manufacturer. However, a TT completely consistent with the OD_{Cal} rarely exists in a clinical setting, especially since commercially available TTs have inner diameter increments of 0.5 mm, resulting in OD differences of approximately 0.7 mm [7]. Even if anesthesiologists use a regression equation and select the TT nearest to the OD_{Cal}, there is a risk of intubating with a TT that is too large and might damage the trachea or the vocal cord. Therefore, we hypothesized that slightly smaller TT sizes might be desirable to prevent an inappropriately large tube selection. The purpose of this study was to validate uncuffed TT size predictions based on the patient's age in days and to investigate a better method to select TTs to decrease the frequency of size reduction and repeated intubation in children under 2 years of age.

Methods

This study was approved by the Ethics Committee at Osaka University Graduate School of Dentistry (approval number: H30-E1). The requirement for written informed consent was waived. Patients aged less than 2 years who underwent oral surgery under general anesthesia and required tracheal intubation between July 2011 and December 2016 at our hospital were included in this study. Exclusion criteria were the use of cuffed TTs and tracheostomies. The anesthesia records of patients were retrospectively investigated. The OD of the used TT (mm) and the age (day) were recorded. We used the OD as the TT size because ODs are different depending on the type and manufacturer of the TT.

Anesthesia and selection of tracheal tube size

Anesthesia was induced with sevoflurane, thiamylal, or propofol. After anesthesia induction, neuromuscular blocking agents were administered before intubation. Although we obtained a regression equation based on our previous data, the TT size on the first attempt was selected at the discretion of the attending anesthesiologists. An adequate TT fit was judged based on air leakage. A leak test was performed after each tracheal intubation by increasing respiratory pressure gradually up to approximately 35 cm H_2O, and 1 or 2 senior anesthetists listened for an audible leak sound near the patient's mouth. At our institution, an uncuffed tube was considered an appropriate size for oral surgery when no air leaks were observed at less than 15 cm H_2O; this threshold prevents intraoral blood from flowing into the trachea. If an air leak was observed with an inflation pressure of less than 15 cm H_2O, the next largest TT size available was chosen. When no air leak was observed at 35 cm H_2O and there was resistance during TT insertion, the intubated TT was exchanged for one with a smaller OD. In cases of no resistance, the original TT choice was used.

Validation analysis

We plotted the scatter diagram between the OD and age and drew the regression line obtained by our previous study. According to this regression equation, an OD was calculated for each patient (OD_{Cal}, $OD_{Cal} = 0.00223 \times$ day + 4.88). However, because a TT with the estimated OD_{Cal} does not always exist, a recommended OD (OD_{Rec}, OD of the first selected TT) was considered. To determine OD_{Rec} values in the range nearest to or below OD_{Cal} values, we also added lines parallel to the regression line at intervals of 0.7 mm because most commercially available uncuffed TTs have OD differences of approximately 0.7 mm [7]. These parallel lines were created using 1 of 2 methods: in the first method, we created lines ±0.7 and ± 1.4 mm from the regression line; in the second method, the parallel lines were created ±0.35 and ± 1.05 mm away from the regression line. The OD_{Rec} value was then compared with the OD of the actual TT used in each patient.

Outcomes

The outcomes were the agreement rate between OD and OD_{Rec} values in the total number of cases, the estimated number of required tubes per patient, and the estimated frequency of size reduction. We defined "average selection" as that in the range nearest to the OD_{Cal} value ($OD_{Cal} - 0.35 < OD_{Rec} \leq OD_{Cal} + 0.35$) and compared it to the "safe selection" calculation, which was in the range nearest to the value below OD_{Cal} ($OD_{Cal} - 0.7 < OD_{Rec} \leq OD_{Cal}$). The standard value provided by the manufacturers was used as the OD of each type and size of TT.

Statistical analysis

The sample size was determined by the study period. The start of the study period was determined as after our previous study period (which was between February 2003 and June 2011) [10]. The end of the study period was December 2016, because cuffed tubes have been used since 2017 at our institution. All statistical analyses were performed with EZR (Saitama Medical Center, Jichi Medical University, Saitama, Japan), which is a graphical user interface for R software (The R Foundation for Statistical Computing, Vienna, Austria). More precisely, this program is a modified version of the R commander that was designed with statistical functions frequently used in biostatistics [11]. Continuous variables are presented as the mean ± standard deviation (SD) with comparisons performed using a paired t-test. Dichotomous or categorical variables are presented as numbers (percentages) and were analyzed using the McNemar's test. A P-value < 0.05 indicated statistical significance.

Table 1 Outer diameters of uncuffed tracheal tubes from different manufacturers according to their inner diameters

Inner diameter (mm)	Outer diameter (mm)			
	SILICONISED	IVORY	RAE	SPIRAL
3.0	4.2	4.4	4.2	4.7
3.5	4.8	5.1	4.8	5.3
4.0	5.5	5.9	5.6	6.0
4.5	6.2	6.6	6.2	6.7
5.0	6.9	7.3	6.9	7.3
5.5	7.6	8.0	7.4	8.0

SILICONISED: Portex siliconized PVC, uncuffed tracheal tube
IVORY: Portex tracheal tube IVORY uncuffed tracheal tube
RAE: Mallinckrodt oral RAE tracheal tube, uncuffed, Murphy eye
SPIRAL: PHYCON wire reinforced uncuffed tube

Results

Uncuffed TTs from different manufacturers were used in this study. The ODs of these TTs with their corresponding inner diameters are shown in Table 1. Although the "Spiral" tube type was not used during the study period, we have stated its parameters in the table because it was included in our previous study [10]. Severe, adverse respiratory events including severe postoperative croup or subglottic edema were not observed.

We reviewed 883 anesthetic records of patients under 2 years of age during the study period. Four cases of tracheostomy and 76 cases with cuffed TT use were excluded. A total of 803 anesthetic records without any missing data were finally analyzed (Fig. 1). Demographic data are presented in Table 2. Patient age in relation to height or body weight are presented in Fig. 2.

Parallel lines to the regression line of OD_{Cal} in the scatter plot of OD are shown in Fig. 3. The estimated numbers of required TTs per patient in the average selection and safe selection groups are shown in Tables 3 and 4, respectively. The agreement rates were 60.8 and 55.1% ($P = 0.001$), the estimated numbers of required TTs per patient were 1.40 ± 0.51 and 1.47 ± 0.55 ($P < 0.001$), and the estimated probabilities of a required size reduction were 13.3 and 4.0% ($P < 0.001$), respectively.

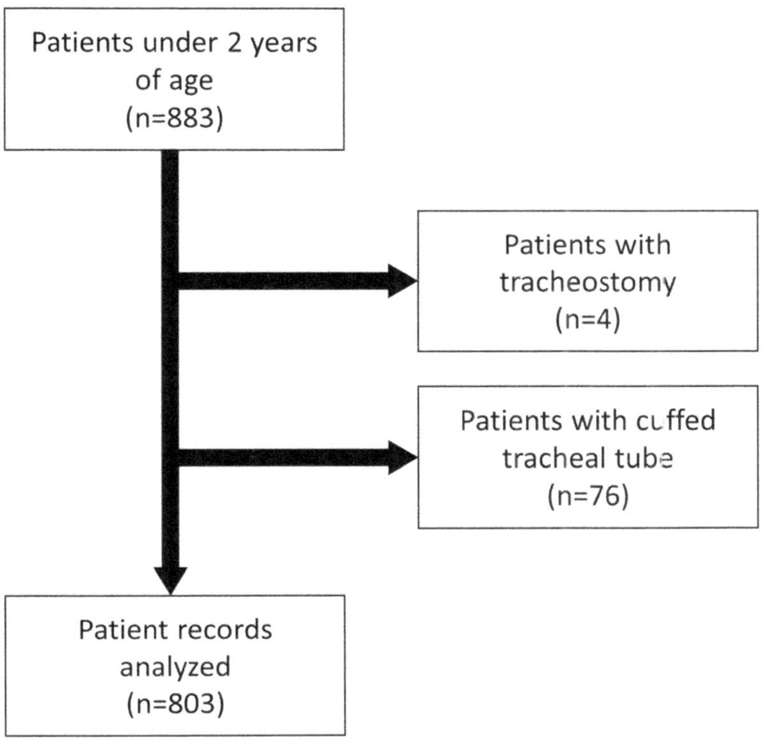

Fig. 1 Flow chart of patient selection

Table 2 Demographic and procedural data

Variables	Values
Age, days	308 ± 182
Body weight, kg	7.8 ± 1.9
Height, cm	69.3 ± 7.6
Sex, M / F	459 / 344
Main operation method	
Cheiloplasty	308 (38.4%)
Palatoplasty	454 (56.5%)
Tongue operation	34 (4.2%)
Lip repair	3 (0.4%)
Other oral surgery	4 (0.5%)
Operation time, min	68 ± 24
Anesthesia time, min	138 ± 27

Data are presented as number of patients (percentage) or mean ± standard deviation. *M* Male, *F* Female

Discussion

Our findings support the selection of an OD_{Rec} in the "safe selection" range (OD_{Cal} - 0.7, OD_{Cal}). Our size reduction probability was 4% with an acceptable estimated number of required TTs per patient, slightly higher than that needed for the "average selection" range (OD_{Cal} - 0.35, OD_{Cal} + 0.35). To our knowledge, this is the first report on the number of required TTs and the probability of a required size reduction after TT selection. Although the estimated number of required TTs was lower in the "average selection" group, we believe that the "safe selection" method is adequate based on intubation times and the probability of a required size reduction.

Previously reported agreement rates were 48% [7], 60% [8], and 98% [6] predicted by ultrasonography, 57% by radiography [9], and 52.6% using middle finger length [12]. Agreement rates of age-based formulae vary widely with values of 53.5% [13], 60% [6], 24–40% [7], and 32–43% [9]. In the present study, the agreement rate was 60.8% when the first selection used the "average selection" approach and 55.1% when predicted by the "safe selection" method; these values are not low compared to other studies. Eck et al., who had conducted one of the few previous studies on the size of uncuffed TTs in patients younger than 2 years, calculated a regression equation to predict TT sizes for infants younger than 1 year [14] with an R^2 value of 0.387, indicating poor correlation.

Uncuffed TT selection should incorporate the patient's benefit, economic factors, and the anesthetist. Considerations for the patient's benefit should include a decreased frequency of laryngoscopy and intubation, as well as preventing intubation with an oversized TT. From an economical perspective, it is better to reduce the number of TTs used. With an OD_{Rec} determined by "safe selection" parameters, the average number of required TTs was 1.47. Uncuffed TTs may have a beneficial economic effect; in fact, a Microcuff™ tube in our country is approximately 2.8-fold more expensive than an uncuffed tube.

Some anesthetists perform re-intubation with the next smallest TT if the primarily selected TT does not exhibit

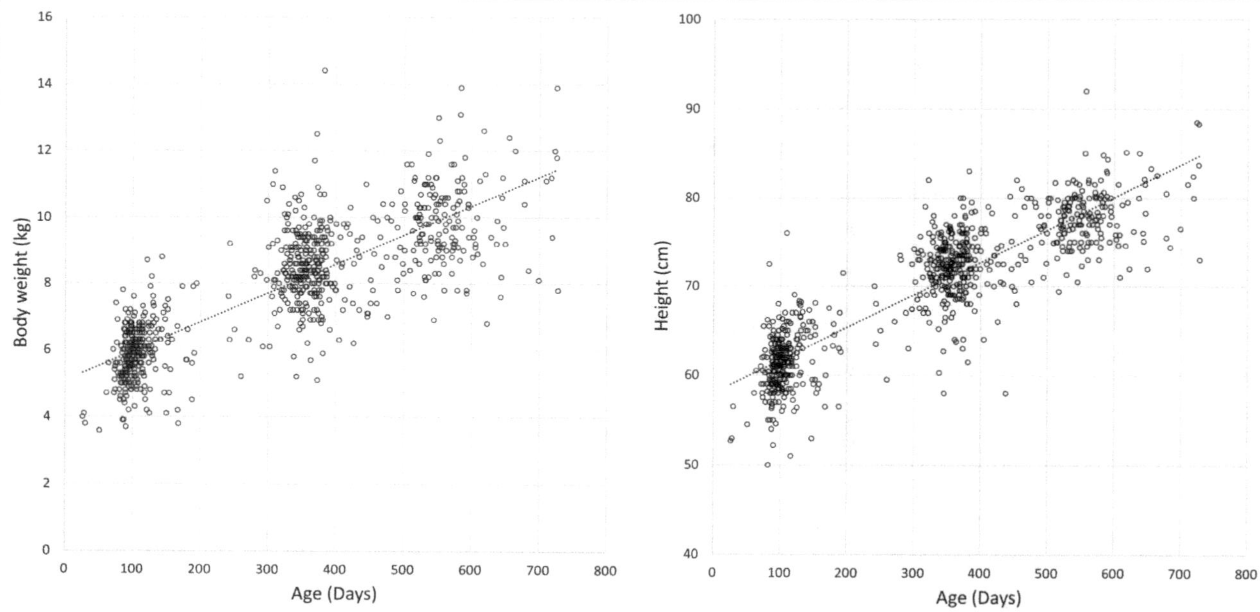

Fig. 2 Scatterplot of age in relation to height and body weight. Line in the scatter plot are as follows: dotted line, regression line

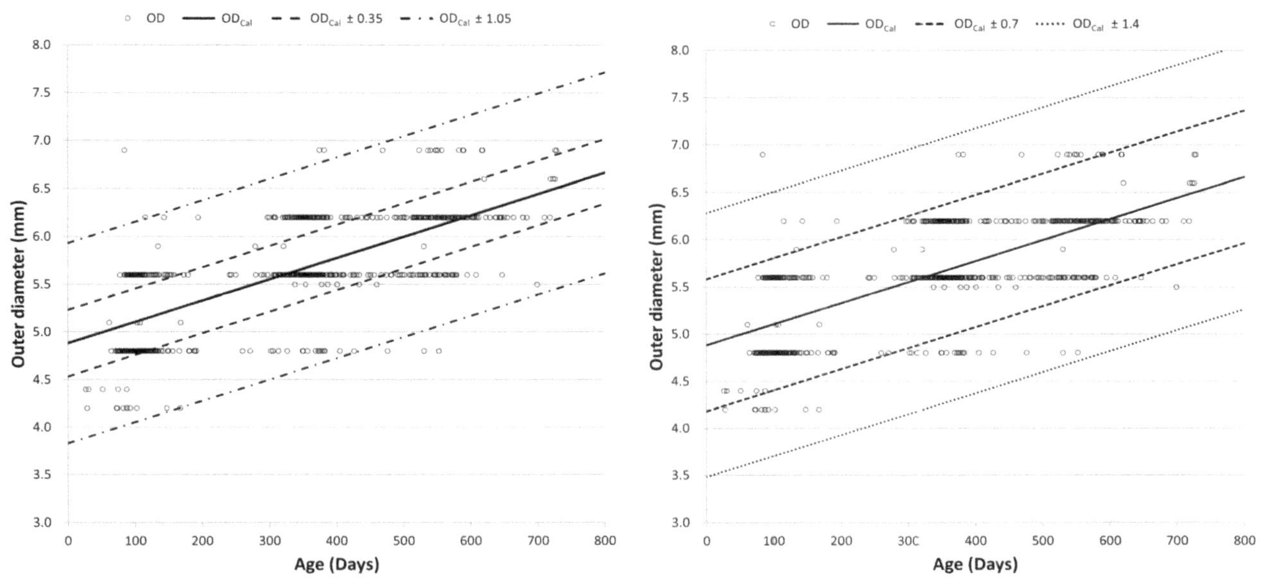

Fig. 3 Scatterplot of age in relation to the outer diameter of the tracheal tube used. Lines in the scatter plot are as follows: solid line, regression line; long-dashed lines, regression line ±0.35 mm; and dashed-dotted lines, regression line ±1.05 mm, regression line ±0.7 mm; and dotted lines, regression line ±1.4 mm. OD, outer diameter of the tube used, mm; OD_{Cal}, calculated outer diameter, mm

an air leak. If the consequent leak is too large and ventilation becomes difficult, re-intubation is performed again using the first TT. In this situation, the anesthetist has confirmed an excessive air leak when using the smaller TT, but the frequency of laryngoscopy and intubation has been increased. Although using an airway catheter is one of the methods for tube exchange and prevention of laryngoscopy, it is difficult to judge the insertion resistance. Another anesthetist may use the first TT to avoid re-intubation if neither an air leak nor insertion resistance is present. In this situation, anesthesia experience is required, and an anesthetist may be apprehensive regarding TT use; therefore, a smaller TT may be optimal. In consideration of these issues, smaller sized TTs based on safe selection parameters should be primarily selected.

Generally, if there is no air leak at an inflation pressure of 25–40 cm H_2O, a TT should be substituted with a smaller sized one [1, 15]. However, we used the criterion of the lack of an air leak at less than 15 cm H_2O as a guide for appropriate TT selection as this threshold prevents intraoral blood from flowing into the trachea during surgery. Therefore, there might be several cases in our study in which an air leak would not have been observed at an inflation pressure of 25–40 cm H_2O. In adults, tracheal mucosal capillary blood flow is compromised above 30 cm H_2O and totally obstructed above 50 cm H_2O [16]. Adverse events increase in children with no air leaks at 25 cm H_2O [17]. In the present study, severe respiratory adverse events were not observed.

Previous studies adopted several ranges as criteria for appropriate leak pressure including 10–30 cm H_2O [9, 14], 10–20 cm H_2O [6], 15–25 cm H_2O [7], 15–30 cm H_2O [8], 10–35 cm H_2O [18], and 5–40 cm H_2O [19]. This indicates that the optimal leak pressure is still controversial. Also, there were some cases in which the

Table 3 Number of cases and estimated number of required tubes per patient with the predicted outer diameter determined by "nearest value to the calculated outer diameter"

OD of tracheal tube	Number of cases (%)	Estimated number of required tubes
$OD \leq OD_{Cal} - 1.05$	4 (0.5)	3
$OD_{Cal} - 1.05 < OD \leq OD_{Cal} - 0.35$	103 (12.8)	2
$OD_{Cal} - 0.35 < OD \leq OD_{Cal} + 0.35$	488 (60.8)	1
$OD_{Cal} + 0.35 < OD \leq OD_{Cal} + 1.05$	204 (25.4)	2
$OD_{Cal} + 1.05 < OD$	4 (0.5)	3

OD Outer diameter of the used tube, mm
OD_{Cal} Calculated outer diameter, mm
Estimated number of required tubes, estimated number of required tubes per patient when the recommended outer diameter of the first selected tracheal tube (OD_{Rec}) was assumed to be in the range "$OD_{Cal} - 0.35 < OD_{Rec} \leq OD_{Cal} + 0.35$"

Table 4 Number of cases and estimated number of required tubes per patient with the predicted outer diameter determined by "nearest value below the calculated outer diameter"

OD of the tracheal tube	Number of cases (%)	Estimated number of required tubes
$OD \le OD_{Cal} - 1.4$	0 (0)	3
$OD_{Cal} - 1.4 < OD \le OD_{Cal} - 0.7$	31 (4.0)	2
$OD_{Cal} - 0.7 < OD \le OD_{Cal}$	442 (55.1)	1
$OD_{Cal} < OD \le OD_{Cal} + 0.7$	312 (38.8)	2
$OD_{Cal} + 0.7 < OD \le OD_{Cal} + 1.4$	17 (2.0)	3
$OD_{Cal} + 1.4 < OD$	1 (0.1)	4

OD Outer diameter of the used tube, mm
OD_{Cal} Calculated outer diameter, mm
Estimated number of required tubes, estimated number of required tubes per patient when the recommended outer diameter of the first selected tracheal tube (OD_{Rec}) was assumed to be in the range "$OD_{Cal} - 0.7 < OD_{Rec} \le OD_{Cal}$"

optimal TT size that met the leak pressure criteria was not found. Furthermore, results may differ according to the chosen air leak pressure range. In the present study, all patients underwent oral surgery accompanied with intraoral bleeding. Therefore, it is important to use a TT with an optimal fit to prevent air leaks into the trachea. This air leak criterion may have led to the selection of slightly larger TTs in our study when compared with other studies. In general intubation situations, a slightly smaller size might be better based on the air leak criteria, although our data are especially applicable to a variety of patients undergoing oral surgery. Particularly in difficult airway situations [20], reduction of TT exchange and selection of excessively large TT are required.

Limitations

This study has several limitations. First, the head position might affect the leak pressure [21]. Our results included surgeries performed with an extended head, such as palatoplasty in cleft palate patients, but the head position during surgery was not the same in all cases. Second, most ODs of commercially available TTs are at increments between 0.6 and 0.8 mm. We calculated the estimated number of required TTs using the value of 0.7 mm as the difference in size between different ODs. Therefore, our results may be subject to error or potential bias. However, we consider such error to be acceptable, because we used a mean value for generalization. The third limitation is the retrospective design of our study; consequently, actual intubation times were not recorded in all cases. Hence, further prospective studies are needed. Although there are some limitations, these study findings can improve TT selection under various conditions. Moreover, if future material improvements make it possible to further decrease the thickness of the TT wall, our results may be directly applicable to the prediction of uncuffed TT sizes.

Conclusions

Uncuffed TT size predictions based on the range "$OD_{Cal} - 0.7 < OD_{Rec} \le OD_{Cal}$" in patients under 2 years of age is easy and comprehensively adequate because the probability of size reduction is less than 4% and the number of required TTs and laryngoscopies are low. Even if their chosen criteria for TT air leaks are different, anesthesiologists should select a TT size for the first attempt based on this "safe selection" approach using the "nearest value below OD_{Cal}" rule according to the regression equation obtained at each institution, as this rule is superior to the "nearest to OD_{Cal}" rule.

Abbreviations

OD: Outer diameter of the tube used; OD_{Cal}: Calculated outer diameter; OD_{Rec}: Recommended outer diameter; TT: Tracheal tube

Acknowledgements

We would like to thank Editage (http://www.editage.jp) for English language editing.

Authors' contributions

HH and HN designed the study. HH, HM, and MI collected the data. AO and CK conducted the statistical analyses. HH and HN wrote the manuscript while HM, MI, AO and CK helped to write and revise the manuscript. All authors read and approved the final manuscript.

References

1. Wheeler M, Cote CJ, Todres ID. The pediatric airway. In: Cote CJ, Lerman J, Todres ID, editors. A practice of anesthesia for infants and children, 4th ed. Philadelphia: Saunders; 2008. p. 237–78.
2. Khine HH, Corddry DH, Kettrick RG, Martin TM, McCloskey JJ, Rose JB, et al. Comparison of cuffed and uncuffed endotracheal tubes in young children during general anesthesia. Anesthesiology. 1997;86:627–31.
3. Weiss M, Dullenkopf A, Fischer JE, Keller C, Gerber AC, European Paediatric Endotracheal Intubation Study Group. Prospective randomized controlled multi-centre trial of cuffed or uncuffed endotracheal tubes in small children. Br J Anaesth. 2009;103:867–73.
4. de Wit M, Peelen LM, van Wolfswinkel L, de Graaff JC. The incidence of postoperative respiratory complications: a retrospective analysis of cuffed vs uncuffed tracheal tubes in children 0-7 years of age. Paediatr Anaesth. 2018; 28:210–7.
5. Keep PJ, Manford ML. Endotracheal tube sizes for children. Anaesthesia. 1974;29:181–5.
6. Shibasaki M, Nakajima Y, Ishii S, Shimizu F, Shime N, Sessler DI. Prediction of pediatric endotracheal tube size by ultrasonography. Anesthesiology. 2010; 113:819–24.
7. Schramm C, Knop J, Jensen K, Plaschke K. Role of ultrasound compared to age-related formulas for uncuffed endotracheal intubation in a pediatric population. Paediatr Anaesth. 2012;22:781–6.
8. Bae JY, Byon HJ, Han SS, Kim HS, Kim JT. Usefulness of ultrasound for selecting a correctly sized uncuffed tracheal tube for paediatric patients. Anaesthesia. 2011;66:994–8.

9. Park HP, Hwang JW, Lee JH, Nahm FS, Park SH, Oh AY, et al. Predicting the appropriate uncuffed endotracheal tube size for children: a radiograph-based formula versus two age-based formulas. J Clin Anesth. 2013;25:384–7.
10. Masawaki A, Hanamoto H, Kitamoto F, Ohnuki T, Murakami S, Inoue M, et al. Uncuffed tracheal tube size in pediatric patients aged below 2 years. J Jpn Dent Soc Anesthesiol. 2012;40:587–91.
11. Kanda Y. Investigation of the freely available easy-to-use software 'EZR' for medical statistics. Bone Marrow Transplant. 2013;48:452–8.
12. Ritchie-McLean S, Ferrier V, Clevenger B, Thomas M. Using middle finger length to determine the internal diameter of uncuffed tracheal tubes in paediatrics. Anaesthesia. 2018;73:1207–13.
13. Takita K, Morimoto Y, Okamura A, Kemmotsu O. Do age-based formulae predict the appropriate endotracheal tube sizes in Japanese children? J Anesth. 2001;15:145–8.
14. Eck JB, De Lisle DG, Phillips-Bute BG, Ginsberg B. Prediction of tracheal tube size in children using multiple variables. Paediatr Anaesth. 2002;12:495–8.
15. Cote CJ. Pediatric anesthesia. In: Miller RD, editor. Miller's anesthesia, 7th ed. Philadelphia: Churchill Livingstone; 2010. p. 2559–97.
16. Seegobin RD, van Hasselt GL. Endotracheal cuff pressure and tracheal mucosal blood flow: endoscopic study of effects of four large volume cuffs. Br Med J (Clin Res Ed). 1984;288:965–8.
17. Suominen P, Taivainen T, Tuominen N, Voipio V, Wirtavuori K, Hiller A, et al. Optimally fitted tracheal tubes decrease the probability of postextubation adverse events in children undergoing general anesthesia. Paediatr Anaesth. 2006;16:641–7.
18. Davis D, Barbee L, Ririe D. Pediatric endotracheal tube selection: a comparison of age-based and height-based criteria. AANA J. 1998;66:299–303.
19. King BR, Baker MD, Braitman LE, Seidl-Friedman J, Schreiner MS. Endotracheal tube selection in children: a comparison of four methods. Ann Emerg Med. 1993;22:530–4.
20. Gruppo di Studio SIAARTI "Vie Aeree Difficili,", Frova G, Guarino A, Petrini F, Merli G, Sorbello M, et al. Recommendations for airway control and difficult airway management in paediatric patients. Minerva Anestesiol. 2006;72:723–48.
21. Finholt DA, Henry DB, Raphaely RC. Factors affecting leak around tracheal tubes in children. Can Anaesth Soc J. 1985;32:326–9.

15

Influence of anesthesia methods on surgical outcomes and renal function in retrograde intrarenal stone surgery

Ohseong Kwon[1], Jung-Man Lee[2], Juhyun Park[3], Min Chul Cho[3], Hwancheol Son[3], Hyeon Jeong[3], Seung Hoon Ryang[4] and Sung Yong Cho[4*]

Abstract

Background: We analyzed the influence of anesthesia methods on surgical outcomes and renal function in retrograde intrarenal surgery (RIRS) in a prospective, randomized controlled study.

Methods: Seventy patients who underwent RIRS from September 2015 to February 2017 were randomly allocated to general anesthesia (GA) or spinal anesthesia (SA) groups. Renal function was assessed using estimated glomerular filtration rate, and separate renal function was evaluated using nuclear medicine tests. Maneuverability and accessibility were evaluated after every surgery. All procedures were performed by a single experienced surgeon (SY Cho).

Results: Stone-free rate was higher in the GA (92.3%, 36 of 39) than the SA (71.0%, 22 of 31) ($P = 0.019$) group. Pain score was higher in the GA than in the SA group on the first postoperative morning ($P = 0.025$), but pain scores of the two groups were similar before discharge ($P = 0.560$). There were no differences in the changes of serum creatinine level ($P = 0.792$) and changes of estimated glomerular filtration rate ($P = 0.807$). Differences of separate renal function between operative and contralateral site increased significantly in patients under GA than under SA at postoperative 3 months ($P = 0.014$). Maneuverability and accessibility were better in SA with sedation than GA ($P < 0.001$).

Conclusions: RIRS under SA showed advantages in renal function change using renogram at postoperative 3 months and in lower pain score on the first postoperative morning. Performance of operator under SA was worse than that under GA and significantly improved with sedation. RIRS under SA showed advantages in lower pain score at postoperative first day.

Keywords: Renal stone, Retrograde intrarenal surgery, Spinal anesthesia

Background

According to the European Association of Urology (EAU) guidelines, retrograde intrarenal surgery (RIRS) is recommended as an alternative treatment option to percutaneous nephrolithotomy (PNL) for renal stones less than 2 cm in size [1]. Routinely, most urologists prefer general anesthesia (GA) during surgery for renal stones. Because the patient's breathing can be controlled, patients can be more comfortable, and the surgeon can be comfortable because of diminished patient movement under general anesthesia. However, some previous studies presented that mortality or major complications are reduced with regional anesthesia than with GA [2–4] and there have been some controversial reports. Although regional anesthesia may be preferred in critically ill patients [5–7], some previous studies, including high quality meta-analyses, suggest that there are no differences in major outcomes or critical complications between GA and spinal anesthesia

* Correspondence: kmoretry@daum.net
[4]Department of Urology, Seoul National University Hospital, 101, Daehak-ro Jongno-gu, 03080 Seoul, Republic of Korea

(SA) [8–10]. Therefore, these two anesthesia methods might be suitable for RIRS in the general population.

Renal function abnormalities or perioperative renal dysfunction due to anesthesia, may be present even in normal patients. A previous study reported that renal dysfunction could happen even in patients who had normal renal function preoperatively [11]. These complications are associated with the type of surgery, baseline renal function, underlying diseases, and the amount of intraoperative bleeding. SA may be free from the toxic effects of muscle relaxants, opioids, and inhalation anesthetics, which may be more beneficial than GA in terms of kidney function [12]. RIRS may increase the risk of electrolyte abnormalities due to absorption of irrigation fluid, and GA presents with limitations in early detection of electrolyte abnormalities. However, there are few previous studies comparing anesthetic methods with respect to renal function [13–15].

Therefore, this study aimed to analyze the influence of anesthesia methods on surgical outcomes and renal function in RIRS.

Methods

Patients and study design

The prospective, randomized study was conducted in compliance with Good Clinical Practices (GCP) and the Declaration of Helsinki, and the study protocol was approved by the Institutional Review Board of Seoul National University Hospital (approval number: 16–2015-75). After receiving written informed consent, 70 patients, classified as American Society of Anesthesiologists (ASA) physical status I-II, registered from September 2015 to February 2017, were recruited. Eligible patients older than 20 years with renal stones greater than 10 mm were included. The decision for active stone removal was based upon the EAU guidelines. Patients were excluded if they had urologic anatomical abnormalities. Patients with ASA status ≥ grade III, a contraindication for spinal anesthesia or RIRS, or unexpected intraoperative renal injury, were also excluded. The CONSORT Statement Extension for Randomized Controlled Trials of Nonpharmacological Trials was closely followed. Following preoperative evaluations, the enrolled patients were randomly allocated to GA or SA groups using the permuted block method. Figure 1 shows the trial design.

Surgical methods

All RIRS procedures were performed by a single surgeon (SY Cho) who performed over one thousand cases according to the same methods described in the same authors' investigations [16, 17]. Ureteral access sheaths (Navigator™, Boston Scientific, MA, USA), 11/13-Fr or 12/14-Fr, were inserted at the level of the ureteropelvic junction. Flexible ureteroscopes, Flex-X2S (Karl Storz, Tuttlingen, Germany) and URF-V or V2 (Olympus, Tokyo, Japan), were inserted through the access sheath. After the distal end of the scope was located in the renal pelvis, a 365- or 200-μm laser fiber was used for stone fragmentation. The renal stones were busted into fragments measuring less than 2 mm. An endoscopy irrigation pump (Stryker, Kalamazoo, MI, USA) was used to maintain continuous intrarenal pressure. A double-J stent was routinely inserted at the time of surgery, and removed at postoperative 5 to 10 days.

Anesthesia methods

Standard monitoring, including non-invasive blood pressure, electrocardiography, oxygen saturation, and body temperature was applied in all patients.

For the GA group, 30 mg lidocaine, 1.5–2.0 mg/kg propofol, 50–100 μg fentanyl was administered to induce anesthesia. Following loss of consciousness, 0.6–0.8 mg/kg rocuronium was administered, and the patients were intubated. Patients were ventilated with a tidal volume of 6–8 ml/kg. Anesthesia was maintained using 1–4 vol% of sevoflurane in oxygen and air.

The patients in the SA group were placed in a lateral decubitus position. An anesthesiologist wearing a sterile gown cleaned the skin on the patient's back with 0.5% chlorhexidine. After the cleaned skin was dried and draped in a sterile manner, the anesthesiologist inserted a 25-gauge spinal needle into the space between 4th spinous process and 5th spinous process or between 3rd spinous process and 4th spinous process. The intrathecal position of the tip of the needle was confirmed by aspiration of clean cerebrospinal fluid, following which 10–17 mg (median: 14 mg) hyperbaric bupivacaine (Marcaine Heavy inj 0.5%, Astrazeneca, France) and 20 μg fentanyl were administrated intrathecally considering operation site and patient's height. After injection, the patients were placed in supine position. The anesthesiologist checked for sensory loss in the dermatome, and motor loss to ensure adequate anesthesia for RIRS. On failure of first trial of spinal anesthesia, spinal anesthesia was repeated after patient approval. If the second trial of spinal anesthesia failed, the patient was dropped from the study and general anesthesia was administered in the routine manner. For the SA group, sedation was applied with 1–3 mg of midazolam according to patient's lead after identifying the level of spinal anesthesia.

Clinical parameters and statistical analysis

Patient characteristics included age, sex, body mass index, laboratory results, and other comorbidities. Stone characteristics included laterality, Hounsfield units, numbers, maximal size, and volume. Primary outcome was renal function change assessed by estimated

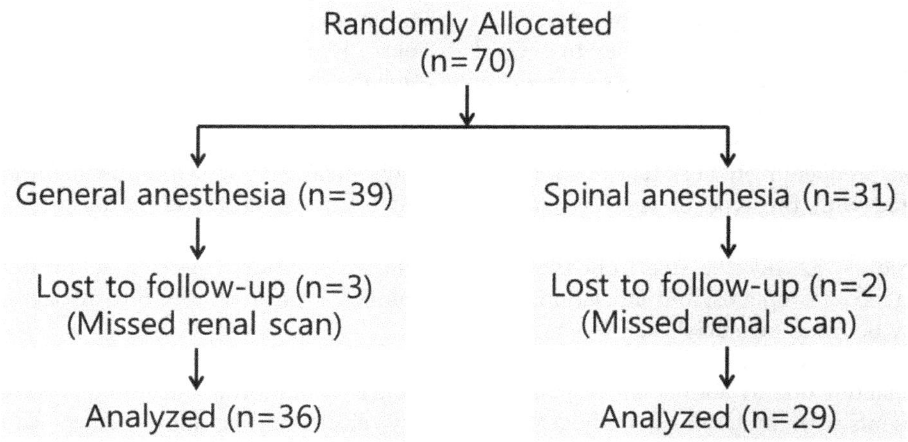

Fig. 1 CONSORT diagram

glomerular filtration rate and separate renal function evaluated by nuclear medicine test. And, secondary outcome was performance of operator evaluated by one experienced surgeon. The computed tomography (CT) scans were acquired preoperatively. Information regarding the presence of hydronephrosis and infundibulopelvic angles was acquired [18], and the stone distribution was analyzed using the Seoul National University Renal Stone Complexity (S-ReSC) scores [19]. Renal function was assessed using the estimated glomerular filtration rate before surgery and on the day after surgery. Separate renal function was evaluated using nuclear medicine tests with diethylenetriamine pentaacetic acid (99 m Tc-DTPA) prior to procedure, and at 3 months after the procedure. The separate renal function was re-assessed postoperatively, when the difference between the separate renal function of the affected and contralateral sides was over 10%. Intraoperative parameters included operative time and stone fragmentation time per surgery. The operative time was defined as the time from endoscopic insertion into the urethra to the insertion of the urethral Foley's catheter. Follow-up images of plain X-ray or non-contrast CT were acquired 1, 7, and 60–90 days postoperatively to assess the absence of residual fragments. Stone-free status was clinically defined as the absence of evidence for remnant stones < 2 mm on the follow-up images. Intraoperative incidents associated with anesthesia (blood pressure fluctuation, nausea, and pain) were documented. Blood pressure fluctuation was defined as a change of more than 20% of the baseline systolic blood pressure in the ward before the surgery in this trial.

One experienced surgeon evaluated maneuverability and accessibility after every operation. Maneuverability and accessibility were graded as 'very poor (1-2)', 'poor (3–4)', 'so so (5-6)', 'good (7–8)' and 'very good (9-10)'. Postoperative pain was evaluated using visual analog scale scores from 1 to 10, with 10 being most severe. Postoperative complications were defined according to modified Clavien classification system [20].

We planned a study of experimental subjects with one control(s) per experimental subject. Primary endpoint was difference of renal function recovery rate and the difference was 6.5% from previous investigation. The recovery rate was defined as the rate of changes of separate renal function into less than 10% between the two kidneys in patients who underwent according to the preoperative functional deterioration [11]. In a previous pilot study, the response within each subject group was normally distributed with standard deviation 9%. If the true difference in the previous investigations between the experimental and control means is 6.5%, we will need to study 31 experimental subjects and 31 control subjects to be able to reject the null hypothesis that the population means of the experimental and control groups are equal with probability (power) 0.8 (non-inferiority test). The Type I error probability associated with this test of this null hypothesis is 0.05. Considering dropout rates about 10%, we decided to include total 70 patients (35 patients each).

All parameters were represented as the mean value ± standard deviation or frequency (percentage). Comparative results were analyzed by using an independent *t*-test or a Mann-Whitney U test between the two groups. Categorical variables were analyzed using the Chi-square and Fisher's exact test. Statistical significance was considered at *P*-value < 0.05. Statistical analyses were performed with IBM SPSS Statistics version 20 (IBM, Chicago, IL, USA) and R version 3.0.1 (http://www.r-project.org).

Results

Patients and stone characteristics

Patient demographics and stone characteristics are shown in Table 1. Thirty-nine patients were assigned to the GA group, and 31 patients were assigned to the SA group. All of them completed this study trial. The blockade level of spinal anesthesia was between T2-T10 (number of T2/T3/T4/T6/T8/T10 in the SA group: 2/5/7/8/7/2). One patient complained mild discomfort of pain sensation during the surgery. His height was 178 cm and we injected 14 mg of bupivacaine and 20 μg of fentanyl intrathecally for spinal anesthesia, which lead to a blockade level at T10. We treated the patient with midazolam 5 mg and fentanyl 100 μg because the patient complained of mild discomfort. Baseline preoperative serum creatinine was significantly higher in the GA group than in the SA group ($P = 0.035$). There were no significant differences between the two groups in terms of age, gender, stone laterality, and incidence of comorbidities, and mean number of stones, mean maximal stone size, mean Hounsfield unit, and distribution of S-ReSC scores.

Surgical outcomes and renal function change

Table 2 shows operative outcomes in the two groups. In the SA group, there were no anesthetic conversions. Stone-free rate (SFR) was higher in the GA (92.3%, 36 of 39) than in the SA (71.0%, 22 of 31) ($P = 0.019$) group. Changes in serum creatinine after surgery were not significantly different between the two groups ($P = 0.792$). Pain score of the GA group was higher than that of the SA group on the first postoperative morning (4.9 ± 2.4 vs. 3.7 ± 1.7, $P = 0.025$); however, pain scores of the two groups were similar before discharge (3.1 ± 1.9 vs. 2.9 ± 1.2, $P = 0.560$) 1 or 2 days postoperatively. There were no differences in postoperative complications between the two groups ($P = 0.841$), and there were no complications of Clavien classification grade III or higher.

Considering parameters of renal function after surgery, there were no differences in changes in serum creatinine level ($P = 0.792$) and changes in estimated glomerular filtration rate ($P = 0.807$) between the GA and SA groups. The preoperative DTPA renal scan was performed in 65 of 70 patients, and 26 (40%) showed a difference greater than 10% in separate renal function. After 3 months, 11 of 12 patients (91.7%) in the SA group showed improvement in separate renal function,

Table 1 Patient characteristics and perioperative findings

	General	Spinal
Patient characteristics		
Number	39	31
Mean age (years)	54.1 ± 14.5 (29-83)	54.7 ± 14.0 (26-80)
Male: female	26 (66.7%) : 13 (33.3%)	20 (64.5%) : 11 (35.5%)
Mean body mass index (kg/㎡)	24.7 ± 2.7 (17.3-31.4)	25.0 ± 3.7 (19.3-34.4)
Side (right/left)	15 (38.5%) : 24 (61.5%)	15 (48.4%) : 16 (51.6%)
History of previous treatment	11 (28.2%) (SWL:11)	15 (48.4%) (SWL:14, RIRS:1)
Diabetes mellitus	5 (12.8%)	7 (22.6%)
Hypertension	9 (23.1%)	12 (38.7%)
Preoperative serum creatinine (㎎/㎗)	1.00 ± 0.45 (0.54-3.10)	0.80 ± 0.22 (0.58-1.38)
Preoperative GFR (㎖/min/㎡)	80.5 ± 22.6 (20.3-118.1)	95.7 ± 21.0 (53.3-151.2)
Stone characteristics		
Mean number of stones	2.3 ± 2.1 (1-13)	2.0 ± 1.4 (1-7)
Mean maximal stone size (㎜)	11.3 ± 3.3 (5-20)	12.0 ± 3.4 (7-20)
Mean total stone volume (㎣)	674.1 ± 552.0 (85-2879)	810.4 = 630.0 (138-3257)
Solitary kidney	1 (2.6%)	0
Staghorn stone	1 (2.6%)	0
Mean Hounsfield unit (HU)	937.0 ± 294.2 (362-1568)	961.1 ± 354.4 (208-1574)
Mean infundibulopelvic angle (°)	51.0 ± 11.2 (31-72)	53.9 ± 13.4 (31-90)
S-ReSC scores: 1-2/3-4/≥5	31 / 4 / 4	27 / 4 / 0
Multiple caliceal stones	16 (41.0%)	14 (45.2%)
Lower caliceal stone	25 (64.1%)	21 (67.7%)
Preoperative fever	1 (2.6%)	0
Preoperative stent placement	1 (2.6%)	1 (3.2%)

SWL extracorporeal shockwave lithotripsy, RIRS retrograde intrarenal surgery, GFR glomerular filtration rate, S-ReSC Seoul National University Renal stone Complexity

Table 2 Operative outcomes of the two groups

	General (n=39)	Spinal (n=31)	*P* value
Anesthesia time (minutes)	108.6 ± 29.4 (65-185)	111.1 ± 44.3 (40-285)	0.775
Operative time (minutes)	57.6 ± 26.8 (15-139)	63.7 ± 39.4 (10-220)	0.445
Stone fragmentation time (minutes)	15.6 ± 13.6 (3-65)	19.0 ± 18.1 (2-70)	0.465
Postoperative serum creatinine (㎎/㎗)	1.02 ± 0.47 (0.58-2.86)	0.83 ± 0.31 (0.31-1.75)	0.061
Serum creatinine change (㎎/㎗)	0.04 ± 0.24	0.03 ± 0.14	0.792
Postoperative GFR (㎖/min/㎡)	76.9 ± 24.9 (22.4-123.7)	94.3 ± 26.9 (38.8-141.2)	0.011*
GFR change (㎖/min/㎡)	-3.6 ± 14.6	-2.6 ± 16.8	0.807
SFR after initial treatment	36 (92.3%)	22 (71.0%)	0.019*
Visual analog scale			
Right after operation	0.9 ± 1.3	1.3 ± 1.6	0.178
Postoperative first day morning	4.9 ± 2.4	3.7 ± 1.7	0.025*
Before discharge	3.1 ± 1.9	2.9 ± 1.2	0.560
Postoperative stent removal (day)	9.7 ± 5.7 (1-32)	9.4 ± 4.9 (4-30)	0.784
Postoperative hospital stay (day)	1.2 ± 0.4 (1-3)	1.4 ± 1.1 (1-6)	0.314
Stone composition			0.992
Uric acid	6	5	
Calcium oxalate monohydrate	30	23	
Struvite	2	2	
Carbonate apatite	1	1	
Intraoperative event	11	5	0.232
Blood pressure fluctuation	10	4	
Others (nausea, pain, etc.)	1	1	
Postoperative complications	3	2	0.841
Grade I			
Postoperative fever	0	2	
Grade II			
Infection needed antibiotics	3	0	
Grade III-V	0	0	
Postoperative painkiller usage	29	23	0.987
Separate renal function data			
Preoperative			
Patients (n)	36	29	
Operative/contralateral (±SD)	43.0% (±11.7)/57.0% (±11.7)	46.5% (±5.0)/53.5% (±5.4)	0.144/0.139
Operative site minus contralateral site (±SD)	-13.9% (±23.5)	-6.9% (±10.3)	0.140
Postoperative 3 months			
Patients (n)	14	12	
Operative/contralateral (±SD)	35.0% (±12.8)/65.0% (±12.8)	45.7% (±6.0)/54.3% (6.0)	0.014/0.014
Operative site minus contralateral site (±SD)	-30.0% (±25.7)	-8.6% (±12.0)	0.014*

GFR glomerular filtration rate, SFR stone-free rate, VAS visual analog scale

whereas 10 of 14 patients (71.4%) in the GA group showed improvement in separate renal function ($P = 0.330$). The difference in separate renal function increased significantly in the GA group than in the SA group ($P = 0.014$).

Maneuverability and accessibility among anesthetic methods

Between GA and SA, scores of maneuverability (5.50 ± 0.00 vs. 5.31 ± 3.44, $P = 0.726$) and accessibility (5.50 ± 0.00 vs. 5.44 ± 3.56, $P = 0.910$) during procedures were not different (Table 3). However, considering sedation during SA, maneuverability and accessibility were better in SA with sedation than in GA, but worse in SA without sedation than in GA. Maneuverability was 'so so' (5.50 ± 0.00) in GA, 'very good' (9.04 ± 1.20) in SA with sedation, and nearly 'poor' (2.61 ± 1.23) in SA without sedation ($P < 0.001$). In addition, accessibility was 'so so' (5.50 ± 0.00) in GA, 'very good' (9.19 ± 0.75) in SA with sedation, and 'poor' (2.72 ± 1.83) in SA without sedation ($P < 0.001$).

Discussion

The present study compared, for the first time, changes in renal function using renogram after GA with those after SA in RIRS for renal stones. There was no difference in postoperative change in serum creatinine level and estimated glomerular filtration rate between the GA and SA groups. However, patients of SA group showed improvements in separate renal function recovery. The difference in separate renal function between the operative and contralateral sites increased significantly in patients under GA than those under SA 3 months postoperatively. So far other studies concluded that renal function did not worsen postoperatively after they evaluated only serum creatinine level. However, we evaluated separate renal function with DTPA renal scan, and there

Table 3 Maneuverability and accessibility among anesthetic methods

	General anesthesia ($n = 39$)	Spinal anesthesia ($n = 31$)	P value
Maneuverability			0.726
Very poor (1–2)	0	9	
Poor (3–4)	0	8	
So so (5–6)	39	2	
Good (7–8)	0	1	
Very good (9–10)	0	11	
Accessibility			0.910
Very poor (1–2)	0	11	
Poor (3–4)	0	4	
So so (5–6)	39	2	
Good (7–8)	0	3	
Very good (9–10)	0	11	

*Some SA patients had sedation

might be some potential negative effect from GA. Postoperative pain after GA was higher than after SA on the first postoperative morning; however, the pain scores were similar prior to discharge. This study also evaluated maneuverability and accessibility during surgery, and SA with sedation showed better maneuverability and accessibility than GA. In addition, some studies reported that surgeries under regional anesthesia could show reduced major complications (for example, mortality, morbidity, and myocardial infarction) than those under GA [2–4]. In general, urologists routinely prefer GA for RIRS in patients with renal stones. Under GA, surgeons can be more comfortable due to decreased patient movement by controlling breathing [21].

Safety and efficacy of SA compared with that of GA during PNL have been reported several times [22–25]. Karacalar and colleagues suggested that spinal-epidural anesthesia along with intravenous patient-controlled sedation could be an alternative to GA [22]. The incidence of nausea and the use of antiemetics were significantly higher in GA ($P = 0.01$ and 0.001, respectively), and patients reported better satisfaction ($P = 0.001$) and lower pain scores ($P = 0.001$) after spinal-epidural anesthesia. Kuzgunbay and colleagues compared surgical outcomes of PNL between GA and SA [23]. There were no significant differences in SFR, and clinically insignificant residue fragments rates were observed between the two groups ($P = 0.543$). Moreover, there were no significant differences among the surgical parameters ($P = 0.439$); thus, it was suggested that SA did not affect the efficacy and safety of PNL. In 2011, Singh and coworkers performed a prospective and randomized study comparing surgical parameters between GA and SA during PNL [24]. There were no significant differences in complete stone clearance. However, patients after SA used lesser doses of analgesics and had shorter hospital stay. Even in treatment of staghorn stone, PNL was performed safely and effectively under SA [25].

Some studies have reported GA as a risk factor for renal dysfunction after non-urologic surgeries as well [26–28]. An overview of randomized trials commented that regional anesthesia reduced postoperative serious complications [26]. There were reductions in overall mortality, cardiopulmonary complications, and renal failure after SA. Hassan and colleagues investigated renal function change after total hip replacement operation [27]. Patients were classified to have renal impairment using relative increase in serum creatinine level. GA was one of significant risk factors for elevation of serum creatinine levels ($P = 0.0083$). The same authors also reported that GA was a risk factor for renal dysfunction after total knee replacement [28].

Until recently, feasibility of SA for RIRS had been rarely reported. In 2015, Zeng and coworkers conducted a prospective randomized trial to evaluate feasibility of SA for patients undergoing RIRS [13]. There were no significant differences in SFR ($P = 0.804$), postoperative pain ($P = 0.146$), and incidence of complications ($P = 0.870$). Patients in the GA group bore higher medical costs; however, the reports made no comments about sedation during SA. Karabulut and colleagues suggested that SA could be an option for RIRS [13]. There were no significant differences in SFR and postoperative complication rates between SA and GA ($P > 0.05$). Moreover, SA had advantages of lesser postoperative pain and lower medical costs ($P < 0.001$). However, both studies did not evaluate renal function change using renogram after RIRS. In our study, changes in serum creatinine and glomerular filtration rate were not significantly different between the two methods ($P = 0.792$ and 0.807, respectively). The immediate postoperative serum creatinine level did not show the serum creatinine changes due to the short postoperative period. However, the difference of separate renal function between the operative and contralateral sites increased in the GA group at postoperative 3 months ($P = 0.014$). Separate renal function might be affected negatively by GA. Therefore, it might be desirable not to conclude that separate renal function is not deteriorated after only serum creatinine level is evaluated. Present study also assessed maneuverability and accessibility of operator, which were better in SA with sedation than GA. However, the maneuverability and accessibility during SA without sedation were poorer than those during GA, so overall SFR after GA was higher than that after SA in this study.

Although this study had some limitations, to the best of our knowledge, our study was the first prospective, randomized study to compare change in renal function using renogram between SA and GA after RIRS, and to evaluate the surgical performance of the operator. First, the small sample size was a limitation of this study; thus, there was an imbalance between the number of patients after permuted block randomization. Moreover, the authors used the Chronic Kidney Disease Epidemiology Collaboration (CKD-EPI) creatinine-based equation or the Modification of Diet in Renal Disease (MDRD) Study equation in patients with a relatively well-preserved kidney function according to patient status [see Appendix]. The tidal volume during GA was independently chosen by the anesthesiologist, and sedation during SA was decided by patients just before surgery. Further studies comparing GA with low tidal volume and SA with sedation would be helpful to determine a better anesthetic strategy. Maneuverability and accessibility were measured subjectively by the operator, but all measurements were carried out by one experienced operator (SY Cho).

Conclusions

There were no significant differences in changes in serum creatinine level and estimated glomerular filtration rate between GA and SA groups immediately. Also, operator performance was better under GA than under SA in general. However, RIRS under SA showed advantages in renal function change using renogram at postoperative 3 months and in lower pain score on the first postoperative morning. In addition, the performance of operator was significantly improved under SA with sedation. Hence, this topic warrants further investigations to evaluate safer and more convenient analgesic settings during RIRS.

Appendix

Modification of Diet in Renal Disease (MDRD) Study equation.

eGFR(ml/min/1.73 m2) = 186 × (serum creatinine) - 1.154 × (age) - 0.203 × (0.742 if female) × (1.212 if black).

Chronic Kidney Disease Epidemiology Collaboration (CKD-EPI) creatinine-based.

Equation.

$\text{eGFR(ml/min/1.73 m2)} = 141 \times \min(\text{Scr}/\kappa,1)^{\alpha} \times \max(\text{Scr}/\kappa,1)^{-1.209} \times 0.993^{\text{Age}} \times (1.018 \text{ if female}) \times (1.212 \text{ if Black})$.

$\kappa = 0.7$ for females and 0.9 for males.

$\alpha = -0.329$ for remales, -0.411 for males.

min: minimum of Scr/κ or 1.

max: maximum of Scr/κ or 1.

Abbreviations

CT: computed tomography; EAU: European Association of Urology; GA: general anesthesia; PNL: percutaneous nephrolithotomy; RIRS: retrograde intrarenal surgery; SA: spinal anesthesia

Acknowledgements

Not applicable.

Authors' contributions

OK wrote the paper. OK, RSH, SYC analyzed the data. JML performed all anesthesia in this study. JP, MCC, HS, HJ all contributed patients. SYC designed this study and contributed in writing this manuscript. All authors read and approved the final manuscript.

Authors' information

Professor Sung Yong Cho, the corresponding author, is one of the core members of Asian Urolithiasis Guideline panel in the Urological Association of Asia (UAA).

Author details

[1]Department of Urology, Hallym University Kangnam Sacred Heart Hospital, Seoul, South Korea. [2]Department of Anesthesiology and Pain Medicine, SMG-SNU Boramae Medical Center, Seoul, South Korea. [3]Department of Urology, SMG-SNU Boramae Medical Center, Seoul, South Korea. [4]Department of Urology, Seoul National University Hospital, 101, Daehak-ro Jongno-gu, 03080 Seoul, Republic of Korea.

References

1. Türk C, Petřík A, Sarica K, Seitz C, Skolarikos A, Straub M, et al. EAU guidelines on interventional treatment for Urolithiasis. Eur Urol. 2016;69: 475–82.
2. Ruppert V, Leurs LJ, Rieger J, Steckmeier B, Buth J, Umscheid T. EUROSTAR Collaborators Risk-adapted outcome after endovascular aortic aneurysm repair: analysis of anesthesia types based on EUROSTAR data. J Endovasc Ther. 2007;14:12–22.
3. Eck DL, Koonce SL, Goldberg RF, Bagaria S, Gibson T, Bowers SP, et al. Breast surgery outcomes as quality measures according to the NSQIP database. Ann Surg Oncol. 2012;19:3212–7.
4. Kfoury E, Dort J, Trickey A, Crosby M, Donovan J, Hashemi H, et al. Carotid endarterectomy under local and/or regional anesthesia has less risk of myocardial infarction compared to general anesthesia: an analysis of national surgical quality improvement program database. Vascular. 2015;23:113–9.
5. Schulz-Stübner S. The critically ill patient and regional anesthesia. Curr Opin Anaesthesiol. 2006;19:538–44.
6. Khan SA, Qianyi RL, Liu C, Ng EL, Fook-Chong S, Tan MG. Effect of anaesthetic technique on mortality following major lower extremity amputation: a propensity score-matched observational study. Anaesthesia. 2013;68:612–20.
7. Guay J, Choi PT, Suresh S, Albert N, Kopp S, Pace NL. Neuraxial anesthesia for the prevention of postoperative mortality and major morbidity: an overview of cochrane systematic reviews. Anesth Analg. 2014;119:716–25.
8. Afolabi BB, Lesi FE. Regional versus general anaesthesia for caesarean section. Cochrane Database Syst Rev. 2012;10:CD004350.
9. Guay J, Parker MJ, Gajendragadkar PR, Kopp S. Anaesthesia for hip fracture surgery in adults. Cochrane Database Syst Rev. 2016;2:CD000521.
10. Johnson RL, Kopp SL, Burkle CM, Duncan CM, Jacob AK, Erwin PJ, et al. Neuraxial vs general anaesthesia for total hip and total knee arthroplasty: a systematic review of comparative-effectiveness research. Br J Anaesth. 2016; 116:163–76.
11. Choo MS, Park J, Cho MC, Son H, Jeong H, Cho SY. Changes in separate renal function in patients who underwent minimally invasive renal stone surgery according to the preoperative functional deterioration. Sci Rep. 2019;9:3610.
12. Alizadeh R, Fard ZA. Renal effects of general anesthesia from old to recent studies. J Cell Physiol. 2019;234:16944–52.
13. Zeng G, Zhao Z, Yang F, Zhong W, Wu W, Chen W. Retrograde intrarenal surgery with combined spinal-epidural vs general anesthesia: a prospective randomized controlled trial. J Endourol. 2015;29:401–5.
14. Bosio A, Dalmasso E, Alessandria E, Agosti S, Pizzuto G, Peretti D, et al. Retrograde intra-renal surgery under spinal anesthesia: the first large series. Minerva Urol Nefrol. 2018;70:333–9.

15. Karabulut I, Koc E, Yilmaz AH, Ahiskali EO, Keskin E, Adanur S, et al. Could spinal anesthesia be a choice for retrograde intrarenal surgery. Urologia. 2018;85:169–73.
16. Kwon O, Park J, Cho MC, Son H, Jeong H, Cho SY. Feasibility of single-session endoscopic combined intrarenal surgery for ipsilateral large renal stones and retrograde intrarenal surgery for contralateral renal stones: initial experience. Int J Urol. 2017;24:377–82.
17. Park J, Oh S, Cho MC, Son H, Jeong H, Jeong CW, et al. The acceptable criterion of stone burden and the significant factors to choose retrograde intrarenal stone surgery or miniaturized percutaneous nephrolithotomy for the treatment of renal stones >10 mm. J Endourol. 2017;31:1012–8.
18. Resorlu B, Oguz U, Resorlu EB, Oztuna D, Unsal A. The impact of pelvicaliceal anatomy on the success of retrograde intrarenal surgery in patients with lower pole renal stones. Urology. 2012;79:61–6.
19. Jeong CW, Jung JW, Cha WH, Lee BK, Lee S, Jeong SJ, et al. Seoul National University Renal Stone Complexity Score for predicting stone-free rate after percutaneous nephrolithotomy. PLoS One. 2013;8:e65888.
20. Dindo D, Demartines N, Clavien PA. Classification of surgical complications: a new proposal with evaluation in a cohort of 6336 patients and results of a survey. Ann Surg. 2004;240:205–13.
21. Emiliani E, Talso M, Baghdadi M, Ghanem S, Golmard J, Pinheiro H, et al. The use of apnea during ureteroscopy. Urology. 2016;97:266–8.
22. Karacalar S, Bilen CY, Sarihasan B, Sarikaya S. Spinal-epidural anesthesia versus general anesthesia in the management of percutaneous nephrolithotripsy. J Endourol. 2009;23:1591–7.
23. Kuzgunbay B, Turunc T, Akin S, Ergenoglu P, Aribogan A, Ozkardes H. Percutaneous nephrolithotomy under general versus combined spinal-epidural anesthesia. J Endourol. 2009;23:1835–8.
24. Singh V, Sinha RJ, Sankhwar SN, Malik A. A prospective randomized study comparing percutaneous nephrolithotomy under combined spinal-epidural anesthesia with percutaneous nephrolithotomy under general anesthesia. Urol Int. 2011;87:293–8.
25. Buldu I, Tepeler A, Kaynar M, Karatag T, Tosun M, Umutogluv T, et al. Comparison of anesthesia methods in treatment of staghorn kidney stones with percutaneous nephrolithotomy. Urol J. 2016;13:2479–83.
26. Rodgers A, Walker N, Schug S, McKee A, Kehlet H, van Zundert A, et al. Reduction of postoperative mortality and morbidity with epidural or spinal anaesthesia: results from overview of randomised trials. BMJ. 2000;321:1493.
27. Hassan BK, Sahlström A, Dessau RB. Risk factors for renal dysfunction after total hip joint replacement; a retrospective cohort study. J Orthop Surg Res. 2015;10:158.
28. Hassan B, Sahlström A, Dessau R. Risk factors for renal dysfunction after total knee joint replacement. Acta Orthop Belg. 2015;81:647–53.

16

Unveiling what is absent with in: Illustrating anesthetic considerations in a patient with hydranencephaly

Alexis R. Tovar and Allison L. Thoeny*

Abstract

Background: Hydranencephaly is a rare and debilitating congenital condition in which most anesthesiologists are unfamiliar. Primary surgical treatment involves CSF diversion, though other palliative procedures requiring anesthesia are often required. With medical advancements and a resulting prolonged life expectancy, caring for these patients is becoming more routine.

Case presentation: We follow an infant with hydranencephaly over three different procedures requiring anesthesia from 5 months of age to 2 years, highlighting the various anesthetic considerations.

Conclusions: Anticipation of difficult positioning, deliberate airway management, and attention to anesthetic recovery were all necessary to safely care for this patient. An understanding of the challenges this particular condition poses will help anesthesiologists provide the most safe and effective care when encountering these patients.

Keywords: Hydranencephaly, Positioning, Airway, Anesthetic recovery, Palliative

Background

Hydranencephaly is a rare congenital condition that occurs in less than 1 in 10,000 births in which brain development is severely restricted [1]. Cerebral structures are often limited to brainstem and thalamus only, with cerebral spinal fluid (CSF) filling a membranous sac normally inhabited by cerebral cortex [2, 3]. Diagnosis can initially be overlooked at birth due to preservation of brainstem functions, or may be confused with simple congenital hydrocephalus [3, 4]. However, within the first few weeks complications such as increased intracranial pressure (ICP), temperature dysregulation, and aspiration will arise along with a progressively enlarging head circumference [2]. As a consequence, neurological prognosis is poor and the life expectancy of these patients is reduced, with the majority dying within a few weeks or months after birth [2, 3, 5].

According to neurosurgical literature, survival in hydranencephaly past age five in the modern treatment era is becoming more common [5]. It is therefore likely that anesthesiologists will encounter such patients surviving into childhood who require anesthesia for cerebral imaging and other palliative procedures. Anesthetic considerations of the infant with hydranencephaly are complex, and pose a permanently greater challenge than hydrocephalus, due to their grave neurologic prognosis. Comprehensive management of these patients including airway, optimal anesthetic choice, safety of muscle relaxants, and postoperative monitoring has yet to be described in the anesthetic literature. We therefore delineate three separate anesthetic encounters in a patient with hydranencephaly from infancy to toddlerhood in an endeavor to augment literature on anesthetic management of such patients. Written HIPAA consent was

* Correspondence: athoeny@email.arizona.edu
University of Arizona, 1501 N Campbell Ave, Room 4401, PO Box 245114, Tucson, AZ 85724, USA

obtained from the patient's parent for the publication of this case report. This manuscript adheres to the applicable EQUATOR guideline.

Case presentation

Our patient was born full-term via cesarean section. At 30 week's gestation, a diagnosis of hydranencephaly was made with fetal ultrasound (US). At the time of delivery, his Appearance, Pulse, Grimace, Activity, and Respiration (APGAR) scores were 7 and 9 at 1 and 5 min. Primitive reflexes were intact, and physical exam was unremarkable with the exception of macrocephaly. His initial head circumference was approximately 40 cm, and his birth weight was 3.6 kg. Palliative care was consulted and helped initiate goals of care discussion and coordination of hospice care with the family. He was made "do not resuscitate" and discharged home with a poor prognosis.

Follow-up with primary care did not happen until he was 5 months of age, as the family reported difficulty with traveling given his worsening head size. They also reported progressive episodes of apnea and seizures. An MRI was ordered to evaluate for presence of cerebral tissues, and Neurosurgery was consulted for palliative shunting.

His MRI took place at 5 months of age. Head circumference measured 64 cm, and his weight was 9.5 kg. General anesthesia with a supraglottic airway device was planned as opposed to endotracheal tube (ETT) intubation due to the brevity of the procedure and intact laryngeal reflexes. Patient was placed on an MRI-compatible bed with a large shoulder roll to optimize sniffing position, given his macrocephaly. Mask induction with 8% sevoflurane followed by supraglottic airway device placement and intravenous (IV) access was uneventful. He was maintained on 2% sevoflurane. Emergence from anesthesia was performed outside the scanner to facilitate ease of access to all airway and emergency equipment. Upon removal of the airway device under low volatile concentration and presumed awake anesthetic depth, the patient went into laryngospasm. This quickly resolved with positive pressure ventilation. He was monitored for several more minutes before being transported to the post-anesthesia care unit (PACU). In PACU, he recovered without any further complications. No seizures were witnessed postoperatively, and he was discharged home.

MRI imaging revealed intact brainstem and a nearly absent cerebral cortex replaced by a large membranous sac of CSF, consistent with hydranencephaly (Fig. 1). The patient underwent palliative ventriculoperitoneal shunt placement at 8 months of age at an outside hospital (Fig. 2).

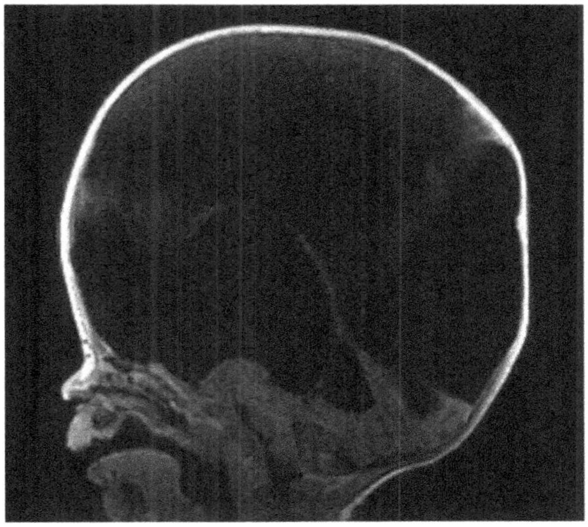

Fig. 1 MRI sagittal view with brain parenchyma in posterior fossa, cerebral falx, thalamus, brainstem, and cerebellum visualized

At 22 months of age, he returned to our institution for laparoscopic gastrostomy tube placement and management of chronic constipation secondary to opioid use as palliative medication. At presentation, he was 14.2 kg with a head circumference of 68 cm. Patient was placed supine, with blue towels underneath his shoulders to act as a shoulder roll. A gel ring was placed underneath his head for stabilization, and mask induction was performed (Fig. 3). A 24-gauge IV was obtained, he was given propofol, and his airway was secured easily using a Miller 1 blade and a 3.5 mm cuffed tube. Due to his significant baseline hypotonia, paralytic was not administered. Sevoflurane was used for maintenance of anesthesia. During the case, he also received 1.2 mg morphine for pain management, which was half of his normal home dose. Temperature was monitored with a nasopharyngeal probe, and he remained normothermic with the use of an underbody forced-air warming device and maintenance of warm ambient temperatures. Upon emergence, when noted to grimace and cry with an undetectable end-tidal volatile concentration, he was extubated. Recovery in PACU was unremarkable, and he was admitted for post-operative monitoring. His post-operative course was remarkable for opioid dependence and agitation, requiring a 24 day inpatient stay for treatment of opioid withdrawal.

Ten months later, the patient returned with stridor and labored breathing. He had several admissions prior to this for recurrent pulmonary infections, concerning for repeated aspiration events. Computed tomography (CT) imaging at this admission revealed tonsillar hypertrophy and concern for pneumonia. He was admitted to the pediatric intensive care unit (PICU) and placed on

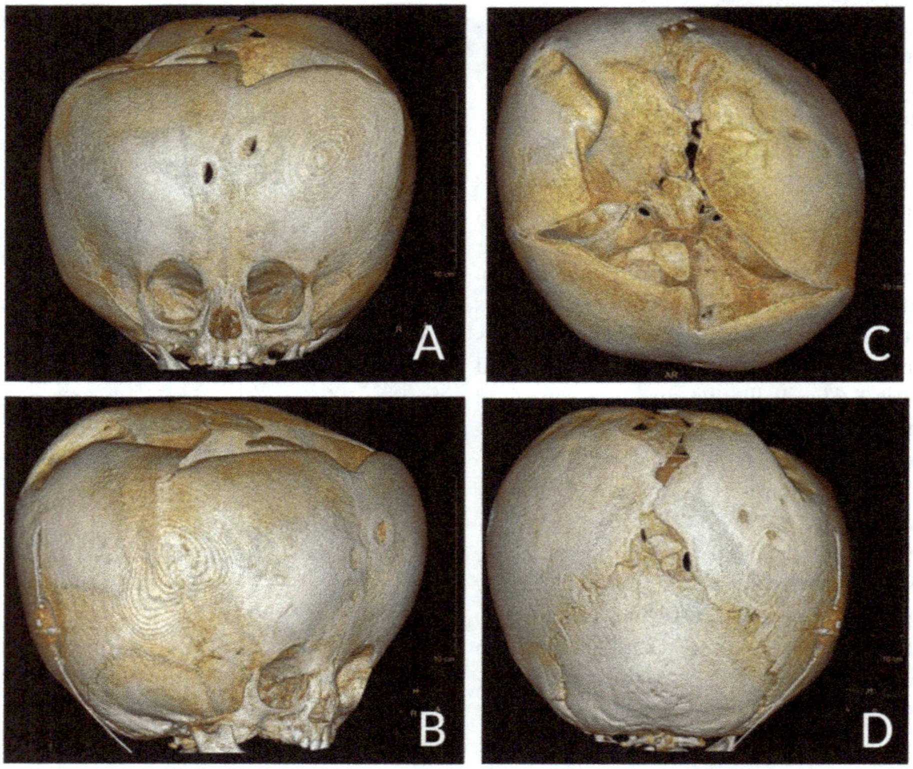

Fig. 2 a-d 3D CT reconstruction of patient's cranium and face after ventriculoperitoneal shunt placement

broad spectrum antibiotics for treatment of community-acquired versus aspiration pneumonia. On day 2 of admission, he underwent direct laryngoscopy and bilateral adenotonsillectomy for diagnostic and potential therapeutic treatment of his stridor. Given concern for increased airway difficulty due to his exaggerated macrocephaly, tonsillar hypertrophy, and reactive airway, spontaneous respirations were maintained during initial direct laryngoscopy with video laryngoscope using a combination of sevoflurane and IV dexmedetomidine and fentanyl. During the initial attempt at endotracheal intubation the patient went into laryngospasm with resulting hypoxia and bradycardia, which persisted despite deepening anesthetic depth and applying positive pressure ventilation. He was immediately given IV succinylcholine as well as IV atropine, with resolution of the laryngospasm. The airway was secured during the second attempt with moderate difficulty due to tonsillar hypertrophy. A 4.0 uncuffed ETT was chosen due to concerns for worsening laryngeal edema and the potential for unresolved stridor, with plans to remain intubated postoperatively. He was transported immediately back to the PICU for post-operative recovery and management, where he was successfully extubated the following day. His hospital course was complicated by returning to the operating room for tonsillar hemorrhage 9 days later, as well as for intermittent hypoxia. After 14 days in the hospital he was discharged home with oxygen.

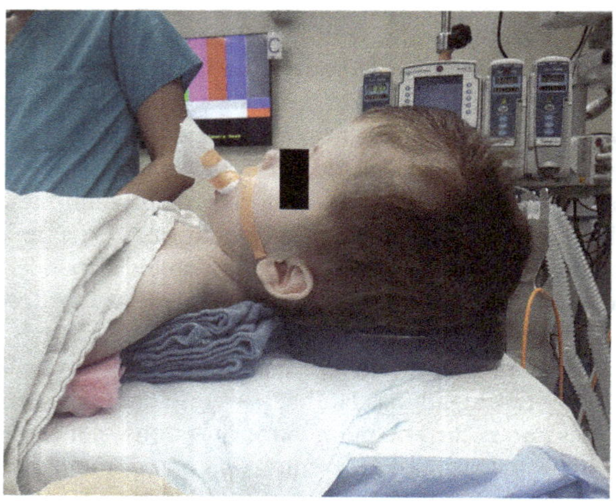

Fig. 3 Patient with large shoulder roll and gel ring to aid in obtaining a sniffing position during induction and emergence

Discussion

Hydranencephaly represents a rare form of disturbance in cerebral development, nevertheless one increasingly encountered by anesthesiologists. The pathogenesis of the destruction of cerebral hemispheres is not well defined, but is generally considered to be due to an occlusion of the bilateral internal carotid arteries between the 8th and 12th weeks of gestation [2]. The cause for this occlusion can be variable (i.e. infectious, iatrogenic, genetic), and thus mirrors the variability seen in brain development and clinical presentation in each child [2, 3].

Prenatal diagnosis has historically been lacking, though increasingly improved with the advent of routine fetal ultrasound [2]. Approximately 1% of infants diagnosed with congenital hydrocephalus actually have hydranencephaly; differentiation between these two diagnoses is critical as congenital hydrocephalus has a significantly better prognosis [1]. However, with the quality of medical care and surgical interventions now available, life expectancy in hydranencephaly can extend once a child survives past their first 2 years of life [6].

Treatment in this population is non-curative and involves ethical and medical considerations of what course may be optimal for each child, as the degree of neurologic impairment is not improved with surgical intervention. Surgical interventions, namely CSF diversion procedures, are being performed around the world however with success in improving quality and duration of life in hydranencephaly [5, 7]. Anesthesiologists are thus tasked with providing care beyond initial palliative shunting, which may include anything from shunt revisions to enteral feeding access.

A careful and deliberate approach to anesthetic care of these rare and poorly affected patients is a daunting task for any anesthesiologist as management is largely unknown. Apart from one report we found demonstrating feasible ketamine use in an infant with hydranencephaly in 1974 [8], the literature is void of anesthetic management in hydranencephaly. Given the irreversible extent of neurologic disturbance in these infants, we believe the considerations for anesthesia in patients with hydranencephaly are in fact complex, and as seen in our patient, may include anticipation of difficult positioning, airway management, optimal anesthetic technique, and anesthetic recovery. Maintaining appropriate hemodynamics and normothermia are also essential as complications from increased intracranial pressure, such as aspiration and seizures, can occur [2].

With any exaggerated macrocephaly, as previously discussed in management of infants with hydrocephalus [9], it is vital to allow proper extension of the head in sniffing position by placing a large shoulder roll and stabilizing the head with a small towel or ring. In anticipation of a difficult airway, maintaining spontaneous ventilation is beneficial. We believe that using sevoflurane for mask induction may be advantageous, given the possible decreased intracranial compliance. With the anticipation of a difficult airway, the use of a video laryngoscope as the initial form of laryngoscopy or as an alternative can also be considered.

If IV induction is feasible and the airway appears favorable, rapid sequence intubation may be considered given the higher aspiration risk to these patients. A non-depolarizing agent is arguably best for paralysis as succinylcholine can result in profound bradycardia in infants with autonomic dysfunction, which is a presumed expectation in this population. Alternatively, if succinylcholine is required for ideal intubating conditions or as an emergency rescue medication, as was the case in our patient for resolution of laryngospasm, one should administer atropine concurrently. Consideration of the risk-benefit balance between aspiration risk and neuromuscular recovery in each patient context is prudent, however. This may lead the clinician to avoid use of neuromuscular relaxants all together, as was the case for our patient during his gastrostomy tube placement.

Maintenance of anesthesia may be accomplished with volatile or IV anesthetics, as an optimal agent for patients with hydranencephaly has not been identified in literature. Though maintenance of cerebral perfusion pressure (CPP) may not be as critical in these children due to lack of cerebral structures, an agent that decreases ICP and maintains hemodynamics is still beneficial to avoid seizures, aspiration, and maintain cardiac output to other vital organs.

Our patient tolerated sevoflurane anesthesia over three different procedures very well. An alternative for shorter procedural sedation may be ketamine. Although ketamine is a relative contraindication with increased ICP due to its ability to increase cerebral metabolic rate, it does preserve cerebral blood flow and mean arterial pressure. In fact, a clinical trial of 30 intensive care pediatric patients receiving ketamine as procedural sedation or as therapy for intracranial hypertension demonstrated an increased CPP and decreased ICP by 30% [10]. Ketamine has been used as a successful alternative in the past in an infant with hydranencephaly [8].

Another challenge is that assessment of recovery from anesthesia may prove difficult, given limited cognitive function and general hypotonia [3]. It is critical to completely reverse any residual paralysis in order to return the patient to baseline neuromuscular tone. Patients with hydranencephaly are at risk for respiratory distress and prolonged mechanical ventilation [5]. If benzodiazepines or narcotics are required, short-acting agents should be chosen to facilitate a rapid recovery and avoid post anesthetic apneic events. To avoid airway complications during emergence as seen in our patient, adequate time should be given for elimination of anesthetic effects and stable respiratory mechanics observed before extubation is attempted.

There are limitations to our observations seen in this case report that merit acknowledgement. Principally, we practice at an academic institution in which a different attending and resident anesthesiologist cared for our patient at each anesthetic encounter, reflecting the variability in anesthetic technique and management between encounters. This further emphasizes the importance of publishing collective observations and recommendations to guide future anesthetic considerations of hydranencephaly. Furthermore, since we did not employ IV drugs such as propofol for maintenance of anesthesia, we are unable to comment if that might constitute a good choice. Lastly, we understand that further study of other children with hydranencephaly is indicated to draw formal conclusions about anesthetic management.

Patients with hydranencephaly are a rare population to encounter, even for a pediatric anesthesiologist. However, with advancing medical capabilities and extended life expectancy, these encounters are becoming more common. Though similar to congenital hydrocephalus in terms of airway management and difficulty with positioning, patients with hydranencephaly distinguish themselves by being a continuing anesthetic challenge throughout their life; this is in part due to their lack of neurological recovery after CSF diversion procedures. With keen preparation and consideration of difficult positioning, airway, and anesthetic recovery, anesthesiologists can provide a safe and efficacious anesthetic for the variety of procedures that these children may require.

Abbreviations

APGAR : Appearance, pulse, grimace, activity, and respiration; CPP : Cerebral perfusion pressure; CSF : Cerebrospinal fluid; CT : Computed tomography; ETT : Endotracheal tube; ICP : Intracranial pressure; IV : Intravenous; MRI : Magnetic resonance imaging; PACU : Post anesthesia care unit; PICU : Pediatric intensive care unit; US : Ultrasound

Acknowledgements

We want to thank Dr. Vance Nielsen for his guidance and advice regarding article composition in preparation for publication.

Authors' contributions

ART helped draft, conceive, and design the written work. ART also obtained informed consent for publication from the patient's mother. ALT helped oversee the drafting and editing of the work. All authors read and approved the final manuscript.

Author's information

ART is a resident physician anesthesiologist at the University of Arizona. ALT is a Clinical Assistant Professor in pediatric anesthesiology at the University of Arizona.

References

1. Wijerathne BT, Rathnayake GK, Ranaraja SK. A rare variation of hydranencephaly: case report. F1000Research. 2014;1:22.
2. Cecchetto G, Milanese L, Giordano R, Viero A, Suma V, Manara R. Looking at the missing brain: hydranencephaly case series and literature review. Pediatr Neurol. 2013;48:152–8.
3. Pavone P, Praticò AD, Vitaliti G, Ruggieri M, Rizzo R, Parano E, et al. Hydranencephaly: cerebral spinal fluid instead of cerebral mantles. Ital J Pediatr. 2014;40:79.
4. Huff N, Naik S. Hydranencephaly in Monochorionic-Diamniotic twins. Pediatr Neurol. 2017;67:107–8.
5. Akutsu N, Azumi M, Koyama J, Kawamura A, Taniguchi M, Kohmura E. Management and problems of prolonged survival with hydranencephaly in the modern treatment era. Childs Nerv Syst. 2020;36:1239–43.
6. Merker B. Life expectancy in hydranencephaly. Clin Neurol Neurosurg. 2008; 110:213–4.
7. Thiong'o GM, Ferson SS, Albright AL. Hydranencephaly treatments: retrospective case series and review of the literature. J Neurosurg Pediatr. 2020. https://doi.org/10.3171/2020.3.PEDS19596.
8. Morse N, Smith PC. Ketamine anesthesia in a hydranencephalic infant. Anesthesiology. 1974;40:407–9.
9. Sharma J, Purohit S, Sharma M, Kumar M. A case of massive hydrocephalus; perioperative challenges and literature review. Anaesth Intensive Care. 2016; 20:353–7.
10. Bar-Joseph G, Guilburd Y, Tamir A, Guilburd JN. Effectiveness of ketamine in decreasing intracranial pressure in children with intracranial hypertension. J Neurosurg Pediatr. 2009;4:40–6.

17

Grisel's syndrome: A case report on this rare pediatric disease and its anesthetic challenges

Kavya N. Reddy[1], Shabaaz M. Baig[2], Meenu Batra[2], Kevin Colodner[3], Uchenna Maduouko[4], Anna Korban[2] and Shridevi Pandya Shah[2*]

Abstract

Background: Grisel's syndrome is a non-traumatic atlantoaxial subluxation associated with inflammatory conditions of the head and neck, which occurs primarily in children. Increased flexibility of the ligaments during inflammation is implicated in the pathogenesis of the subluxation between the axis and atlas. The potential sequelae may be severe, and early diagnosis and treatment of Grisel's syndrome can prevent tragic outcomes.

Case presentation: We present a case of torticollis in an 8-year-old child. She had a two-week history of a streptococcal throat infection. The patient was treated with several different methods of conservative care, including muscle relaxation, cervical halter traction, and Halo application. However, the torticollis persisted. The patient then required surgical correction involving cervical spine fusion. She had no complications and experienced no reoccurrence of the torticollis to date.

Conclusion: Grisel's syndrome is a pathology for which conservative management is successful in most cases. Cases requiring surgical intervention are rarely documented in the literature. Our case is significant, as in spite of aggressive conservative management, the patient required surgical correction. Patients requiring surgical management of Grisel's syndrome may require additional anesthetic exposure for diagnostic interventions like magnetic resonance imaging or neck manipulations for closed reduction. We discuss the features of Grisel's syndrome and specific anesthetic management considerations for procedures such as magnetic resonance imaging, application of cervical traction, and surgical correction of torticollis.

Keywords: Grisel's syndrome, Atlantoaxial subluxation (AAS), Pediatric anesthesia, Airway management, Positioning, Cervical spine

* Correspondence: pandyas1@njms.rutgers.edu
[2]Department of Anesthesiology, Rutgers New Jersey Medical School, 185 South Orange Ave, MSB-E 577, Newark, NJ 07103, USA

Background

Nontraumatic atlantoaxial subluxation (AAS) is a rare complication of upper respiratory tract infections and otolaryngologic surgeries first described by Sir Charles Bell in 1830 in a patient with syphilis, pharyngitis, and lethal spinal compression. A century later, a French physician, Grisel, described two cases of pharyngitis and nontraumatic AAS and named it Grisel's syndrome [1]. Grisel's syndrome refers only to non-traumatic AAS, and most commonly occurs after an upper respiratory infection, though some unusual causes include mumps, tuberculosis, and Kawasaki disease [2]. It may also be seen after certain otolaryngologic operations such as adenoidectomies, tonsillectomies, and ear surgeries.

Grisel's syndrome is most often seen in children but may also be seen in adults. Originally, Grisel theorized that the subluxation occurs secondary to muscular spasm. The most recent explanation is the two-hit hypothesis, which posits that hyperemia following infection or trauma leads to decalcification of the anterior arch of C1 and laxity of the transverse ligament [3]. Fielding has characterized four different types of rotatory AAS (see Table 1) [4].

Types I and II are most often seen without any neurological deficits and are typically resolved conservatively with oral non-steroidal anti-inflammatory drugs (NSAIDs), antibiotics, physical therapy, and the collar. Types III and IV are more severe and are associated with neurological deficits and serious complications and are managed with surgical fusion. The most definitive imaging modalities for AAS are computed tomography (CT) and magnetic resonance imaging (MRI) studies.

In our study, we review the literature published so far, which indicates the most common etiologies, diagnostic modalities, and management of these patients. There is, however, a paucity of literature regarding the anesthetic management of this pathology. We present the case of our patient with Grisel's syndrome who failed conservative management and had to undergo surgical fixation with a discussion on the anesthetic management and challenges we faced in this case.

Informed consent was obtained from the patient's parents for this clinical case report.

Case presentation

We report a case of an 8-year-old female with a 2-week history of recent streptococcal throat infection who presented to the emergency room with torticollis. She was treated conservatively with antibiotics, muscle relaxation, and physiotherapy. Neither an otolaryngology consult nor radiological tests were ordered. A month later, her torticollis persisted, for which she received a CT scan. It showed a C1-C2 AAS, which was consistent with a diagnosis of Grisel's syndrome. At this point, conservative management was continued with cervical halter traction of 5 lbs., which was subsequently increased to 8 lbs. during her month-long stay in the pediatric intensive care unit (PICU). Post manual reduction, she had full range of motion of her neck, and CT showed complete resolution of subluxation. However, she returned with persistent torticollis 3 months later. An MRI at this time showed C1-C2 rotatory subluxation with associated narrowing of the cervico-medullary junction. She underwent Halo application under anesthesia, which was uneventful. After a week, however, the patient showed no improvement. The next step was C1-C2 cervical fusion under general anesthesia in the operating room.

The patient was brought to the operating room and standard monitors were placed. Total intravenous anesthesia was requested by the surgeon as motor and somatosensory evoked potentials would be monitored during surgery. The patient was induced with 200 ml of propofol, 100 mcg of fentanyl, and 2 mg of versed through a preexisting intravenous (IV) line. No muscle relaxants or inhalational agents were used during induction or maintenance of anesthesia. The patient was intubated endotracheally using the video laryngoscope while maintaining inline stabilization of the neck and spinal cord. Patient had been intubated with use of conventional direct laryngoscopy during her previous anesthetic. And so fiberoptic bronchoscope was not required. A second large bore IV and arterial line were placed after intubation. Total intravenous anesthesia (TIVA) was used for maintenance with an infusion of 0.1–0.2 mcg/k/min remifentanil and 100–120 mcg/kg/min propofol as tolerated intraoperatively. Somatosensory evoked potentials and motor evoked potentials remained unchanged throughout the surgery. Duration of surgery was about 10 h. The estimated blood loss was one liter. The patient received 2 l of crystalloids, 250 cc of albumin, one unit of packed red blood cells, one unit of fresh frozen plasma, and 500 cc of cell saver. The patient had a foley placed prior to the surgery which showed a urine output of 800 ml. Given that the length of surgery was 10 h, the major fluid shift, and the need

Table 1 Types of Rotary Atlantoaxial Subluxation (AAS)

Type I	The atlas is rotated on the odontoid, and there is no anterior displacement of the atlas
Type II	The atlas is rotated on one lateral articular process with 3 to 5 mm of anterior atlas displacement
Type III	Rotation of the atlas with an anterior displacement greater than 5 mm
Type IV	Rotation and posterior displacement of the atlas

for immobilization, the patient was left intubated after surgery. The propofol infusion was continued postoperatively for sedation and she was transferred to the care of the PICU. She was extubated the next day. A follow-up CT scan showed a complete resolution of subluxation. Based upon follow up imaging (see Fig. 1), there were no adverse or unexpected outcomes.

Discussion

A PubMed search was performed using the phrases "Grisel's syndrome," "spontaneous AAS," and "ENT surgery complications." We made an extraction form focusing on the etiology, diagnostic modalities, treatment received (conservative or surgical), and follow-up outcomes. Single case reports and case series of both pediatric and adult cases were included. We identified 115 papers, of which 15 papers were excluded as they were not in English. We were able to analyze 100 papers evaluated by three independent reviewers. After an analysis of those 100 papers, we found 80 papers that met the inclusion criteria of nontraumatic AAS, Grisel's syndrome, and torticollis. Of those 80 papers included in the study, 62 were case reports (62 cases), 14 were case series (37 cases), and 4 were retrospective reviews (1 case report, 3 case series (20 cases)), making a total of 119 cases for our purposes. Out of these 119 cases, 55% described infection as the causative factor, and 45% had a post-surgical cause as the etiology. Adenoidectomy (30%), oto-surgery (15%), adenotonsillectomy (13%), and tympanoplasty (7%) were the most common surgical procedures established as the primary cause of AAS in the category of post-surgical AAS.

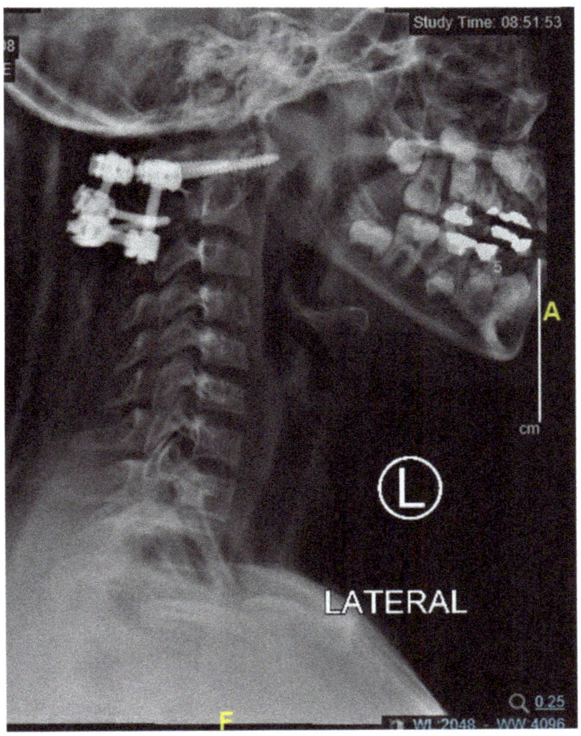

Fig. 1 lateral view of C1-C2 postsurgical fixation

Diagnosis of the disease process was by CT scan (55%) followed by X-ray only (19%), X-ray diagnosis with CT confirmation (18%), and direct MRI confirmation (8%). In our analysis, treatment for cases of infectious origin were successful mainly through conservative methods such as antibiotics, NSAIDs, cervical collars, or Halo application. Surgical fusion was employed in 17% of cases due to failed conservative treatment. In post-surgical patients, conservative treatment was successful in 93% of cases. The remainder had to undergo surgical fusion. The most likely reason for an increased failure of conservative management and the necessity of surgical fusion in the cohort of patients with an infectious etiology is the duration of symptoms and delayed diagnosis.

Grisel's syndrome is a diagnosis of exclusion. Differential diagnoses such as traumatic head posture and developmental torticollis that must be ruled out first. Congenital conditions that involve ligamentous laxities, such as Marfan syndrome and Down syndrome, are more susceptible to AAS [5]. Rare causes of AAS include tuberculosis [6] and Kawasaki disease [7]. Case reports have linked Grisel's to the use of monopolar suction electrocautery in adenoidectomy for bleeding control [5]. Karkos et al. reported 96 cases, of which 48% were due to infections [8]. Bocciolini et al. described 100 cases, of which 77 cases were caused by infection [9]. CT with 3D reconstruction proved to be an excellent method of documenting the presence and degree of AAS [5].

Neurological complications are infrequent but can be devastating and are seen in 15% of cases. They can range from radiculopathy to quadriplegia and death from respiratory failure due to medullary compression. Diagnosis of AAS should be based on a high degree of clinical suspicion as early detection and treatment are critical factors in preventing severe neurological complications. Post-surgical neck pain and torticollis are early signs of AAS and should not merely be attributed to the usual post-surgical pain and malaise.

Administration of anesthesia, especially airway management, in these patients presents a significant challenge. This is due to the abnormal laxity/inflammatory distention of cervical ligaments. These patients are at high risk of neurological injury during laryngoscopy, and tracheal intubation as a head extension or any sudden movements of the cervical spine may cause subluxation of the atlas over the axis, resulting in spinal cord compression. Therefore, one needs to maintain inline cervical stabilization, preferably using a video laryngoscope, and be prepared with a difficult airway cart including need for fiberoptic bronchoscope [10]. Gupta et al. also suggests using fentanyl for analgesia to prevent the general anesthetic complications of respiratory depression and myocardial depression [10]. Postoperatively patients with AAS must be carefully monitored for signs of neurological complications. Keeping the patient immobilized postoperatively and under close watch in the intensive care unit is one strategy to prevent these issues from arising. When patients require continued ventilation after surgery, consideration should be given to allow them to awaken after the procedure, to test for signs of myelopathy.

Positioning for otolaryngologic procedures such as tonsillectomies, direct laryngoscopies, or ear procedures also deserves deliberation. As positioning is an important part of anesthetic management, being aware of the optimal position for a patient with AAS is critical. This will help alleviate the chances of postoperative neurological complications commonly associated with AAS. For myringotomies, it is recommended to strap the patient to the operating room table securely, place supports alongside the head, and roll the table side to side, rather than turning the head. For airway procedures that usually involve head extension, it is crucial to communicate with the surgeon preoperatively about minimizing head and neck movement. It may be possible for the surgeon to perform the laryngoscopy or tonsillectomy without using suspension.

For urgent surgeries, the patient should be treated with cervical spine precautions. An unstable cervical spine will require neurological and electrophysiological monitoring. TIVA and delivery of anesthesia to patients with cervical traction and halo outside the operating room in MRI and CT suites can also be considered.

Grisel's syndrome remains a rare disease with little in the literature regarding its implications in anesthesia. If we review the literature, we may be able to find principles of anesthetic management for similar types of spine surgery. However, anesthetic management of Grisel's syndrome has its unique implications. Challenges include, but are not limited to, the usage of TIVA, airway management, positioning, and anesthesia outside of the operating room. The practicing anesthesiologist would be well served by being aware of this disease and its management to ensure the safety and health of their patients.

Abbreviations

AAS: Atlantoaxial Subluxation; NSAIDs: Non-steroidal Inflammatory Drugs; CT: Computed Tomography; MRI: Magnetic Resonance Imaging; IV: Intravenous; PICU: Pediatric Intensive Care Unit; TIVA: Total Intravenous Anesthesia

Acknowledgments

Not applicable.

Authors' contributions

KN functioned as the resident involved in the case, created a poster to be presented at annual IARS conference, worked on designing manuscript, reviewing the literature, and writing of the manuscript. SB was involved in writing, editing, and redesigning the manuscript as well as additional literature review and analysis. MB helped with editing the manuscript, redesigning, and journal search. KC reviewed the literature and assisted in the preparation of the poster. UM helped with the literature review and preparing statistics. AK was involved in the clinical care during anesthesia, reviewed literature, and helped with editing. SPS performed all required anesthetics on the patient. This is her original research. She contributed at every level, reviewing the literature, editing the article, and designing the manuscript. All authors have read and approved the manuscript.

Author details

Saint Louis University, St. Louis, USA. [2]Department of Anesthesiology, Rutgers New Jersey Medical School, 185 South Orange Ave, MSB-E 577, Newark, NJ 07103, USA. [3]University of Maryland, College Park, USA. [4]New York Medical College, Valhalla, USA.

References

1. Robinson PH, de Boer A. La maladie de Grisel: a rare occurrence of "spontaneous" atlanto-axial subluxation after pharyngoplasty. Br J Plast Surg. 1981;34(3):319–21.
2. Clark WC, Coscia M, Acker JD, Wainscott K, Robertson JT. Infection-related spontaneous atlantoaxial dislocation in an adult. Case report. J Neurosurg. 1988;69(3):455–8.
3. Battiata AP, Pazos G. Grisel's syndrome: the two-hit hypothesis--a case report and literature review. Ear Nose Throat J. 2004;83(8):553–5 PMID: 15487635.
4. Fielding JW, Hawkins RJ, Ratzan SA. Spine fusion for atlanto-axial instability. J Bone Joint Surg Am. 1976;58(3):400–7 PMID: 1262375.
5. Kraft M, Tschopp K. Evaluation of persistent torticollis following adenoidectomy. J Laryngol Otol. 2001;115(8):669–72.
6. Diom ES, Ndiaye C, Djafarou AB, Ndiaye IC, Faye PM, Tall A, et al. A case of cervical Pott's disease revealed by parapharyngeal abscess. Eur Ann Otorhinolaryngol Head Neck Dis. 2011;128(3):151–3. Available from. https://doi.org/10.1016/j.anorl.2010.12.005.
7. Nozaki F, Kusunoki T, Tomoda Y, Hiejima I, Hayashi A, Kumada T, et al. Grisel syndrome as a complication of Kawasaki disease: a case report and review of the literature. Eur J Pediatr. 2013;172(1):119–21.
8. Karkos PD, Benton J, Leong SC, Mushi E, Sivaji N, Assimakopoulos DA. Grisel's syndrome in otolaryngology: a systematic review. Int J Pediatr Otorhinolaryngol. 2007;71(12):1823–7.
9. Bocciolini C, Dall'Olio D, Cunsolo E, Cavazzuti PP, Laudadio P. Grisel's syndrome: a rare complication following adenoidectomy. Acta Otorhinolaryngol Ital. 2005;25(4):245.
10. Gupta A, Prakash J, Kumar P, Singh N. Anesthetic issues and difficult airway management in a case of grisel's syndrome. Anesth Essays Res. 2017;11(4):1094.

1-1-8 one-step sevoflurane wash-in scheme for low-flow anesthesia: Simple, rapid and predictable induction

Sirirat Tribuddharat, Thepakorn Sathitkarnmanee*, Naruemon Vattanasiriporn, Maneerat Thananun, Duangthida Nonlhaopol and Wilawan Somdee

Abstract

Background: Sevoflurane is suitable for low-flow anesthesia (LFA). LFA needs a wash-in phase. The reported sevoflurane wash-in schemes lack simplicity, target coverage, and applicability. We proposed a one-step 1-1-8 wash-in scheme for sevoflurane LFA to be used with both N_2O and Air. The objective of our study was to identify time for achieving each level of alveolar concentration of sevoflurane (F_AS) from 1 to 3.5% in both contexts.

Methods: We recruited 199 adults requiring general anesthesia with endotracheal intubation and controlled ventilation—102 in group N_2O and 97 in group Air. After induction and intubation, a wash-in was started using a fresh gas flow of O_2:N_2O or O_2:Air at 1:1 L·min^{-1} plus sevoflurane 8%. The ventilation was controlled to maintain end-tidal CO_2 of 30–35 mmHg.

Results: The rising patterns of F_AS and inspired concentration of sevoflurane (F_IS) are similar, running parallel between the groups. The F_AS/F_IS ratio increased from 0.46 to 0.72 within 260 s in group N_2O and from 0.42 to 0.69 within 286 s in group Air. The respective time to achieve an F_AS of 1, 1.5, 2, 2.5, 3, and 3.5% was 1, 1.5, 2, 3, 3.5, and 4.5 min in group N_2O and 1, 1.5, 2, 3, 4, and 5 min in group Air. The heart rate and blood pressure of both groups significantly increased initially then gradually decreased as F_AS increased.

Conclusions: The 1-1-8 wash-in scheme for sevoflurane LFA has many advantages, including simplicity, coverage, swiftness, safety, economy, and that it can be used with both N_2O and Air. A respective F_AS of 1, 1.5, 2, 2.5, 3, and 3.5% when used with N_2O and Air can be expected at 1, 1.5, 2, 3, 3.5, and 4.5 min and 1, 1.5, 2, 3, 4, and 5 min.

Keywords: Wash-in, Low flow anesthesia, Nitrous oxide, Air, Sevoflurane

Background

Low-flow anesthesia (LFA; fresh gas flow (FGF) ≤ 1 L·min^{-1}) is gaining in popularity because it has a relatively lower cost, causes less environmental burden, and medically because it increases the humidity and temperature of inspired gas, leading to improved mucociliary function of the patient [1]. Since use of low FGF leads to a long time constant, a wash-in phase using a high FGF and high vaporizer concentration of volatile anesthetic (F_V) is warranted in order to rapidly achieve the required concentration of inhalation anesthetic in the breathing system. Sevoflurane—when used with strong base-free CO_2 absorbent—is suitable for use in LFA because it has low blood-gas solubility. The minimum alveolar concentration (MAC) of sevoflurane varies with patient age—from 1.4% at age 80 to 2.3% at age 1 year [2]. The optimal alveolar concentration of sevoflurane (F_AS) to prevent motor movement and autonomic response during anesthesia is MAC-Bar which approximates 1.5 MAC. Thus, the target of F_AS during anesthesia in daily practice varies between 1 to 3.5%, depending on the adjuvant drugs used. A good wash-in scheme should be able to precisely and promptly achieve every target of F_AS. There are a few reports regarding wash-in schemes of sevoflurane LFA but those studies

* Correspondence: thepakorns@gmail.com
Department of Anesthesiology, Faculty of Medicine, Khon Kaen University, 123 Mitrapap road, Ampur Muang, Khon Kaen 40002, Thailand

achieved only one or two targets of F_AS [3–5]. In highly developed healthcare areas—where an anesthetic gas monitor is placed in every operating theatre—a wash-in scheme would be unnecessary. By contrast, in less developed areas where anesthetic gas monitors are rare or nonexistent, a precise and reliable wash-in scheme is mandatory for sevoflurane LFA. Since the carrier gases used in anesthesia comprise both O_2 plus N_2O and O_2 plus Air, we propose a simple one-step 1-1-8 wash-in scheme for sevoflurane LFA using FGF of 2 L·min^{-1} by combining O_2 with N_2O or Air at 1:1 L·min^{-1} and a F_V of sevoflurane (F_VS) 8%, which can be used to estimate the time to achieve each F_AS in daily practice. The hypothesis is that this scheme can precisely and promptly achieve every F_AS from 1 to 3.5% within 5 min.

The primary outcome of the current study was the time to achieve a F_AS of 1, 1.5, 2, 2.5, 3, and 3.5% in both contexts. The secondary outcomes were to identify the changes in heart rate and blood pressure during wash-in.

Methods

The current study was approved by the Khon Kaen University Ethics Committee in Human Research (HE601228) and was registered with ClinicalTrials.gov (NCT03510013). The study was conducted in accordance with Declaration of Helsinki and the ICH GCP. All participants gave written informed consent before being recruited into the study.

This was a prospective, descriptive study. We aimed to recruit two groups of patients: group N_2O and group Air. We calculated the sample size from a pilot study on 20 patients, which identified a standard deviation of 40 s at an F_AS of 3.5%. With the total width of the expected confidence interval of 16 s, and a significance criterion of 0.05, the total number of patients required was 96. The inclusion criteria were adult patients, between 18 and 64, with an American Society of Anesthesiologists (ASA) physical status of 1–2, undergoing elective surgery under general anesthesia at Srinagarind Hospital, Khon Kaen University, Khon Kaen, Thailand. The exclusion criteria were patients with a BMI > 30 kg·m^{-2}; a contraindication for N_2O or succinylcholine; having pulmonary or cardiac disease; or, being pregnant.

All patients received standard intra-operative anesthetic monitoring and care. The monitoring included electrocardiogram, pulse oximetry, non-invasive blood pressure measurement, capnography, and MAC value. The anesthetic machine—with an integrated anesthetic gas analyzer used in this study was the Dräger Primus (Dräger AG, Lübeck, Germany). We used a standard circle circuit with Litholyme as the CO_2 absorbent. Heart rate and blood pressure were recorded as baseline parameters before induction of anesthesia. After pre-oxygenation for 3 min, each patient was premedicated with fentanyl 1–2 µg·kg^{-1}, then propofol 2 mg·kg^{-1} was given as the induction agent. Endotracheal intubation was facilitated with succinylcholine 1.5 mg·kg^{-1}. After a correct endotracheal tube position was confirmed, cisatracurium 0.15 mg·kg^{-1} was given.

Group N_2O

The ventilation was controlled using O_2:N_2O at 1:1 L·min^{-1} and F_VS of 8%. The ventilator was set at volume-control with an inspiratory:expiratory (I:E) ratio of 1:2, a positive end-expiratory pressure (PEEP) of 0, and a tidal volume of 8 mL·kg^{-1} with a respiratory rate of 12 min^{-1}—which was adjusted periodically to achieve an end-tidal CO_2 of 30–35 mmHg. The times to achieve a respective F_AS of 1, 1.5, 2, 2.5, 3, and 3.5% were recorded as the primary outcome. The inspired concentration of sevoflurane (F_IS), heart rate, and blood pressure at each F_AS were recorded as the secondary outcomes. When the F_AS reached 3.5%, the FGF was reduced to 1 L·min^{-1} and the F_VS readjusted at the discretion of the attending anesthesiologist. Surgery started after completion of recording the study parameters.

Group air

The same procedure was used except using O_2:Air at 1:1 L·min^{-1} and F_VS of 8%.

Statistical analysis

Continuous data were presented as means ± standard deviation (SD) while categorical data were presented as numbers (%). The primary outcomes were presented as means ± SD with a 95% confidence interval (CI). The secondary outcomes (viz., heart rate and blood pressure at different time points) were compared using repeated measures analysis of variance. A $P < 0.05$ was considered statistically significant. All data were analyzed using SPSS 16.0 (SPSS Inc., Chicago, IL, USA).

Results

A total of 199 patients were recruited between September and December 2018—102 in group N_2O and 97 in group Air. The patient and clinical characteristics are presented in Table 1. The trajectories of time to achieve each F_AS for all patients of group N_2O and group Air are presented in Figs. 1 and 2. The gradual rising pattern of F_AS and F_IS are similar and parallel in both groups (Fig. 3). The ratio of F_AS/F_IS of both groups rises rapidly from 0.46 to 0.72 within 260 s for group N_2O and 0.42 to 0.69 within 286 s in group Air (Fig. 4). The respective time to achieve a F_AS of 1, 1.5, 2, 2.5, 3, and 3.5% (in sec) with 95% CI and the approximate upper limit of the 95% CI (in min) of group N_2O and group Air are presented in Tables 2 and 3. A F_AS of 3.5% can be achieved within 4.5 min in group N_2O and 5 min in group Air. The heart rate and blood pressure

Table 1 Patient and clinical characteristics

Parameter	Nitrous oxide ($n = 102$)	Air ($n = 97$)
Age (years)	42.5 ± 12.7	46.0 ± 12.1
Weight (kg)	58.6 ± 10.0	58.4 ± 9.9
Height (cm)	159.8 ± 6.4	160.3 ± 7.7
Sex		
Male	22 (21.6)	24 (24.7)
Female	80 (78.4)	73 (75.3)
ASA classification		
1	71 (69.6)	57 (58.8)
2	31 (30.4)	40 (41.2)
Systolic blood pressure (mmHg)	135.6 ± 20.2	128.7 ± 17.5
Diastolic blood pressure (mmHg)	80.9 ± 10.2	77.0 ± 11.7
Heart rate (beat/min)	80.2 ± 14.5	76.2 ± 11.3

Data are presented as means ± SD or numbers (%)
ASA American Society of Anesthesiologists

significantly increased initially (albeit slightly) then gradually decreased as the F_AS increased in both groups ($p < 0.001$ for all parameters) (Fig. 5).

Discussion

Sevoflurane is a popular and widely used volatile anesthetic because it does not irritate the airway, hence it can be used as an induction agent, especially in children. Moreover, its low blood and fat solubility leads to rapid onset, easy depth of anesthesia adjustment, and early recovery [6]. Due to its high cost, however, LFA is used to reduce the amount needed [7]. The more important reasons to implement sevoflurane LFA are benefits to environment and mucociliary function of the patient [1]. Previously, the recommended lowest FGF to be used with sevoflurane was 1 L·min^{-1} for exposures up to 1 h and 2 L·min^{-1} for exposures > 1 h because of compound A concern [8]. With the introduction of strong base-free CO_2 absorbents (e.g., Amsorb Plus and Litholyme), the issue with compound A from sevoflurane has been resolved and sevoflurane can be safely used in LFA [9]. LFA, however, needs a wash-in phase to rapidly build up F_AS to the required target concentration. The wash-in can be achieved by (a) increasing FGF to reduce the time constant [10]; (b) increasing F_VS to induce a concentration effect [11]; or (c) integrating both methods.

A few studies have addressed the wash-in technique for sevoflurane LFA. Lindqvist et al. reported a 2-step wash-in technique to achieve a F_AS of 1.2%; starting with FGF 1 L·min^{-1} and F_VS 8% for 1 min, then reducing FGF to 1, 0.7, 0.5, and 0.3 L·min^{-1}. They found that the respective time to achieve the target F_AS was 1.8, 1.5, 2.5, and 3.6 min [3]. Horwitz et al. reported that by using a FGF of 1.0 or 0.5 L·min^{-1} with a F_VS 6% during the wash-in, the respective time to reach 1 MAC was 6.2 ± 1.3 and 15.2 ± 2.4 min and up to 1.5 MAC at 7.5 ± 2.5 and 19 ± 4.4 min [4]. The limitation of these two schemes is that they cover only 1 or 2 F_AS targets, and hence cannot be applied for other required F_AS targets.

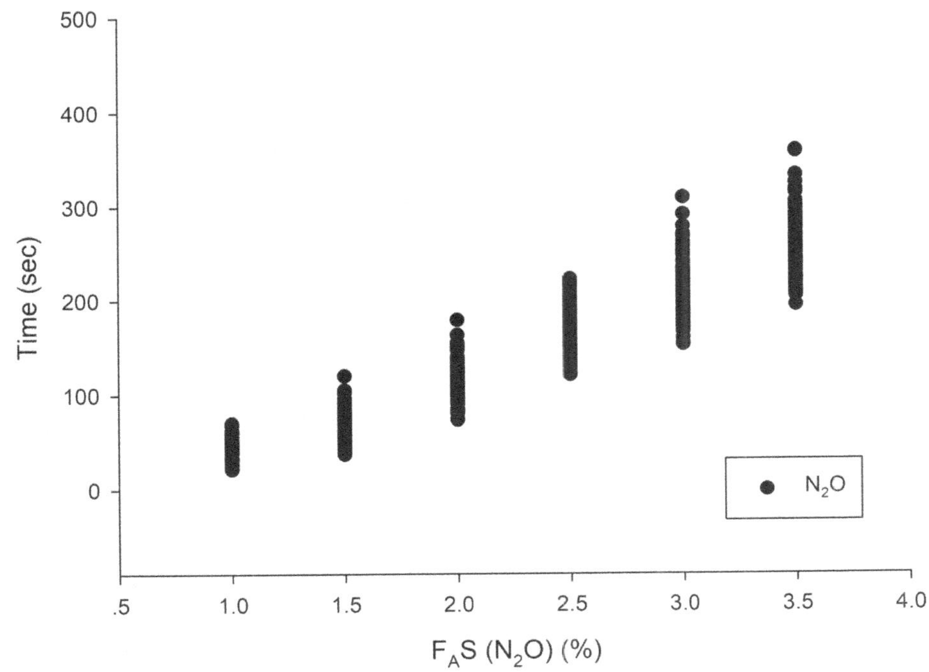

Fig. 1 Trajectories of F_AS vs. time to achieve each F_AS during wash-in of group N_2O. F_AS, alveolar concentration of sevoflurane

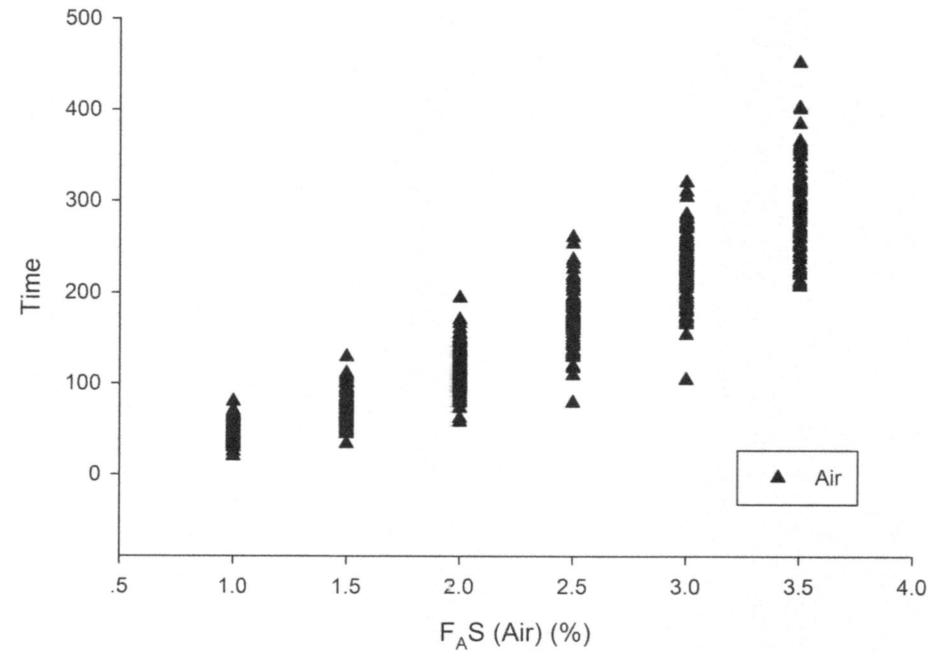

Fig. 2 Trajectories of F_AS vs. time to achieve each F_AS during wash-in of group Air. F_AS, alveolar concentration of sevoflurane

Jakobsson et al. reported a wash-in in a test-lung model with a respective FGF of 0.3 and 4 L·min^{-1} and a F_VS of 8%. They found that the F_AS reached 1 MAC (2.1%) at 547 ± 83 and 38 ± 6 s, respectively [5]. Leijonhufvud et al reported a wash-in in a test-lung using a respective FGF of 1, 2, 4, 4.8, 6, and 8 L·min^{-1} and a F_VS 6% in a Flow-I and a Aisys anesthetic machine. They found that the respective mean time to achieve 1 MAC was 431.3, 185.6, 66, 53.6, 53.6, and 52.6 s for the Flow-I and 262.7, 144.3, 57.7, 52.3, 57.7, and 58.3 s for the Aisys [12]. Finally, Shin

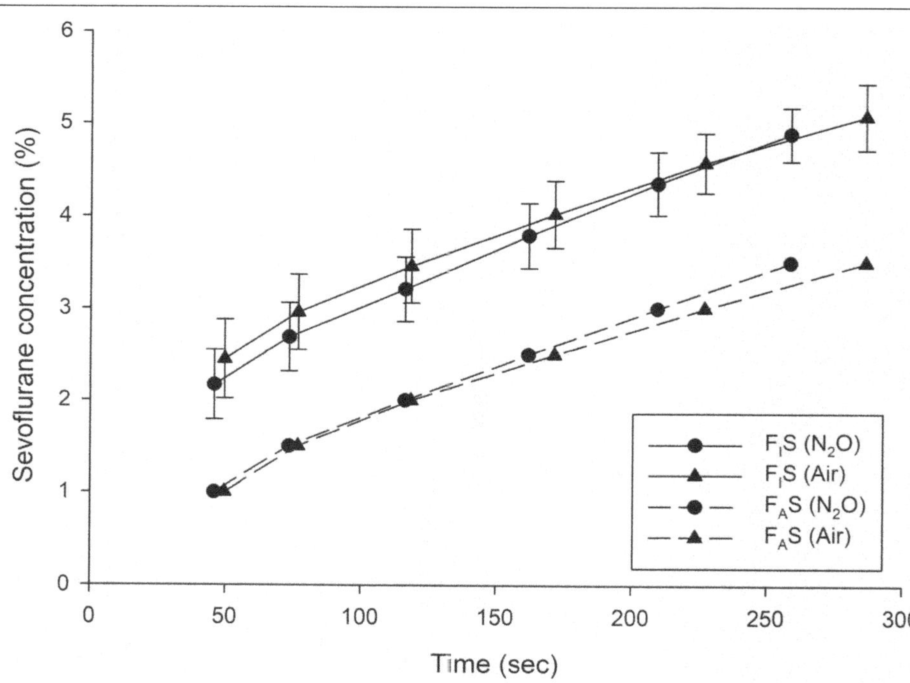

Fig. 3 Rising pattern of F_AS and F_IS of group N_2O and group Air. F_AS, alveolar concentration of sevoflurane; F_IS, inspired concentration of sevoflurane

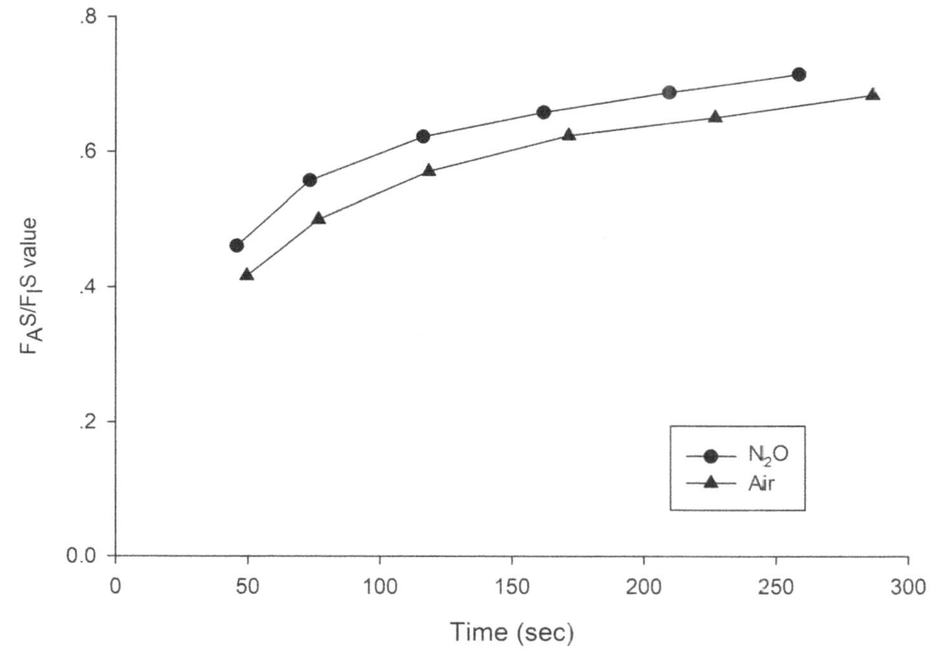

Fig. 4 Rising pattern of F_AS/F_IS ratio of group N_2O and group Air. F_AS, alveolar concentration of sevoflurane; F_IS, inspired concentration of sevoflurane

et al. performed a wash-in study using a Primus anesthetic machine connected to a test-lung, using a FGF of 0.5, 1, and 3 L·min^{-1} and setting the F_VS to 6%. The respective mean time to reach a F_AS of 4% for each FGF was 1165, 534, and 155 s [13]. The latter 3 studies were, however, all performed in test-lungs such that the uptake of sevoflurane by body tissues was not considered, so the results cannot be generalized to clinical practice.

The current study proposed a 1-1-8 wash-in scheme for sevoflurane LFA using N_2O or Air—which can rapidly and predictably achieve each F_AS (i.e., 1 to 3.5% as is used in daily practice within 4.5 and 5 min, respectively). The time to achieve every F_AS was identical for both groups except at F_AS of 3 and 3.5% where the time in group Air was a nominally longer than group N_2O because of the second gas effect of N_2O [11]. When this wash-in scheme uses O_2: N_2O 1:1 L·min^{-1} as the carrier gases, 50% N_2O provides 0.5 MAC in addition to the MAC of sevoflurane [14], hence this protocol can further reduce the use of sevoflurane. When N_2O is contraindicated or Air is preferred, a higher F_AS is required, and yet this wash-in scheme consistently, precisely, and promptly achieves the required target.

Comparing with a similar 1-1-12 wash-in scheme for desflurane LFA which uses desflurane 12% (2 MAC) [15, 16], the current 1-1-8 sevoflurane wash-in scheme uses a higher MAC (8% or 4 MAC) of sevoflurane. The reasons are that (a) sevoflurane has greater blood and fat solubility than desflurane, leading to higher body tissue uptake, which results in a longer time to achieve an equivalent MAC; and, (b) sevoflurane has a 3 times lower MAC value, hence 4 MAC of sevoflurane was used to augment a concentration effect [11].

The trajectories of the times to achieve each F_AS in both groups (Figs. 1 and 2) suggests that the tested wash-in

Table 2 Actual time in seconds with 95% CI and approximate upper CI limit time in minutes to achieve each F_AS in group N_2O ($n = 102$)

F_AS (%)	F_IS (%)	Time (sec)	95%CI (sec)	Approximated upper CI limit time (min)
1	2.2	45.8 ± 9.8	43.9–47.8	1
1.5	2.7	73.5 ± 14.5	70.7–76.4	1.5
2	3.2	116.3 ± 20.4	112.3–120.3	2
2.5	3.8	161.9 ± 23.3	157.3–166.4	3
3	4.4	208.4 ± 30.6	202.4–214.4	3.5
3.5	4.9	258.5 ± 35.0	251.7–265.4	4.5

Data are presented as means ± SD or ranges
F_IS inspired concentration of sevoflurane, *F_AS* alveolar concentration of sevoflurane, *CI* confidence interval

Table 3 Actual time in seconds with 95% CI and approximate upper CI limit time in minutes to achieve each F_AS in group Air (n = 97)

F_AS (%)	F_IS (%)	Time (sec)	95%CI (sec)	Approximated upper CI limit time (min)
1	2.4	49.6 ± 10.9	47.4–51.8	1
1.5	3.0	76.8 ± 16.5	73.5–80.2	1.5
2	3.5	118.5 ± 24.0	113.6–123.3	2
2.5	4.0	171.5 ± 30.5	165.4–177.7	3
3	4.6	226.9 ± 38.4	219.1–234.6	4
3.5	5.1	286.4 ± 48.1	276.7–296.1	5

Data are presented as means ± SD or ranges
F_IS inspired concentration of sevoflurane, *F_AS* alveolar concentration of sevoflurane, *CI* confidence interval

scheme has acceptable intra- and inter-subject variability. The parallel rising pattern of F_AS and F_IS (Fig. 3) shows that the wash-in scheme has enough power to drive both F_AS and F_IS to the desired target of both groups within 4.5 and 5 min, as reflected in the rising F_AS/F_IS ratio pattern (Fig. 4). The rising F_A/F_I ratio pattern reflects the onset of volatile anesthetic: the more rapid the rise the shorter the onset. The rapidly rising F_AS/F_IS ratio of the 1-1-8 wash-in scheme in both groups underscores the efficacy of this scheme. The higher F_AS/F_IS ratio of the group N_2O reflects the second gas effect [11].

The changes in heart rate and blood pressure during the wash-in process are similar to the 1-1-12 wash-in scheme for desflurane [15, 16] (i.e., slightly increasing initially then gradually decreasing as presented in Fig. 5). The changes are statistically but not clinically significant.

The 1-1-8 wash-in scheme has many advantages: (a) simplicity – just a one-step setting; (b) coverage – includes every F_AS target from 1 to 3.5% used in daily practice both in balanced anesthesia and pure inhalation anesthesia; (c) swiftness – accomplishing the desired target within 1 to 4.5 or 5 min; (d) safety – no clinically significant change in heart rate and blood pressure; (e) economy – just 2 $L{\cdot}min^{-1}$ of FGF; and (f) applicability – can be applied with both N_2O and Air. When the target F_AS is achieved, the FGF can be reduced to 1 $L{\cdot}\,min^{-1}$ and the F_AS can simply be maintained by setting the F_VS above the desired F_AS by 50 to 60% [17]. The current study used Litholyme as the CO_2 absorbent to guarantee the safety of sevoflurane LFA.

Most hospitals in developed countries have an anesthetic gas analyzer in the operating theatre, making any wash-in scheme unnecessary during low-flow

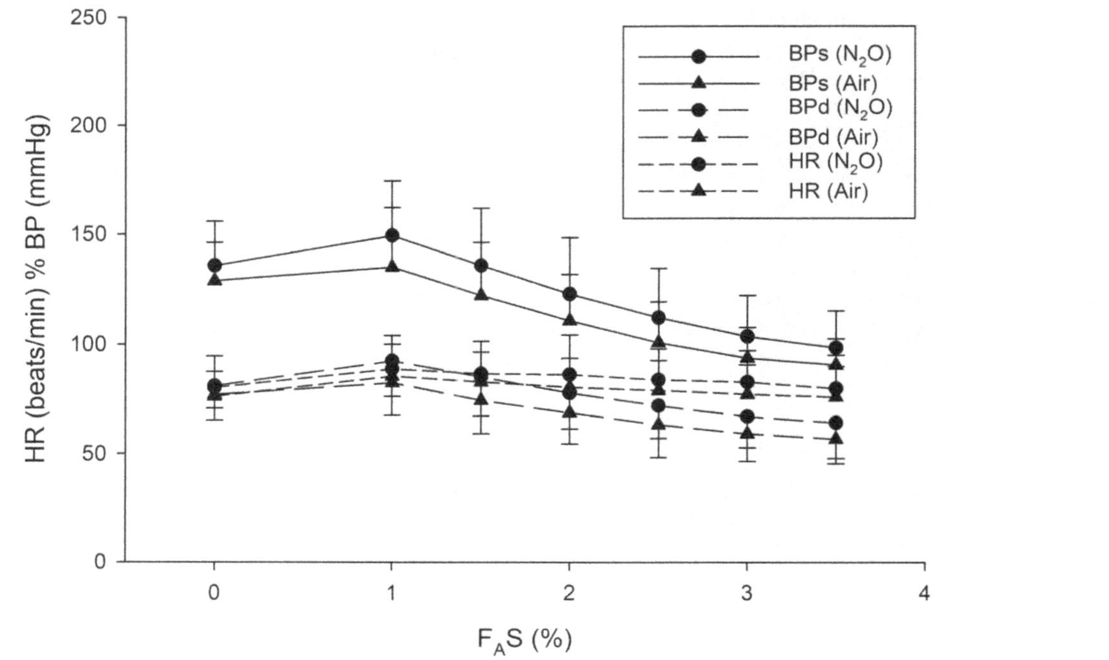

Fig. 5 Pattern of changes in heart rate and blood pressure of group N_2O and group Air at each F_AS. $p < 0.001$ for all values. F_AS, alveolar concentration of sevoflurane; BPs, systolic blood pressure; BPd, diastolic blood pressure; HR, heart rate

anesthesia. Many operating theatres in less developed areas, however, still lack such equipment. The tested wash-in scheme may thus be applied as guidance to perform sevoflurane LFA provided that an inspired oxygen concentration monitor is available.

Limitations

Since we excluded patients with a BMI > 30 kg m^{-2}; having pulmonary or cardiac disease; or, being pregnant, this wash-in scheme may not be applied in those groups of patients. Further studies are required.

Conclusions

In patients requiring general anesthesia with endotracheal intubation and controlled ventilation, the 1-1-8 wash-in scheme for sevoflurane LFA yields a respective F_AS of 1, 1.5, 2, 2.5, 3, and 3.5% at 1, 1.5, 2, 3, 3.5, and 4.5 min when used with N_2O and at 1, 1.5, 2, 3, 4, and 5 min when used with Air. This technique uses a one-step setting for O_2:N_2O or O_2:Air 1:1 L·min^{-1} with sevoflurane 8%. There were statistically but not clinically significant changes in heart rate and blood pressure during the wash-in process.

Abbreviations

ASA: American Society of Anesthesiologists; CI: Confidence interval; CO_2: Carbon dioxide; F_AS: Alveolar concentration of sevoflurane; FGF: Fresh gas flow; F_IS: Inspired concentration of sevoflurane; F_V: Vaporizer concentration of volatile anesthetic; F_VS: Vaporizer concentration of sevoflurane; N_2O: Nitrous oxide; O_2: Oxygen; SD: Standard deviation

Acknowledgments

We thank Bryan Roderick Hamman for assistance with the English-language presentation of the manuscript under the aegis of the Publication Clinic KKU, Thailand.

Authors' contributions

ST and TS designed the study, performed the study, performed the statistical analysis and wrote the manuscript. NV, MT, DN, and WS performed the study and collected data. All authors read and approved the final manuscript.

References

1. Baum JA. Low-flow anesthesia: theory, practice, technical preconditions, advantages, and foreign gas accumulation. J Anesth. 1999;13:166–74.
2. Nickalls RW, Mapleson WW. Age-related iso-MAC charts for isoflurane, sevoflurane and desflurane in man. Br J Anaesth. 2003;91:170–4.
3. Lindqvist M, Jakobsson J. Minimal flow anesthesia for short elective day case surgery; high vaporiser settings are needed but still cost-effective. Ambul Surg. 2011;17:27–9.
4. Horwitz M, Jakobsson JG. Desflurane and sevoflurane use during low- and minimal-flow anesthesia at fixed vaporizer settings. Minerva Anestesiol. 2016;82:180–5 PMID: 26198766.
5. Jakobsson P, Lindgren M, Jakobsson JG. Wash-in and wash-out of sevoflurane in a test-lung model: A comparison between Aisys and FLOW-i. F1000Res. 2017;6:389.
6. Young CJ, Apfelbaum JL. Inhalational anesthetics: desflurane and sevoflurane. J Clin Anesth. 1995;7:564–77.
7. Ryu HG, Lee JH, Lee KK, Gil NS, Kim CS, Sim SE, et al. The effect of low fresh gas flow rate on sevoflurane consumption. Korean J Anesthesiol. 2011;60:75–7.
8. Gentz BA, Malan TP Jr. Renal toxicity with sevoflurane: a storm in a teacup? Drugs. 2001;61:2155–62.
9. Marini F, Bellugi I, Gambi D, Pacenti M, Dugheri S, Focardi L, et al. Compound A, formaldehyde and methanol concentrations during low-flow sevoflurane anesthesia: comparison of three carbon dioxide absorbers. Acta Anaesthesiol Scand. 2007;51:625–32.
10. Honemann C, Hagemann O, Doll D. Inhalational anesthesia with low fresh gas flow. Indian J Anesth. 2013;57:345–50.
11. Korman B, Mapleson WW. Concentration and second gas effects: can the accepted explanation be improved? Br J Anesth. 1997;78:618–25.
12. Leijonhufvud F, Joneby F, Jakobsson JG. The impact of fresh gas flow on wash-in, wash-out time and gas consumption for sevoflurane and desflurane, comparing two anesthesia machines, a test-lung study. F1000Res. 2017;6:1997.
13. Shin HW, Yu HN, Bae GE, Huh H, Park JY, Kim JY. The effect of fresh gas flow rate and type of anesthesia machine on time to reach target sevoflurane concentration. BMC Anesthesiol. 2017;17:10.
14. Vereecke HEM, Proost JH, Heyse B, Eleveld DJ, Katoh T, Luginbühl M, et al. Interaction between nitrous oxide, sevoflurane, and opioids: a response surface approach. Anesthesiology. 2013;118:894–902.
15. Sathitkarnmanee T, Tribuddharat S, Suttinarakorn C, Nonlhaopol D, Thananun M, Somdee W, et al. 1-1-12 one-step wash-in scheme for desflurane-nitrous oxide low-flow anesthesia: rapid and predictable induction. Biomed Res Int. 2014;2014:867504.
16. Sathitkarnmanee T, Tribuddharat S, Nonlhaopol D, Thananun M, Somdee W. 1-1-12 one-step wash-in scheme for desflurane low flow anesthesia: performance without nitrous oxide. Drug Des Devel Ther. 2015;9:977–81.
17. Hargasser S, Hipp R, Breinbauer B, Mielke L, Entholzner E, Rust M. A lower solubility recommends the use of desflurane more than isoflurane, halothane, and enflurane under low-flow conditions J Clin Anesth. 1995;7:49–53.

19

Anesthetic management of a patient with limb-girdle muscular dystrophy 2B

X. Q. Cao[1], K. Joypaul[2], F. Cao[3], L. L. Gui[1], J. T. Hu[4] and W. Mei[1*]

Abstract

Background: Limb-girdle muscular dystrophies (LGMDs) belong to few neuromuscular disorders mainly involving pelvic and shoulder girdle muscles. Also, cardiac or pulmonary complications, increased rhabdomyolysis risk when exposed to volatile anesthetics and succinylcholine may increase anesthesia related risks. However, current reports about the anesthesia management of these patients are limited.

Case presentation: We described our anesthetic management of a 36 years old woman with LGMD 2B receiving arthroscopic knee surgery. In consideration of the high risk of rhabdomyolysis, total intravenous anesthesia (TIVA) was selected for her surgery. Considering the unpredictable respiratory depression, opioid based patient-controlled intravenous analgesia was replaced with an intra-articular cocktail therapy consisting of 20 ml of 0.2% ropivacaine. Also, we reviewed the literatures on anesthetic management of LGMD through searching PubMed, in order to provide a comprehensive and safe guidance for the surgery.

Conclusions: Carefully conducted general anesthesia with TIVA technique is a good choice for LGMD patients. Neuraxial anesthesia may be used if general anesthesia needs to be avoided. To warrant safe anesthesia for surgery, any decision must be well thought out during perioperative period.

Keywords: Limb-girdle muscular dystrophy 2B, Anesthesia, Surgery

Background

Limb-girdle muscular dystrophies (LGMDs) belong to few very rare neuromuscular disorders mainly involving pelvic and shoulder girdle muscles [1]. The estimated incidence of this disease is 1 to 6.5 in 100,000 [2]. Although named as the typical muscle, LGMDs are actually a group of systemic diseases and may be complicated with cardiac or pulmonary involvements [3]. Increased risk of rhabdomyolysis and malignant hyperthermia (MH) when exposed to volatile anesthetics and succinylcholine are life-threatening complications [1]. However, the current reports about anesthetic management of LGMD patients are limited. We aimed to present our clinic experience about a patient with LGMD 2B receiving arthroscopic knee surgery. Then, we reviewed literatures on anesthetic management of LGMD published in PubMed, in order to provide a comprehensive and safe guidance for surgery. The reporting of this case was approved by the Research and Ethics Committee of Tongji Hospital at Tongji Medical College, Huazhong University of Science and Technology (TJ-IRB20180902). The patient had gave written informed consent for reporting and publishing her clinical data and images.

Case presentation

A 36 years old woman, 54 kg in weight, 1.60 m tall, BMI 21.09, was hospitalized with left knee joint injury and was scheduled for arthroscopy of left knee (Fig. 1). She had a history of LGMD type 2B diagnosed in 2013 by muscle biopsy. Genetic testing showed homozygous DYSF mutation on 11 and 33 exons, and MRI revealed fat infiltration and fluid collection within the lower limb muscles. Her symptoms predominantly affected her lower limbs. Her initial symptom presented as difficulty in climbing stairs at 24 years old. During her admission, she did not have any muscle weakness in the upper

* Correspondence: wmei@hust.edu.cn
[1]Department of Anesthesiology and Pain Medicine, Tongji Hospital, Tongji Medical College, Huazhong University of Science and Technology, 1095 Jiefang Road, Wuhan 430030, People's Republic of China

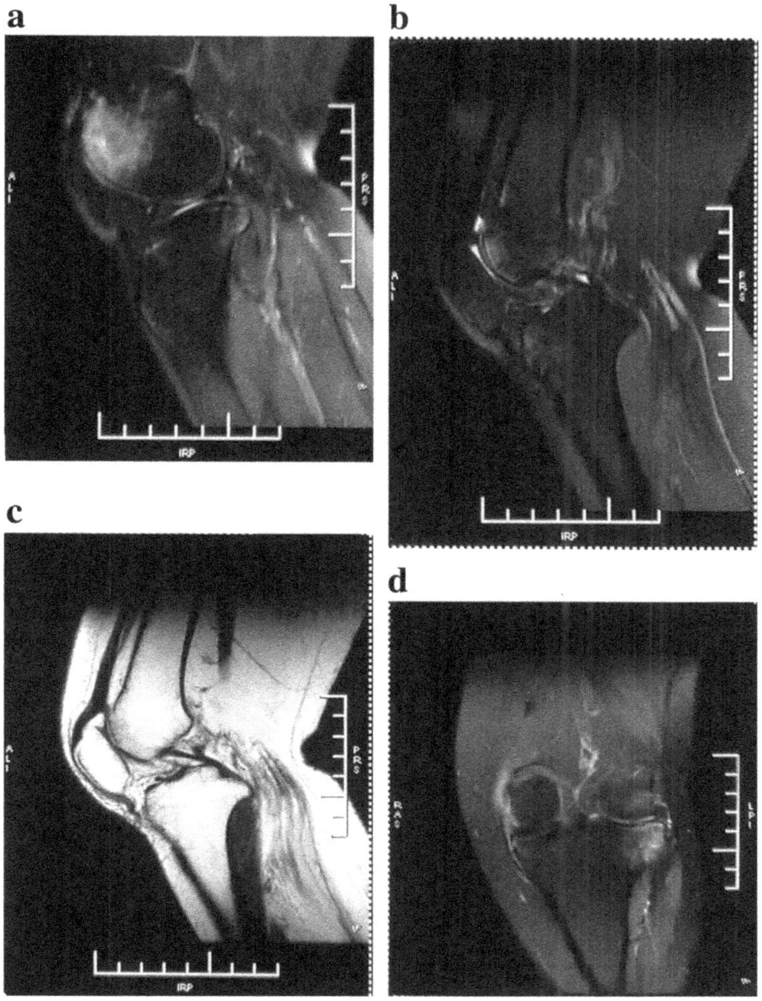

Fig. 1 Left knee joint magnetic resonance imaging. It revealed left knee joint injury. **a** Osteoedema of distal femur; **b** Rupture of anterior cruciate ligament; **c** Relaxation of quadriceps femoris tendon and patellar ligament; **d** Posterolateral osteoedema of tibial plateau

limbs, dysphagia, or other clinical manifestations. Her symptoms were slow in progression, with inability to climb the stairs by 2011. She underwent multiple examinations for muscle enzyme levels, electromyography (EMG), etc., and she was also once misdiagnosed as 'polymyositis'. Aspartate aminotransferase (AST), alanine aminotransferase (ALT) and creatine kinase (CK) levels were high. She underwent an uneventful cesarean section under spinal anesthesia in February of 2017. Her younger brother was also diagnosed with LGMD type 2B.

Her current physical examination was remarkable, muscle strength, muscle tension, and muscular volume of the upper limbs were all found to be normal. Muscle strength of the lower limbs was at level 4, whereas muscle tension was decreased (Fig. 2). MRI of lower limbs revealed atrophy of quadriceps femoris, adductor muscles, semimembranosus, and hypertrophy of gracilis as well as the long head of biceps femoris. Her complete blood count, blood chemistry and urinalysis were unremarkable. Abnormal laboratory findings were listed as follows: aspartate aminotransferase 83 U/L, alanine transaminase 43 U/L and creatine kinase 3479 U/L. The electrocardiogram (ECG) showed T wave anomaly in the anterior wall. Chest X-ray revealed increased lung markings. After entering the operating room, the patient underwent transthoracic echocardiography and revealed good left ventricular functions and no evidence of cardiomyopathy or pulmonary hypertension.

The patient received adequate explanation about the increased risk of anesthesia and gave her informed consent. In consideration of the high risk of rhabdomyolysis and malignant hyperthermia, we decided to proceed with total intravenous anesthesia (TIVA) for her elective surgery.

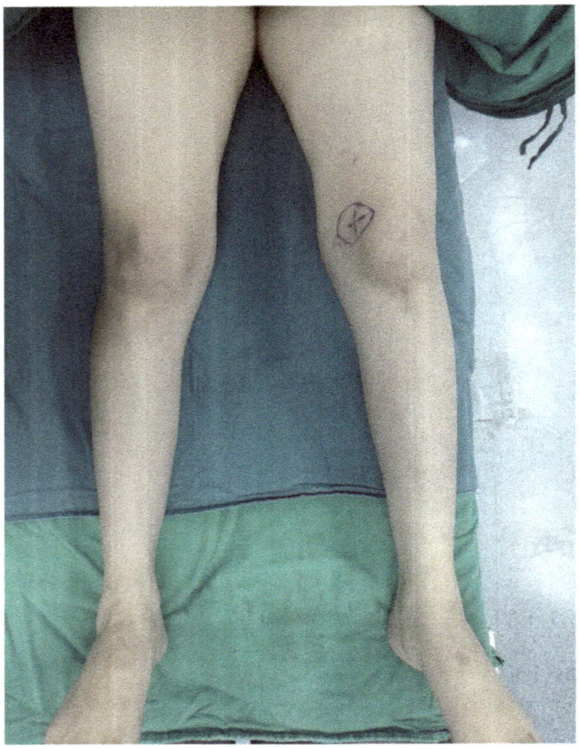

Fig. 2 photograph of patient's lower limbs. It showed muscles of lower limbs atrophy slightly. Muscle strength of the lower limbs was at level 4, whereas muscle tension was decreased

Before the patient was transferred to operating room, the anesthesia apparatus was substituted by a respirator connected with a new breath circuit for necessary isolation from volatile anesthetics. After the patient arrived in the operation room, electrocardiogram and pulse oximetry saturation (SpO_2) monitoring was immediately started. Heart rate was 74 bpm, SpO_2 was 98% in room air. Noninvasive blood pressure (NIBP) was 113/62 mmHg. To avoid the potential muscular damage caused by repeated cuff pressure measurements, invasive blood pressure monitoring was used. Except for the standard monitoring, end-tidal CO_2 ($EtCO_2$) and nasopharyngeal temperature monitoring were also important. Flurbiprofen 50 mg was given intravenously as preventive analgesia regime. Anesthesia induction was performed with 50 mg propofol and 20 mg etomidate after 30μg sufentanil, a size 3# laryngeal mask airway was inserted 2 min later to secure the airway. Muscle relaxant was not used to avoid the delayed recovery of muscular strength. Propofol (6-12 $mg.kg^{-1}.h^{-1}$) and remifentanil (0.1–0.2 $\mu g.kg^{-1}.min^{-1}$) were pumped to maintain anesthesia. Non-tourniquet technology was adopted during the operation to avoid potential muscle damage caused by tourniquet, and controlled hypotension was used to reduce the risk of bleeding. During the operation, heart beat was between 55 and 82 bpm, while the mean blood pressure remained between 70 and 83 mmHg. $EtCO_2$ was maintained at around 40 mmHg. Nasopharyngeal temperature was monitored at 36.2–36.4 °C. After the surgical intervention which lasted around 1 h and 48 min, the patient recovered rapidly approximately within 2 min after cessation of TIVA. Considering the unpredictable respiratory depression, opioid based patient-controlled intravenous analgesia was not used. Instead an intra-articular cocktail therapy consisting of 20 ml of 0.2% ropivacaine was injected at the end of surgery acting as a substitute for postoperative analgesia.

During the follow-up on the second postoperative day, the resting visual analog scale (VAS) pain score was 2 and the VAS pain score at movement was 4. The patient could be mobilized out-of-bed, didn't complain of any significant discomfort during movement of the lower limbs. She was discharged on the fifth day after surgery.

Then, we reviewed relevant literatures published in PubMed as of September 2018. The search was limited to studies about humanity. Only English cases were included. The keywords used for the search included ["limb-girdle muscular dystrophy" OR "limb-girdle muscular dystrophy" OR "LGMD"] and ["anesthetic management" OR "anesthesia" OR "anaesthetic management" OR "anaesthesia"].

Discussion and conclusion

LGMD constitutes a group of genetic disorders originally devided into autosomal dominant (LGMD type 1) and autosomal recessive (LGMD type 2) [4–6], 8 subtypes of LGMD1 and 26 subtypes of LGMD2 are currently recognized [3]. Successive letters of the alphabet have been used to name the LGMDs according to the identification chronology of genetic locus. The pathogenesis of LGMD is the mutation of causative genes leading to abnormal protein synthesis localized to various parts of the muscle fiber [2]. Degeneration and necrosis of muscle fibers, which are replaced by connective tissue and fat is the classic pathologic change [7]. However, the biopsy findings among the various LGMDs lack in specificity and significant overlap. Also, Serum creatine kinase (CK) levels couldn't reflect the severity of LGMD [3]. Genetic testing is necessary for diagnosis of LGMD.

The mutations of dysferlin gene (DYSF, MIM*603009) located on chromosome 2p13.3 induces abnormal dysferlin protein synthesis is the reason of LGMD 2B [8]. The symptom onset ranges from adolescence to late adulthood (17–30 years of age), the disease progresses fairly slowly, and approximately 10% of patients may be confined to a wheelchair [9].

Serum CK levels are considerably high, usually up to 40 times of the normal [10, 11].

The use of inhalation anesthetics and succinylcholine may lead to threatening hyperkalemia and rhabdomyolysis, and should be avoided [12–14]. Propofol, etomidate and opioids are proved to be trigger-free agents [15, 16]. However, myopathic patients are more sensitive to anesthetics, opioids and muscle relaxants [17]. In order to minimize the risk of postoperative respiratory depression, short acing anesthetic agents are the optimum selection [14]. Propofol, as it's short-acting, easiness in titration, is suitable for LGMD [1]. Remifentanil was also unlikely to cause postoperative respiratory failure and prolonged sedation. Therefore, we chose total intravenous anesthesia (TIVA) by infusing propofol and remifentanil for anesthetic maintenance of this patient. Sufentanil 30μg was also used in this patient to provide adequate analgesia. Considering the high sensitivity and prolonged duration of action to muscle relaxants in these patients, muscle relaxants were avoided in our case. Therefore, for this patient laryngeal mask airway is more beneficial as compared to an endotracheal intubation. Intravenous patient-controlled analgesia (iv-PCA) based on opioids may lead to unpredictable respiratory depression, and was not considered in our case. Instead, intra-articular injection of cocktail therapy with 0.2% ropivacaine 20 ml had been used with an excellent outcome.

Previous reports were searched through PubMed as of September 2018 using the following key words: ["limb-girdle muscular dystrophy" OR "limb girdle muscular dystrophy" OR "LGMD"] and ["anesthetic management" OR "anesthesia" OR "anaesthetic management" OR "anaesthesia"]. Only English reports were included. Six cases were reviewed. Time of publication, LGMD type, symptoms, complications, operative procedures, preoperative examinations, intraoperative monitoring, anesthesia method, anesthesia machine preparation, anesthesia induction, anesthesia maintenance, pain management after operation are summarized in Table 1.

Through literature review, we found that respiratory impairment was common in LGMD [10],, and thus the high risk of respiratory compromise should be considered when we administer any anesthesia to a patient with LGMD. Additionally, cardiac impairment should be noticed as well [10]. ECG and Chest X-ray should be performed routinely before surgery, and then for any positive finding, echocardiography and pulmonary function test are suggested. In six previous case reports, two patients underwent laparoscopic cholecystectomy, one patient had appendectomy, one patient underwent caesarean section, one patient had an adenoidectomy, and the last patient went through replacement of ascending aorta. Four operations were performed under TIVA, and the other two operations were performed under neuraxial anesthesia including one laparoscopic cholecystectomy and one caesarean section. Propofol and remifentanil were also adopted as primary anesthetics. If muscle relaxants must be used during operation, neuromuscular blockade monitoring was routinely recommended and sugammadex was used to reverse the blockade at the end of the operation. Among previous case reports, no patient received patient-controlled opioid infusion pumps for postoperative analgesia, and no patient experienced respiratory depression. Our anesthetic strategy was basically in parallel with the regime used in these reports. However, we should keep in mind that the use of TIVA couldn't completely avoid the risk of MH [22]. Therefore, regional anesthetic techniques should be considered as an alternative plan. Gerbershagen MU et al. suggested regional anesthetic techniques should be chosen whenever possible in myopathic patients [14, 23]. When using regional anesthesia for patients with LGMD, the myotoxic effects of local anesthetic is unfortunately a primary concern. Wolfgang Zink et al. found that continuously infusing bupivacaine and ropivacaine for femoral nerve block could induce acute muscle damage with similar histological patterns [24]. They also found that both agents induced ineversible skeletal muscle damage [25], and the complex pathophysiology of local anesthetic myotoxicity had also been reviewed correspondingly [26]. This phenomenon was also demonstrated by other studies [27–29]. Though many of these studies were experimental in animals, and almost all these studies showed some local muscle damages after continuous peripheral nerve blocks, there were also some case reports in clinic about mytoxicity of local anesthetic [30–32]. In this respect, it might be necessary for a LGMD patient to avoid continuous peripheral nerve block with higher concentration of local anesthetics. In contrast, both epidural and combined spinal-epidural anesthesia have been safely used for LGMD patients receiving cesarean section [1, 20]. So far there was no study about myotoxicity after neuraxial anesthesia. It's preferred to use neuraxial anesthesia in LGMD patients whenever general anesthesia had to be avoided or carried an increased risk of complication.

In summary, carefully conducted general anesthesia with TIVA technique is a good choice for LGMD patients. Neuraxial anesthesia may be used if general anesthesia needs to be avoided. To warrant safe anesthesia for surgery in LGMD patients, a comprehensive preoperative evaluation, advanced intraoperative monitoring, thoughtful choice of anesthetic technique and pain management strategy, as well as with cooperation of a multidisciplinary team including pulmonologist, critical care physicians, and neuromuscular disease specialists is mandatory.

Table 1 literature review of anesthetic management of patients with LGMD

Title	Author/ year	Age/ gender	LGMD type	Complication	Operative procedure	Pre-operational examinations	Anesthesia method	Anesthesia machine preparing	Anesthesia induction	Anesthesia maintenance	Intraoperativemonitoring	Pain management after surgery
Anaesthetic management of a patient with limb-girdle muscular dystrophy for laparoscopic cholecystectomy [18]	Freda C. Richa/ 2010	A 57-year-old man	LGMD1	severe restrictive lung disease	laparoscopic cholecystectomy/ 45 min	ECG, Chest X-ray, echocardiography	General anaesthesia (TIVA)	A disposable circuit, fresh CO2-absorbent, disconnecting the vaporisers, flushing with O2 at a rate of 10 L. min^{-1} for 20 min	1 $mg.kg^{-1}$ $.min^{-1}$remifentanil infusing for 1 min, 3 mg. kg^{-1} propofol iv	TIVA by using 0.1–0.4 $mg.kg^{-1}$ min^{-1} remifentanil and 6–9 mg. kg^{-1} $.h^{-1}$ Propofol infusion	ECG, pulse oximetry, end-tidal CO_2, invasive arterial pressure, rectal temperature, BIS	40 ml 0.125% bupivacaine aerosolised intra-peritoneally and 1 g paracetamol given intravenously
Anaesthetic Management of a Child with Limb-Girdle Muscular Dystrophy [19]	Gamze Sarkılar/ 2014	An 8-year old boy	–	–	Appendectomy/ 16 min	–	General anaesthesia (TIVA)	a disposable patient circuit, flushing soda lime with a fresh gas flow rate of 15 L $.min^{-1}$	3 mg kg^{-1} propofol, 0.5 g. kg^{-1} Sufentanil, 0.6 mg kg^{-1} Rocuronium iv	TIVA with propofol infusion (total dose = 100.6 mg) and bolus doses of sufentanil (total dose = 10 mcg)	invasive blood pressure, ECG, pulse oximetry, nasopharyngeal temperature, end-tidal CO_2	2 mg kg^{-1} Tramadol iv
Anaesthetic management of a woman with autosomal recessive limb-girdle muscular dystrophy for emergency caesarean section [20]	T. Allen/ 2007	A 28-year-old woman	autosomal recessive limb-girdle muscular dystrophy (AR-LGMD)	severe restrictive lung disease	caesarean section	ECG, echocardiogram, Pulmonary function tests	combined spinal-epidural (CSE)	–	–	0.5% hyperbaric bupivacaine 1.8 mL and fentanyl 20 μg injected intrathecally	ECG, pulse oximetry and non-invasive blood pressure	continuous epidural infusion of 0.125% plain bupivacaine, oral paracetamol 1 g Q6h and diclofenac 50 mg Q8h.
Anesthetic management for a child with unknown type of limb-girdle muscular dystrophy [1]	Aysu Kocum/ 2010	A 4-year-old girl	unknown	–	Adenoidectomy/ 50 min	–	general anesthesia	–	100 mg propofol, 10 mg Fentanyl iv	6–12 $mg.kg^{-1}.h^{-1}$ propofol continuous infusion	ECG, pulse oximetry and non-invasive blood pressure, end-tidal CO2, axillary body temperature	10 mg Meperidine iv
Laparoscopic cholecystectomy under spinal anesthesia in a patient with limb-girdle muscular dystrophy [21]	Michael C. Chuang/ 2013	A 61-yr-old man	LGMD 2A	dyspneic	laparoscopic cholecystectomy	Echocardiogram, spirometry test	spinal anesthesia	–	–	0.75% hyperbaric bupivacaine 21 mg (2.8 mL) and fentanyl 20 μg. for subarachnoid block, 0.05–0.15 $μg.kg^{-1}.min^{-1}$ remifentanil infusion,	Invasive blood pressure	–
Total intravenous anesthesia for aortic aneurysm replacement surgery in a patient with limb-girdle dystrophy [11]	A. López Álvarez/ 2013	A 61-year-old male	–	shortness of breath	replacement of ascending aorta /330 min	Echocardiogram	General anesthesia (TIVA)	–	TCI at a target dose 3 - 5 μg/ml for propofol and 2–3 ng/mL for remifentanil, and 1.2 mg/Kg bolus of rocuronium	TCI at a target dose 3 — 5 μg/ml for propofol and remifentanil 1 — 3 ng/mL for infusion,	invasive arterial pressure, CVP, 5 lead ECG, pulse oximetry, end-tidal -CO2, BIS, central temperature, NMB, hourly diuresis	fentanyl 300 μg and paracetamol 1 g were administered 30 min before the end of the procedure

Abbreviations

$EtCO_2$: End-tidal CO_2; Iv-PCA: Intravenous patient-controlled analgesia; LGMD: Limb-girdle muscular dystrophy; MH: Malignant hyperthermia; TIVA: Total intravenous anesthesia; VAS: Visual analog scale

Acknowledgements

Not applicable.

Authors' contributions

Concept- MW; Design- MW, CXQ; Supervision-MW; Materials- CXQ, HJT; Data Collection and Processing – CXQ; Analysis and /or Interpretation –MW, CXQ; Literature Review- MW, CXQ; Draft- CXQ; Critical Review- MW, K. J, CF, GLL. All authors gave their comments on the article and approved the final version.

Author details

[1]Department of Anesthesiology and Pain Medicine, Tongji Hospital, Tongji Medical College, Huazhong University of Science and Technology, 1095 Jiefang Road, Wuhan 430030, People's Republic of China. [2]Department of Anesthesiology, Flacq Hospital, Hospital Road, Centre-de-Flacq, Mauritius. [3]Department of Psychiatry, University of Missouri-Kansas City, 5100 Rockhill Road, Kansas City 64110, MO, USA. [4]Department of Anesthesiology, Wuhan No.4 Hospital, 473 Hanzheng Road, Wuhan 430033, People's Republic of China.

References

1. Kocum A, Sener M, Caliskan E, Aribogan A. Anesthetic management for a child with unknown type of limb-girdle muscular dystrophy. Pediatr Int. 2010;52(1):e37–8.
2. Iyadurai SJ, Kissel JT. The Limb-Girdle Muscular Dystrophies and the Dystrophinopathies. Continuum (Minneap Minn). 2016;22(6, Muscle and Neuromuscular Junction Disorders):1954–77.
3. Chu ML, Moran E. The limb-girdle muscular dystrophies: is treatment on the horizon? Neurotherapeutics. 2018;15:849–62.
4. Patel NJ, Van Dyke KW, Espinoza LR. Limb-girdle muscular dystrophy 2B and Miyoshi presentations of Dysferlinopathy. Am J Med Sci. 2017;353(5):484–91.
5. Bushby KM, Beckmann JS. The limb-girdle muscular dystrophies--proposal for a new nomenclature. Neuromuscul Disord. 1995;5(4):337–43.
6. Joyce NC, Oskarsson B, Jin LW. Muscle biopsy evaluation in neuromuscular disorders. Phys Med Rehabil Clin N Am. 2012;23(3):609–31.
7. Liu J, Aoki M, Illa I, Wu C, Fardeau M, Angelini C, Serrano C, Urtizberea JA, Hentati F, Hamida MB, et al. Dysferlin, a novel skeletal muscle gene, is mutated in Miyoshi myopathy and limb girdle muscular dystrophy. Nat Genet. 1998;20(1):31–6.
8. Oh SH, Kang SW, Lee JG, Na SJ, Kim TS, Choi YC. Clinical and pathological characteristics of four Korean patients with limb-girdle muscular dystrophy type 2B. J Korean Med Sci. 2004;19(3):447–52.
9. Domingos J, Sarkozy A, Scoto M, Muntoni F. Dystrophinopathies and limb-girdle muscular dystrophies. Neuropediatrics. 2017;48(4):262–72.
10. Murphy AP, Straub V. The classification, natural history and treatment of the limb girdle muscular dystrophies. J Neuromuscul Dis. 2015;2(s2):S7–S19.
11. Lopez AA, Roman FA, Vilanova VV, Corujeira RM, Arean GI, Valino HC. Total intravenous anesthesia for aortic aneurysm replacement surgery in a patient with limb-girdle dystrophy. Rev Esp Anestesiol Reanim. 2014;61(7):385–7.
12. Yemen TA, McClain C. Muscular dystrophy, anesthesia and the safety of inhalational agents revisited; again. Paediatr Anaesth. 2006;16(2):105–8.
13. Schieren M, Defosse J, Bohmer A, Wappler F, Gerbershagen MU. Anaesthetic management of patients with myopathies. Eur J Anaesthesiol. 2017;34(10):641–9.
14. Wappler F. Anesthesia for patients with a history of malignant hyperthermia. Curr Opin Anaesthesiol. 2010;23(3):417–22.
15. Kim TW, Nemergut ME. Preparation of modern anesthesia workstations for malignant hyperthermia-susceptible patients: a review of past and present practice. Anesthesiology. 2011;114(1):205–12.
16. Muenster T, Forst J, Goerlitz P, Schmitt HJ. Reversal of rocuronium-induced neuromuscular blockade by pyridostigmine in patients with Duchenne muscular dystrophy. Paediatr Anaesth. 2008;18(3):251–5.
17. Shapiro F, Athiraman U, Clendenin DJ, Hoagland M, Sethna NF. Anesthetic management of 877 pediatric patients undergoing muscle biopsy for neuromuscular disorders: a 20-year review. Paediatr Anaesth. 2016;26(7):710–21.
18. Richa F C. Anaesthetic management of a patient with limb-girdle muscular dystrophy for laparoscopic cholecystectomy[J]. Eur J Anaesthesiol. 2011;28(1):72-73.
19. Sarkilar G, Mermer A, Yucekul M, Ceken EM, Altun C, Otelcioglu S. Anaesthetic Management of a Child with Limb-Girdle Muscular Dystrophy. Turk J Anesth Reanim. 2014;42(2):103-105
20. T. Allen, S. Maguire. Anaesthetic management of a woman with autosomal recessive limb-girdle muscular dystrophy for emergency caesarean section. Int J Obstet Anesth. 2007;16(4):370-374
21. Michael C. Chuang, Laura V. Duggan, Rardi D. van Heest, Wendy MacLeod. Laparoscopic cholecystectomy under spinal anesthesia in a patient with limb-girdle muscular dystrophy. Can J Anesth/J canadien d'anesthésie. 2013; 60(12):1276-1277
22. Gerbershagen MU, Wappler F. Anesthesia with neuromuscular diseases. Anaesthesist. 2010;59(10):953–965 966–967.
23. Zink W, Seif C, Bohl JR, Hacke N, Braun PM, Sinner B, Martin E, Fink RH, Graf BM. The acute myotoxic effects of bupivacaine and ropivacaine after continuous peripheral nerve blockades. Anesth Analg. 2003;97(4):1173–9.
24. Zink W, Bohl JR, Hacke N, Sinner B, Martin E, Graf BM. The long term myotoxic effects of bupivacaine and ropivacaine after continuous peripheral nerve blocks. Anesth Analg. 2005;101(2):548–54.
25. Zink W, Graf BM. Local anesthetic myotoxicity. Reg Anesth Pain Med. 2004; 29(4):333–40.
26. Otsuki S, Yasuda T, Mukaida K, Noda Y, Kanzaki R, Miyoshi H, Kondo T, Hamada H, Kawamoto M. Myotoxicity of local anesthetics is equivalent in individuals with and without predisposition to malignant hyperthermia. J Anesth. 2018;32(4):616–23.
27. Nouette-Gaulain K, Sirvent P, Canal-Raffin M, Morau D, Malgat M, Molimard M, Mercier J, Lacampagne A, Sztark F, Capdevila X. Effects of intermittent femoral nerve injections of bupivacaine, levobupivacaine, and ropivacaine on mitochondrial energy metabolism and intracellular calcium homeostasis in rat psoas muscle. Anesthesiology. 2007;106(5):1026–34.
28. Nouette-Gaulain K, Bellance N, Prevost B, Passerieux E, Pertuiset C, Galbes O, Smolkova K, Masson F, Miraux S, Delage JP, et al. Erythropoietin protects against local anesthetic myotoxicity during continuous regional analgesia. Anesthesiology. 2009;110(3):648–59.
29. Neal JM, Salinas FV, Choi DS. Local anesthetic-induced myotoxicity after continuous Adductor Canal block. Reg Anesth Pain Med. 2016;41(6):723–7.
30. Capdevila X, Pirat P, Bringuier S, Gaertner E, Singelyn F, Bernard N, Choquet O, Bouaziz H, Bonnet F. Continuous peripheral nerve blocks in hospital wards after orthopedic surgery: a multicenter prospective analysis of the quality of postoperative analgesia and complications in 1,416 patients. Anesthesiology. 2005;103(5):1035–45.
31. Mather C, McSwiney M. Anaesthesia-related diplopia after cataract surgery. Br J Anaesth. 2003;91(1):152, 152–3.
32. Ranjan RV, Ramachandran TR, Manikandan S, John R. Limb-girdle muscular dystrophy with obesity for elective cesarean section: anesthetic management and brief review of the literature. Anesth Essays Res. 2015;9(1):127–9.

No radiographic index predicts difficult intubation using the Optiscope™ in cervical spine surgery patients

Hyongmin Oh, Hansol Kim, Hyun-Kyu Yoon, Hyung-Chul Lee and Hee-Pyoung Park*

Abstract

Background: The Optiscope™ can be used for intubation with minimal neck motion. We retrospectively investigated radiographic predictors of difficult intubation using the Optiscope™ by analyzing preoperative radiographic images.

Methods: One hundred eighty-four patients who were intubated with the Optiscope™ under manual in-line cervical stabilization for cervical spine surgery were enrolled. Radiographic indices were measured on preoperative cervical spine lateral X-ray and magnetic resonance imaging images. Difficult intubation was defined as failure or time consumption more than 90 s on the first attempt. To identify significant predictors of difficult intubation using the Optiscope™ and evaluate their diagnostic value, multivariable logistic regression and receiver operating characteristic analyses were used.

Results: Fourty-seven patients showed difficult intubation. There was no significant difference in radiographic indices between the difficult and easy intubation groups, but higher body mass index (BMI) (26.5 [3.0] vs. 24.6 [3.5] kg/m^2, $P = 0.001$), shorter sternomental distance (SMD) (122.0 [104.0 to 150.0] vs. 150.0 [130.0 to 170.0] mm, $P = 0.001$), shorter interincisor gap (40.0 [35.0 to 45.0] vs. 43.0 [40.0 to 50.0] mm, $P = 0.006$), and higher incidence of excessive oral secretions (10.6% vs. 2.9%, $P = 0.049$) were observed in patients with difficult intubation. In multivariable analysis, BMI (odds ratio [95% confidence interval]; 1.15 [1.03 to 1.28], $P = 0.011$) and SMD (odds ratio [95% confidence interval]; 0.98 [0.97 to 1.00], $P = 0.008$) were associated with difficult intubation with the Optiscope™. In receiver operating characterstic analysis, the area under the curve for body mass index was 0.68 (95% confidence interval; 0.60 to 0.77, $P < 0.001$) and that for sternomental distance was 0.66 (95% confience interval; 0.57 to 0.75, $P = 0.001$).

Conclusions: The incidence of difficult intubation using the Optiscope™ under manual in-line cervical stabilization was 25.5% in cervical spine surgery patients. No significant predictor of difficult intubation with the Optiscope™ was identified among the measured radiographic indices. Although high BMI and short SMD were predictive of difficult intubation with the Optiscope™, their discrimination power was weak.

Keywords: Optiscope™, Videostylet, Difficult intubation, Predictor, Cervical spine surgery

* Correspondence: hppark@snu.ac.kr
Department of Anesthesiology and Pain Medicine, Seoul National University Hospital, Seoul National University College of Medicine, 101, Daehak-ro, Jongno-gu, Seoul 03080, South Korea

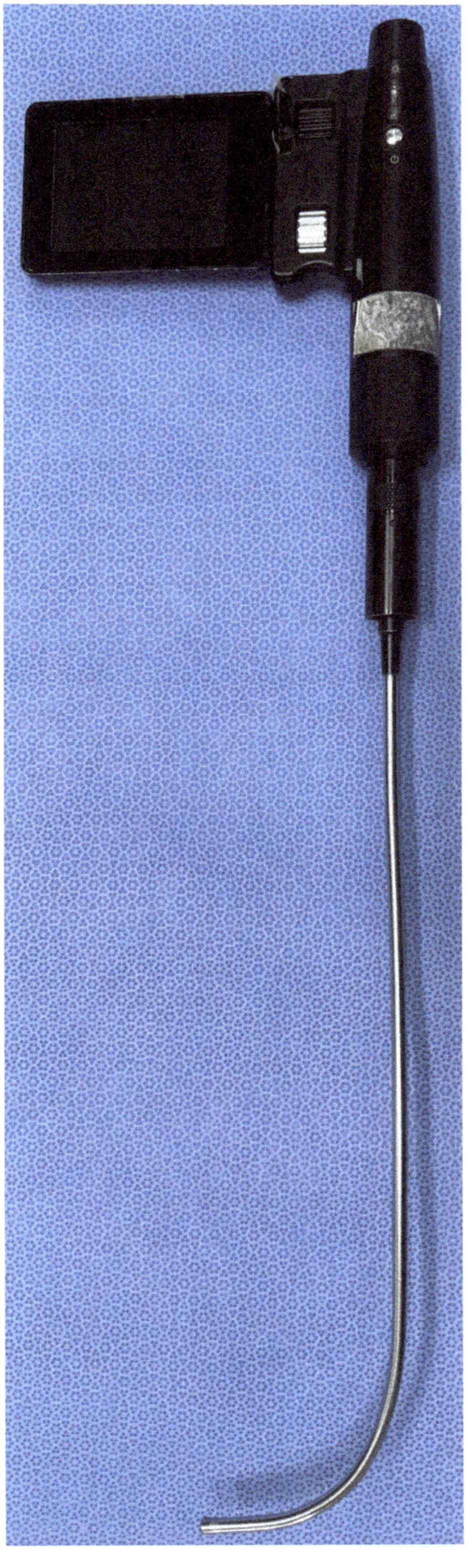

Fig. 1 The Optiscope™ used in this study. This videostylet has a rigid stylet that angled 90 degrees,with a camera lens at the bottome end and a handle and monitor at the top end

Introduction

In patients undergoing cervical spine surgery, endotracheal intubation with direct laryngoscopy is challenging. Application of neck collar or manual in-line cervical stabilization during intubation is necessary to prevent secondary neurologic injury due to excessive neck extension [1]. This maneuver hinders mouth opening and neck extension, resulting in difficult laryngoscopy [2, 3]. For this reason, intubation devices such as videolaryngoscopes, lightwands, flexible fiberoptic bronchoscopes, and videostylets are often used instead of direct laryngoscopes to increase the success rate of intubation and minimize neck motion [4–8].

The Optiscope™ (Clarus Medical LLC, Minneapolis, MN, USA) is a videostylet consisting of a rigid fiberscope with an attached monitor; it is possible to indirectly visualize a patient's larynx on the monitor during intubation (Fig. 1). Unlike direct laryngoscopes, when intubating with the Optiscope™, alignment of the three airway axes is not necessary. Therefore the Optiscope™ is especially useful in patients with neck motion that must be minimized during intubation. In previous studies comparing the Optiscope™ with other intubation devices, use of the Optiscope™ resulted in less cervical spine motion than was observed with videolaryngoscopes, as well as a shorter intubation time than flexible fiberoptic bronchoscopes, and fewer scooping movements than lightwands [4, 9, 10].

In clinical practice, it is important for anesthesiologists to recognize the factors predicting difficult intubation before anesthetic induction. Numerous studies have shown that body mass index (BMI), Mallampati score, and mouth opening predict difficult intubation with intubation devices such as direct laryngoscopes, videolaryngoscopes, and lightwands [11–14]. Regarding radiographic indices associated with difficult intubation, tongue area, atlanto-occipital gap, mandibulohyoid distance, and the angle of the anterior-inferior point of the upper incisor with the neck in extension are related to difficult laryngoscopy, while epiglottis length is associated with increased intubation time when using lightwands [15–18]. Despite the aforementioned advantages of videostylets, no clinical investigation has yet been performed to identify radiographic predictors of difficult intubation with videostylets.

In this study, we aimed to identify radiographic indices associated with difficult intubation with the Optiscope™ in patients undergoing cervical spinal surgery, by analyzing preoperative cervical spine lateral X-ray and magnetic resonance imaging (MRI) images.

Methods

Ethic and approval

Ethical approval for this retrospective study (1909–021-1060) was provided by the Institutional Review Board

(101, Daehak-ro, Jongno-gu, Seoul, Korea, 03080) of Seoul National University Hospital (SNUH) on 6 September 2019. The requirement for written informed consent was waived because of the retrospective nature of the study.

Subject

Patients who underwent cervical spine surgery and were intubated with the Optiscope™ at SNUH from June 2016 to August 2018 were included (Fig. 2). The participants were previously enrolled in a randomized controlled trial previously conducted at our institution to compare the clinical performance of the Optiscope™ and the McGrath™ MAC videolaryngoscope (Medtronic, Minneapolis, MN, USA) in patients undergoing cervical spine surgery [19]. Patients who were intubated with other intubation devices, and those who had any missing radiographic data, were excluded. Based on the number of intubation attempts and time required for intubation, patients were assigned to either the easy or difficult intubation group. Difficult intubation (the primary outcome measure) was defined as failed intubation or intubation requiring more than 90 s on the first attempt [10].

Data collection

General data, including demographic data, American Society of Anesthesiologists physical status, comorbidities, diagnosis, and cervical level operation site were collected. Airway-related variables including the Mallampati score, retrognathia, sternomental distance (SMD), thyromental distance (TMD), and interincisor gap (IIG) were also collected. Twenty-one radiographic indices thought to be associated with difficult intubation with the Optiscope™ were measured three times on preoperative cervical spine lateral X-ray and MRI images, and averaged for analysis by an investigator who was blinded to the group assignments. The radiographic data are shown in Fig. 3 and Table 1. When taking cervical spine X-ray and MRI images, the body and head postions were protocolized in our hospital. In brief, cervical spine lateral X-ray was taken in the standing position with the neutral neck position while MRI images were taken in the supine position with the neutral neck position. When cervical lateral x-ray was taken in the neck extension position, patients were asked to extend the neck without pain or neurologic signs as much as they can. To address potential sources of bias, events that could interfere with intubation with Optiscope™, such as the presence of

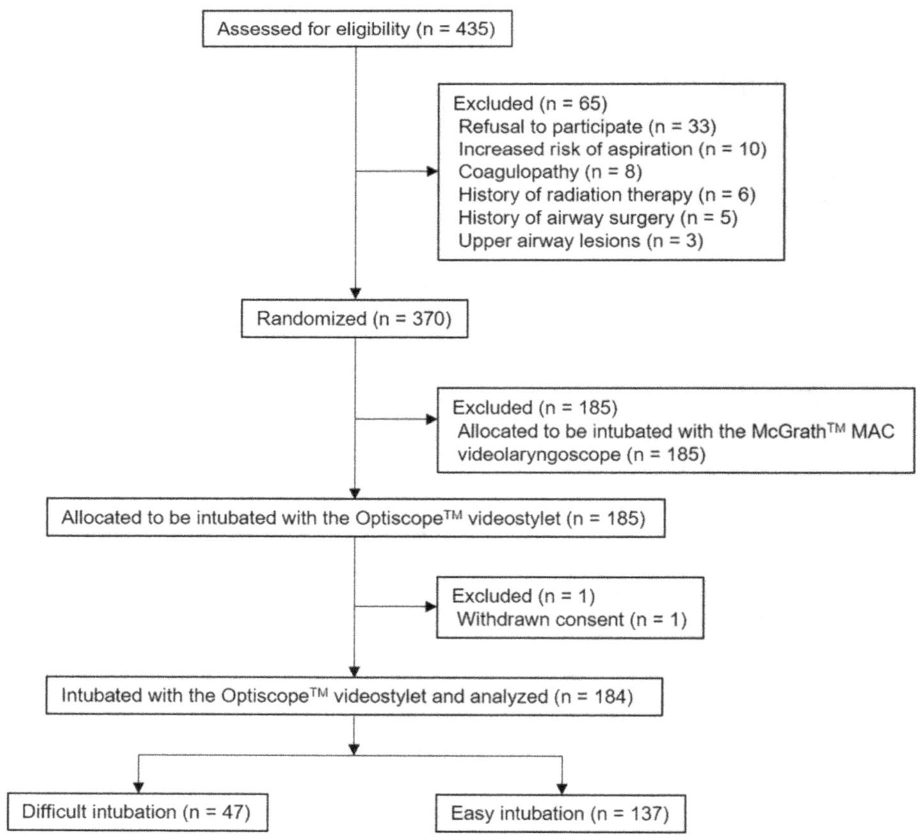

Fig. 2 CONSORT flow diagram

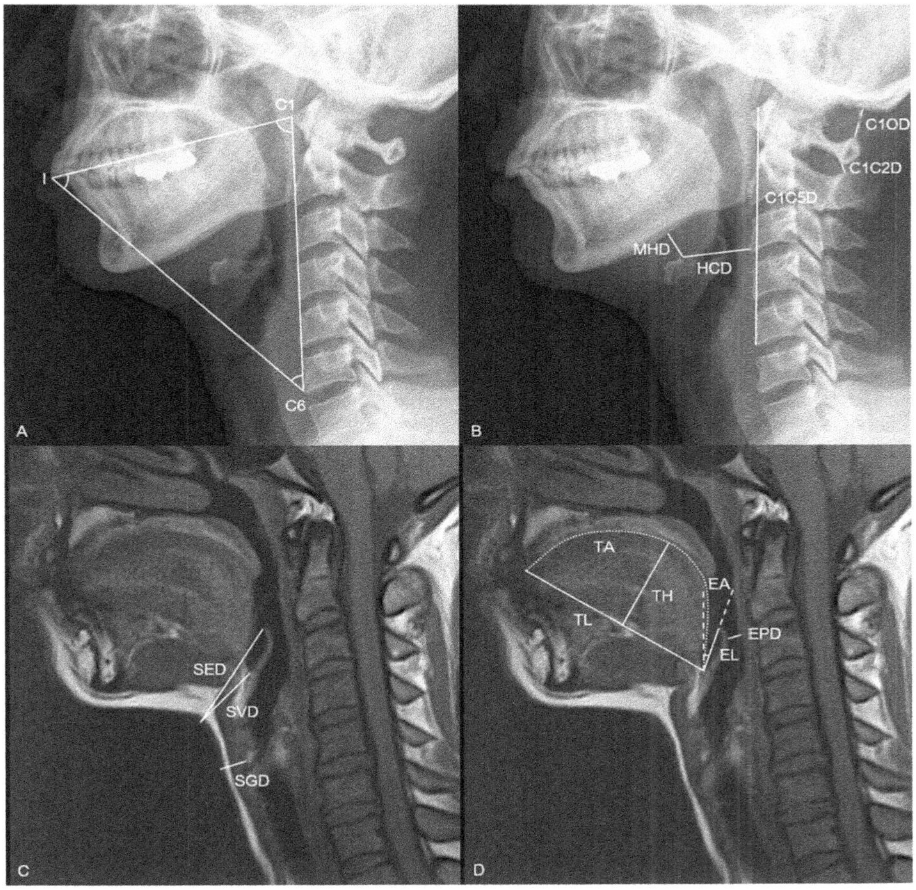

Fig. 3 Measurements of radiographic indices investigated in this study. Radiographic indices were measured on cervical spine lateral X-ray (**a** and **b**) and magnetic resonance imaging (**c** and **d**) images in neutral neck position. I. incisor; C1, atlas; C5, the 5th cervical spine; MHD, mandibulohyoid distance; C1C5D, atlanto-the 5th cervical vertebral distance; C1OD, atlanto-occipital distance; HCD, hyoidocervical distance; C1C2D, atlanto-axial distance; SVD, skin-vallecular distance; SED, skin-epiglottic distance; SGD, skin-glottic distance; TL, tongue length; TH, tongue height; TA: tongue area; EL, epiglottis length; EPD, epiglottic-pharyngeal distance, EA, epiglottis angle

excessive oral secretions and loose incisor, were also recorded.

Anesthetic management

All patients entered the operating room without any premedication. Following routine monitoring, including noninvasive blood pressure, electrocardiography, and pulse oximetry, anesthesia was induced by target-controlled infusion of remifentanil (effect site concentration, 4 ng mL^{-1}) and propofol (effect site concentration, 4 μg mL^{-1}). Rocuronium was administered at 0.6 mg kg^{-1} after loss of consciousness to facilitate endotracheal intubation. At least 120 s after rocuronium administration, intubation was performed with the Optiscope™ by one of two attending anesthesiologists, who had each carried out more than 50 successful intubations with the Optiscope™. To decrease inter-intubator variability, only two skilled attending anesthesiologists participated in intubation with the Optiscope™. A reinforced endotracheal tube (internal diameter = 7.0 mm for females and 7.5 mm for males) was used and manual in-line cervical stabilization was performed by another anesthesiologist during intubation of all patients. The endotracheal tube mounted on the Optiscope™ was inserted along the midline and jaw thrust maneuver was performed if entry into the hypopharynx was difficult. Successful intubation was confirmed by continuous end-tidal carbon dioxide monitoring.

Statistical analysis

Data are presented as number (percent) for categorical variables, mean ± standard deviation for normally distributed variables, and median [interquartile range] for skewed variables. Categorical variables were compared using the chi-square test or Fisher's exact test. Student's t test or the Mann–Whitney U test were used to compare continuous variables based on the normality of the data distribution, as assessed by the Shapiro–Wilk test.

Table 1 Definitions of radiographic indices investigated in this study

	Detailed description	Meaning
Cervical spine lateral X-ray		
MHD (mm)	Linear distance from the inferior border of the mandibular body to the highest point of the hyoid bone	Tongue size
C1C5D (mm)	Linear distance from the antero-superior border of atlas to the antero-inferior border of the fifth cervical vertebra	Neck length
C1OD (mm)	Linear distance from upper margin of posterior tubercle of atlas to occiput	Neck extension
HCD (mm)	Linear distance from the highest point of the hyoid bone to the anterior border of the nearest cervical vertebra	Tongue size
C1C2D (mm)	Linear distance from lower margin of the spinous processes of atlas to upper margin of the spinous processes of axis in the neutral position	Neck extension
C1-I-C6 (°)	The angle between the line from the anterior border of atlas to the tip of upper incisors and the line from the antero-inferior border of C6 vertebral body to the tip of upper incisors in the neutral position	Cervical range of motion
I-C6-C1 (°)	The Angle between the line from the tip of upper incisors to the antero-inferior border of C6 vertebral body and the line from the anterior border of atlas to the antero-inferior border of C6 vertebral body in the neutral position	Cervical range of motion
I-C1-C6 (°)	The Angle between the line from the tip of upper incisors to the anterior border of atlas and the line from the antero-inferior border of C6 vertebral body to the anterior border of atlas.	Cervical range of motion
C1-I-C6′ (°)	Same as C1-I-C6 in the extension position of the cervical spine	Cervical range of motion
I-C6-C1′ (°)	Same as I-C6-C1 in the extension position of the cervical spine	Cervical range of motion
I-C1-C6′ (°)	Same as I-C1-C6 in the extension position of the cervical spine	Cervical range of motion
Cervical spine MRI		
TL (mm)	Linear distance from the vallecula to the tip of the tongue	Tongue size
TH (mm)	Perpendicular height from the line of tongue length to the top of the tongue	Tongue size
TA (mm^2)	Tongue area above the line of tongue length from the tip of the upper incisors to the vallecula in the mid-sagittal plane	Tongue size
EL (mm)	Linear distance from the vallecular to the tip of the epiglottis	Epiglottis size
EPD (mm)	Distance between the epiglottis and the posterior wall of the pharynx	Pharyngeal space
EA (°)	Angle of epiglottis from perpendicular line	Epiglottis angle
CVLVC	Anatomical position of the vocal cords in relation to the cervical vertebrae	Anatomical position of vocal cord
SVD (mm)	Linear distance from skin to the vallecula	Pre-epiglottic area
SED (mm)	Linear distance from skin to the tip of the epiglottis	Pre-epiglottic area
SGD (mm)	Linear distance from skin to the anterior tip of vocal cords	Pre-cord area

MHD Mandibulohyoid distance, *C1C5D* Atlanto-the 5th cervical vertebral distance, *C1OD* Atlanto-occipital distance, *HCD* Hyoidocervical distance, *C1C2D* Atlanto-axial distance, *C1-I-C6* C1-incisor-C6 angle in the neck neutral position, *I-C6-C1* Incisor-C6-C1 angle in the neck neutral position, *I-C1-C6* Incisor-C1-C6 angle in the neck neutral position, *C1-I-C6′* C1-incisor-C6 angle in the neck extension position, *I-C6-C1′* Incisor-C6-C1 angle in the neck extension position, *I-C1-C6′* Incisor-C1-C6 angle in the neck extension position; *MRI* Magnetic resonance imaging, *TL* Tongue length, *TH* Tongue height, *TA* Tongue area, *EL* Epiglottis length, *EPD* Epiglottic-pharyngeal distance, *EA* Epiglottis angle, *CVLVC* Cervical vertebral level of vocal cords, *SVD* Skin-vallecular distance, *SED* Skin-epiglottic distance, *SGD* Skin-glottic distance

To identify predictors of difficult intubation with the Optiscope™, univariable and multivariable logistic regression analyses were conducted. Variables with P values lower than 0.1 in univariable analysis were included in the multivariable analysis. Receiver operating characteristic (ROC) analysis was performed to assess the diagnostic value of significant variables in multivariable analysis. The predictive accuracy of significant variables was classified into five grades according to their area under the ROC curve (0.5–0.6; fail, 0.6–0.7; poor, 0.7–0.8; fair, 0.8–0.9; good, 0.9–1.0; excellent) [20]. The optimal cutoff point was set to a value that maximized the

Youden index (sensitivity + specificity − 1). Subgroup analyses were conducted by dividing into two groups based on the optimal cutoff points. Two-sided *P* values less than 0.05 were considered statistically significant. All statistical analyses were performed using SPSS statistical software (version 25.0; SPSS Inc., Chicago, IL, USA).

In a previous study, difficult intubation as defined in the present study was observed in 10% of patients who were intubated using the Optiscope™ with cervical spine immobilization [10]. To reproduce the proportion of cases of difficult intubation with the Optiscope™ with a 95% confidence interval (CI) and a margin of error of 0.05, at least 159 patients were required in this study.

Results

A total of 184 patients who underwent cervical spine surgery from June 2016 to August 2018 were enrolled in this study. Among them, 47 (25.5%) and 137 (74.5%) patients experienced difficult and easy intubation with the Optiscope™, respectively.

As shown in Table 2, there was no significant difference in general characteristics between the difficult and easy intubation groups, except for a higher BMI (26.5 ± 3.0 vs. 24.6 ± 3.5 kg m^{-2}, $P = 0.001$) and a greater incidence of excessive oral secretions [5 (10.6%) vs. 4 (2.9%), $P = 0.049$] in difficult intubation group. Among airway-related variables, the difficult intubation group had a significantly shorter SMD [122.0 (104.0 to 150.0) vs. 150.0 (130.0 to 170.0) mm, $P = 0.001$] and shorter IIG [40.0 (35.0 to 45.0) vs. 43.0 (40.0 to 50.0) mm, $P = 0.006$] compared to the easy intubation group. None of the radiographic indices differed significantly between the two groups (Table 3).

The results of multivariable logistic regression analysis are summarized in Table 4. BMI [odds ratio (95% CI); 1.15 (1.03 to 1.28), $P = 0.011$] and SMD [odds ratio (95% CI); 0.98 (0.97 to 1.00), $P = 0.008$] were related to difficult intubation with the Optiscope™.

In ROC analysis, the area under the curve for BMI was 0.68 (95% CI; 0.60 to 0.77, $P < 0.001$) and that for SMD was 0.66 (95% CI; 0.57 to 0.75, $P = 0.001$), both showing poor predictive accuracy. The optimal cutoff points for BMI and SMD were 25.3 kg m^{-2} and 123.5 mm, respectively. Difficult intubation was observed more frequently in patients whose BMI was higher than 25.3 kg m^{-2} [odds ratio (95% CI); 3.07 (1.54 to 6.12), $P = 0.001$], or whose SMD was shorter than 123.5 mm [odds ratio (95% CI); 3.89 (1.92 to 7.85), $P < 0.001$].

Discussion

This clinical study was performed to identify radiographic predictors of difficult intubation with the Optiscope™ in patients undergoing cervical spine surgery with manual in-line cervical stabilization during intubation. Although high BMI and short SMD were associated with difficult intubation using the Optiscope™, no radiographic index measured on preoperative radiographic images predicted difficult intubation with the Optiscope™.

Many radiographic predictors of difficult laryngoscopy have been identified in previous studies. In one such study, a large tongue area measured on preoperative computed tomography was associated with difficult laryngoscopy in acromegaly patients [16]. In another study conducted in patients with cervical spondylosis, a long mandibulohyoid distance and large angle of the anterior-inferior point of the upper incisor in the extended neck position were related to difficult laryngoscopy [17]. A short atlanto-occipital distance has also been reported to make laryngoscopy difficult [15]. However, these radiographic indices did not predict difficult intubation with the Optiscope™ in the current study. This difference may be due to a difference in intubation method between direct laryngoscopes and the Optiscope™. Because alignment of the three airway axes is not necessary when intubating with the Optiscope™, radiographic indices representing neck extension were not predictive of difficult intubation with the Optiscope™. In addition, the Optiscope™ has a slim body compared to direct laryngoscopes. Therefore, when intubating with the Optiscope™, the impact of an enlarged tongue on intubation is less significant.

In this study, BMI was significantly related to difficult intubation with the Optiscope™ based on multivariable analysis. Patients with a BMI higher than 25.3 kg m^{-2} had a 3.1-fold higher risk of difficult intubation with the Optiscope™. In a previous study investigating the collapsibility index of the upper airway in patients with obstructive sleep apnea, the collapsibility indices in the high and low retroglossal areas were higher in obese versus non-obese patients during sleep, suggesting that obese patients had an increased likelihood of downward movement of the tongue after anesthetic induction [21]. The narrow space between the posterior pharyngeal wall and tongue base can make intubation with the Optiscope™ difficult by hindering its advancement into the hypopharynx. Obesity is known to predict difficult intubation with rigid fiberscopes and lightwands as well as direct laryngoscopes [11]. Although its retromolar or paraglossal aprroach is different from the Optiscope™, the Bonfils™ (Karl Storz Endoscopy, Tuttlingen, Germany), a rigid fiberscope, is similar to the Optiscope™ in terms of its J-shaped structure and scooping movements. In a previous study, the intubation time with the Bonfils™ was longer in patients with small mouth openings, a long TMD, high BMI, and high Cormack and Lehane grade [22]. Lightwand devices also

Table 2 Comparisons of general characteristics and airway-related variables between the difficult and easy intubation groups

	Difficult ($n = 47$)	Easy ($n = 137$)	P value
Male (n)	31 (66.0%)	93 (67.9%)	0.808
Age (yr)	57.8 ± 12.1	54.5 ± 14.0	0.154
Weight (kg)	70.5 ± 11.5	67.0 ± 12.7	0.103
Height (cm)	166.0 (158.5 to 171.0)	164.0 (156.0 to 171.0)	0.253
BMI (kg m^{-2})	26.5 ± 3.0	24.6 (3.5)	0.001
BMI > 25 kg m^{-2}	33 (70.2%)	60 (43.8%)	0.002
BMI > 30 kg m^{-2}	8 (17.0%)	8 (5.8%)	0.019
ASA physical status (n)			0.334
1	18 (38.3%)	60 (43.8%)	
2	23 (48.9%)	66 (48.2%)	
3	6 (12.8%)	11 (6.0%)	
Co-morbidity (n)			
Diabetes	10 (21.3%)	21 (15.3%)	0.347
Hypertension	16 (34.0%)	40 (29.2%)	0.533
Cardiac	1 (2.1%)	6 (4.4%)	0.680
Pulmonary	2 (4.3%)	3 (2.2%)	0.603
Neurologic	4 (8.5%)	6 (4.4%)	0.280
Hepatic	0 (0.0%)	9 (6.6%)	0.114
Renal	1 (2.1%)	4 (2.9%)	1.000
Thyroid	0 (0.0%)	2 (1.5%)	1.000
Rheumatoid arthritis	3 (6.4%)	4 (2.9%)	0.374
Diagnosis (n)			
Degenerative	37 (78.7%)	103 (75.2%)	0.623
Tumor	7 (14.9%)	29 (21.4%)	0.349
Trauma	1 (2.1%)	0 (0.0%)	0.255
Congenital	2 (4.3%)	5 (3.6%)	1.000
Operation site (n)			0.961
Above C2	7 (14.9%)	20 (14.6%)	
Below C3	40 (85.1%)	117 (85.4%)	
Mallampati score (n)			0.084
1	8 (17.0%)	37 (27.0%)	
2	20 (42.6%)	58 (42.3%)	
3	15 (31.9%)	37 (27.0%)	
4	4 (8.5%)	5 (3.6%)	
Retrognathia (n)	2 (4.3%)	1 (0.7%)	0.161
TMD (mm)	80.0 (70.0 to 90.0)	80.0 (70.0 to 90.0)	0.485
RHTMD	20.9 (18.9 to 23.4)	21.0 (18.4 to 23.2)	0.785
SMD (mm)	122.0 (104.0 to 150.0)	150.0 (130.0 to 170.0)	0.001
IIG (mm)	40.0 (35.0 to 45.0)	43.0 (40.0 to 50.0)	0.006
Excessive oral secretions (n)	5 (10.6%)	4 (2.9%)	0.049
Loose upper or lower incisor (n)	0 (0.0%)	3 (2.2%)	0.571

BMI Body mass index, *ASA* American society of anesthesiologists, *TMD* Thyromental distance; *RHTMD* Ratio of height to thyromental distance, *SMD* Sternomental distance, *IIG* Interincisor gap

Table 3 Comparisons of radiographic indices between the difficult and easy intubation groups

	Difficult (*n* = 47)	Easy (*n* = 137)	*P* value
MHD (mm)	14.5 ± 6.2	16.6 ± 9.5	0.080
C1C5D (mm)	103.8 ± 9.6	104.1 ± 10.1	0.835
C1OD (mm)	7.4 (5.1 to 9.2)	7.4 (5.3 to 9.4)	0.720
HCD (mm)	40.4 (36.3 to 44.3)	39.2 (35.8 to 42.8)	0.196
C1C2D (mm)	5.1 (3.0 to 7.1)	4.9 (3.7 to 6.7)	0.956
C1-I-C6 (°)	52.0 (49.0 to 55.1)	52.9 (49.5 to 55.4)	0.296
I-C6-C1 (°)	40.8 (38.7 to 45.0)	41.6 (38.7 to 45.1)	0.845
I-C1-C6 (°)	86.9 ± 9.2	85.4 ± 8.0	0.293
C1-I-C6′ (°)	38.3 (34.8 to 41.2)	37.7 (34.8 to 42.1)	0.866
I-C6-C1′ (°)	30.8 (29.2 to 32.5)	30.8 (27.7 to 33.9)	0.582
I-C1-C6′ (°)	111.2 (107.2 to 115.6)	111.8 (104.7 to 117.2)	0.775
TL (mm)	69.6 (65.7 to 76.2)	69.8 (64.5 to 74.2)	0.634
TH (mm)	36.9 ± 4.6	37.2 ± 5.3	0.743
TA (cm^2)	19.4 ± 4.0	19.3 ± 3.3	0.810
EL (mm)	18.5 ± 2.2	18.6 ± 2.3	0.810
EPD (mm)	7.0 (5.3 to 9.1)	6.6 (4.8 to 8.2)	0.205
EA (°)	31.1 ± 9.6	34.0 ± 11.4	0.126
CVLVC (n)			0.315
C4 level	6 (12.8%)	14 (10.2%)	
C5 level	38 (80.9%)	107 (78.1%)	
C6 level	3 (6.4%)	16 (11.7%)	
SVD (mm)	30.6 ± 4.9	29.4 ± 5.4	0.200
SED (mm)	49.5 ± 7.4	47.4 ± 6.3	0.059
SGD (mm)	12.2 (10.5 to 14.2)	11.5 (9.5 to 13.3)	0.131

MHD Mandibulohyoid distance, *C1C5D* Atlanto-the 5th cervical vertebral distance, *C1OD* Atlanto-occipital distance, *HCD* Hyoidocervical distance, *C1C2D* Atlanto-axial distance, *C1-I-C6* C1-incisor-C6 angle in the neck neutral position, *I-C6-C1* Incisor-C6-C1 angle in the neck neutral position, *I-C1-C6* Incisor-C1-C6 angle in the neck neutral position, *C1-I-C6′* C1-incisor-C6 angle in the neck extension position, *I-C6-C1′* Incisor-C6-C1 angle in the neck extension position, *I-C1-C6′* Incisor-C1-C6 angle in the neck extension position, *MRI* Magnetic resonance imaging, *TL* Tongue length, *TH* Tongue height, *TA* Tongue area, *EL* Epiglottis length; *EPD* Epiglottic-pharyngeal distance, *EA* Epiglottis angle, *CVLVC* Cervical vertebral level of vocal cords

resemble the Optiscope™ in terms of their shape and manipulation type, although they cannot visualize a patient's larynx during intubation. Previous studies demonstrated that BMI, the Mallampati score, neck circumference, and epiglottis length were positively correlated with intubation time with lightwands [12, 18].

SMD is an indicator of neck length and neck extension. Full extension of the neck makes it easy to align the three airway axes during direct laryngoscopy. A short SMD has thus been identified as a predictor of difficult laryngoscopy [23, 24]. In this study, patients with an SMD shorter than 123.5 mm had a 3.9-fold higher risk of difficult intubation with the Optiscope™. A short SMD can make intubation with the Optiscope™ difficult by impeding its insertion into the oral cavity, due to the hyperacute insertion angle; this increases the chance of lens contamination due to oral secretions. However, in predicting difficult intubation with the Optiscope™, the area under the curve for SMD and BMI was 0.66 and 0.68 respectively. This suggests that their discrimination power is so weak that their role as important predictors of difficult intubation with the Optiscope™ may be clinically insignificant.

Based on our clinical experience, one of the most common difficult situations encountered during intubation with the Optiscope™ is non-visibility of the vocal cord due to the tongue base or epiglottis being in contact with the posterior pharyngeal wall. In several cases, this problem was resolved by the jaw thrust maneuver. Therefore, we expected that radiographic indices related to tongue or epiglottis would be associated with difficult intubation, but that was not the case in this study, possibly due to differences in consciousness and muscle tone at the time of radiographic examination and intubation. In general, the tongue and epiglottis tend to move toward the posterior pharyngeal wall in the supine position in anesthetized patients [25]. We think that the upper airway configuration at the time of intubation may be different from that at the time of radiographic examination.

Until now, there is no consensus definition of difficult intubation using videostylets. In this study, difficult intubation with the Optiscope™ was defined as an

Table 4 Factors for difficult intubation with Optiscope™ on univariable and multivariable logistic regression analyses

	Univariable			Multivariable		
	OR	95% CI	*P* value	OR	95% CI	*P* value
BMI (kg m^{-2})	1.17	1.06 to 1.30	0.003	1.15	1.03 to 1.28	0.011
Excessive oral secretions (n)	3.96	1.02 to 15.42	0.047	4.38	0.88 to 21.90	0.072
IIG (mm)	0.95	0.91 to 0.99	0.024	0.97	0.93 to 1.02	0.238
SMD (mm)	0.98	0.97 to 0.99	0.002	0.98	0.97 to 1.00	0.008
SED (mm)	1.05	1.00 to 1.10	0.064	1.03	0.98 to 1.10	0.257

All variables with $P < 0.1$ in univariable logistic regression analysis were shown in this table and all of them were entered into multivariable logistic regression analysis. Nagelkerke R^2 statistic was 0.199 and Hosmer and Lemeshow goodness of fit test was not significant at 5% ($P = 0.814$) in multivariable analysis. *OR* Odds ratio, *CI* Confidence interval, *BMI* Body mass index; *IIG* Interincisor gap, *SMD* Sternomental distance, *SED* Skin-epiglottic distance intubation duration of more than 90 s or failed intubation on the first attempt. In a previous study comparing clinical performance between the Optiscope™ and Surch-Lite™ lightwand (Aaron Medical, St. Petersburg, FL, USA), [10] an intubation duration of 90 s corresponded to the 95th percentile. Therefore, we set the cutoff point of difficult intubation with the Optiscope™ as 90 s.

This study had several limitations. First, there may have been biases that affected the results due to its retrospective design. Second, there were several cases of difficult intubation with the Optiscope™ due to poor visualization caused by oral secretions. No medication, such as glycopyrrolate, was used routinely before intubation to reduce oral secretions. A previous study reported that glycopyrrolate shortened the intubation time with the Optiscope™, by reducing oral secretions and providing better visualization [26]. Third, since this study was performed in patients who were intubated using the Optiscope™ with manual in-line cervical stabilization for cervical spinal surgery, caution should be taken when applying the results of this study to general patients. In addition, this is a single center study, which also can potentially limit generalizability. Lastly, our predictive model of difficult intubation with the Optiscope™ had relatively weak explanatory power. It is possible that other factors predicting difficult intubation with the Optiscope™ were omitted from the analysis. Further research is needed to identify other significant predictors of difficult intubation with the Optiscope™.

Conclusion

The incidence of difficult intubation with the Optiscope™ was 25.5% in patients undergoing cervical spine surgery with manual in-line cervical stabilization during intubation. No significant radiographic predictor of difficult intubation with the Optiscope™ was identified on preoperative cervical spine lateral X-ray or MRI images. Although high BMI and short SMD were associated with difficult intubation with the Optiscope™, they had poor predictive accuracy.

Abbreviations

BMI: Body mass index; C1: Atlas; C1C2D: Atlanto-axial distance; C1C5D: Atlanto-the 5th cervical vertebral distance; C1-I-C6: Atlas-incisor-the 6th cervical vertebra angle in the neck neutral position; C1-I-C6': Atlas-incisor-the 6th cervical vertebra in the neck extension position; C1OD: Atlanto-occipital distance; C5: The 5th cervical spine; CI: Confidence interval; CVLVC: Cervical vertebral level of vocal cords; EA: Epiglottis angle; EL: Epiglottis length; EPD: Epiglottic-pharyngeal distance; HCD: Hyoidocervical distance; I: Incisor; I-C1-C6: Incisor-atlas-the 6th cervical vertebra angle in the neck neutral position; I-C1-C6': Incisor-atlas-the 6th cervical vertebra angle in the neck extension position; I-C6-C1: Incisor-the 6th cervical vertebra-atlas angle in the neck neutral position; I-C6-C1': Incisor-the 6th cervical vertebra-atlas angle in the neck extension position; IIG: Interincisor gap; IRB: Institutional review board; MHD: Mandibulohyoid distance; MRI: Magnetic resonance imaging; ROC: Receiver operating characteristic; SED: Skin-epiglottic distance; SGD: Skin-glottic distance; SMD: Sternomental distance; SNUH: Seoul national university hospital; SVD: Skin-vallecular distance; TA: Tongue area; TH: Tongue height; TL: Tongue length; TMD: Thyromental distance

Acknowledgements

Not applicable.

Authors' contribution

OH designed the study, collected, analyzed and interpreted the data and drafted the manuscript. KH designed the study, collected the data and drafted the manuscript. YHK designed the study, collected the data and drafted the manuscript. LHC designed the study, analyzed and interpreted the data and critically revised the manuscript. PHP designed the study, analyzed and interpreted the data, drafted and critically revised the manuscript. All authors read and approved the final manuscript.

References

1. Austin N, Krishnamoorthy V, Dagal A. Airway management in cervical spine injury. Int J Crit Illn Inj Sci. 2014;4:50–6.
2. Yuk M, Yeo W, Lee K, Ko J, Park T. Cervical collar makes difficult airway: a simulation study using the LEMON criteria. Clin Exp Emerg Med. 2018;5:22–8.
3. Hastings RH, Wood PR. Head extension and laryngeal view during laryngoscopy with cervical spine stabilization maneuvers. Anesthesiology. 1994;80:825–31.
4. Nam K, Lee Y, Park HP, Chung J, Yoon HK, Kim TK. Cervical spine motion during tracheal intubation using an Optiscope versus the McGrath Videolaryngoscope in patients with simulated cervical immobilization: a prospective randomized crossover study. Anesth Analg. 2019;129:1666–72.
5. Turkstra TP, Craen RA, Pelz DM, Gelb AW. Cervical spine motion: a fluoroscopic comparison during intubation with lighted stylet, GlideScope, and Macintosh laryngoscope. Anesth Analg. 2005;101:910–5 table of contents.
6. Houde BJ, Williams SR, Cadrin-Chenevert A, Guilbert F, Drolet P. A comparison of cervical spine motion during orotracheal intubation with the trachlight(r) or the flexible fiberoptic bronchoscope. Anesth Analg. 2009;108: 1638–43.
7. Kill C, Risse J, Wallot P, Seidl P, Steinfeldt T, Wulf H. Videolaryngoscopy with glidescope reduces cervical spine movement in patients with unsecured cervical spine. J Emerg Med. 2013;44:750–6.
8. Yang KH, Jeong CH, Song KC, Song JY, Song JH, Byon HJ. Comparison between Glidescope and Lightwand for tracheal intubation in patients with a simulated difficult airway. Korean J Anesthesiol. 2015;68:22–6.
9. Amir SH, Ali QE, Bansal S. A comparative evaluation of video Stylet and flexible fibre-optic bronchoscope in the performance of intubation in adult patients. Indian J Anaesth. 2017;61:321–5.
10. Seo H, Kim E, Son JD, Ji S, Min SW, Park HP. A prospective randomised study of a rigid video-stylet vs conventional lightwand intubation in cervical spine-immobilised patients. Anaesthesia. 2016;71:1341–6.
11. Wang T, Sun S, Huang S. The association of body mass index with difficult tracheal intubation management by direct laryngoscopy: a meta-analysis. BMC Anesthesiol. 2018;18:79.
12. Lee Y, Lee S, Yon JH, Lee JH. Factors affecting difficult lightwand intubation: a prospective double-blind trial. Korean J Anesthesiol. 2009;56:18–24.
13. Shiga T, Wajima Z, Inoue T, Sakamoto A. Predicting difficult intubation in apparently normal patients: a meta-analysis of bedside screening test performance. Anesthesiology. 2005;103:429–37.
14. Aziz MF, Bayman EO, Van Tienderen MM, Todd MM, St AGEIG, Brambrink AM. Predictors of difficult videolaryngoscopy with GlideScope(R) or C-MAC(R) with D-blade: secondary analysis from a large comparative videolaryngoscopy trial. Br J Anaesth. 2016;117:118–23.
15. Nichol HC, Zuck D. Difficult laryngoscopy--the "anterior" larynx and the atlanto-occipital gap. Br J Anaesth. 1983;55:141–4.
16. Lee HC, Kim MK, Kim YH, Park HP. Radiographic predictors of difficult laryngoscopy in acromegaly patients. J Neurosurg Anesthesiol. 2019;31:50–6.
17. Han YZ, Tian Y, Zhang H, Zhao YQ, Xu M, Guo XY. Radiologic indicators for prediction of difficult laryngoscopy in patients with cervical spondylosis. Acta Anaesthesiol Scand. 2018;62:474–82.
18. Kim J, Im KS, Lee JM, Ro J, Yoo KY, Kim JB. Relevance of radiological and clinical measurements in predicting difficult intubation using light wand

(Surch-lite) in adult patients. J Int Med Res. 2016;44:136–46.
19. Yoon HK, Lee HC, Park JB, Oh H, Park HP. McGrath MAC Videolaryngoscope versus Optiscope video Stylet for tracheal intubation in patients with manual inline cervical stabilization: a randomized trial. Anesth Analg. 2019. https://doi.org/10.1213/ANE.0000000000004442.
20. Tape TG. Interpreting diagnostic tests. In: University of Nebraska Medical Center; 2004. http://gim.unmc.edu/dxtests/Default.htm. Accessed 11 Feb 2020.
21. Kim TH, Chun BS, Lee HW, Kim JS. Differences of upper airway morphology according to obesity: study with Cephalometry and dynamic MD-CT. Clin Exp Otorhinolaryngol. 2010;3:147–52.
22. Nowakowski M, Williams S, Gallant J, Ruel M, Robitaille A. Predictors of difficult intubation with the Bonfils rigid fiberscope. Anesth Analg. 2016;122: 1901–6.
23. Savva D. Prediction of difficult tracheal intubation. Br J Anaesth. 1994;73: 149–53.
24. Al Ramadhani S, Mohamed LA, Rocke DA, Gouws E. Sternomental distance as the sole predictor of difficult laryngoscopy in obstetric anaesthesia. Br J Anaesth. 1996;77:312–6.
25. Nandi PR, Charlesworth CH, Taylor SJ, Nunn JF, Dore CJ. Effect of general anaesthesia on the pharynx. Br J Anaesth. 1991;66:157–62.
26. Cho EA, Hwang SH, Lee SH, Ryu KH, Kim YH. Does glycopyrrolate premedication facilitate tracheal intubation with a rigid video-stylet?: a randomized controlled trial. Medicine (Baltimore). 2018;97:e11834.

21

Anesthesia departments' readiness for the COVID-19 pandemic

Barak Cohen[1,2*], Yuval Baar[1], Shai Fein[3] and Idit Matot[1]

Abstract

Background: The Coronavirus infectious disease 2019 (COVID-19) brings anesthesiologists and intensive care physicians to the mainstay of clinical workload and healthcare managements' focus. There are approximately 900 anesthesiologists in Israel, working in non-private hospitals. This nationwide cross-sectional study evaluated the readiness and involvement of anesthesia departments in Israel in management of the COVID-19 pandemic. The impact on anesthesiologists' health, workload, and clinical practices were also evaluated.

Methods: An online questionnaire was distributed to all of anesthesia department chairs in Israel on April 14th. Each response was identifiable on the hospital level only. Informed consent was waived since no patient data were collected.

Results: Response rate was 100%. A decrease of at least 40% in operating-room activity was reported by two-thirds of the departments. Anesthesiologists are leading the treatment of COVID-19 patients in 19/28 (68%) Israeli hospitals. Israel Society of Anesthesiologists' recommendations regarding intubation of COVID-19 patients were strictly followed (intubations performed by the most experienced available physician, by rapid-sequence induction utilizing video-laryngoscopy, while minimizing the number of people in the room - about 90% compliance for each). Anesthesiologists in most departments use standard personal protective equipment when caring for COVID-19 patients, including N95 masks, face shields, and water-proof gowns. Only one anesthesiologist across Israel was diagnosed with COVID-19 (unknown source of transmission). All department chairs reported emerging opportunities that advance the anesthesia profession: implementation of new technologies and improvement in caregivers' clinical capabilities (68% each), purchase of new equipment (96%), and increase in research activity (36%).

Conclusions: This nationwide cross-sectional study had a complete response rate and therefore well-represents the anesthesia practice in Israel. We found that Israeli anesthesia departments are generally highly involved in the health system efforts to cope with the COVID-19 pandemic. Anesthesia and airway management are performed in a remarkably comparable manner and with proper protection of caregivers. Ambulatory anesthesia activity has dramatically decreased, but many departments find opportunities for improvement even in these challenging times.

Keywords: Cross-sectional, Anesthesia department, Crisis management, COVID-19, Israel

* Correspondence: barakc@tlvmc.gov.il
[1]Division of Anesthesia, Intensive Care, and Pain Management, Tel-Aviv Medical Center, 6 Weizmann St., 6423906 Tel-Aviv, Israel
[2]Outcomes Research Consortium, Cleveland Clinic, Cleveland, OH, USA

Background

The current coronavirus infectious disease 2019 (COVID-19) pandemic brings many challenges to the healthcare system. Since COVID-19 is primarily a respiratory disease, it often leads to respiratory failure, prolonged dependency on mechanical ventilation, and need for high intensity medical care [1]. Anesthesiologists are considered experts in airway management, mechanical ventilation, and intensive care. Although the critical role anesthesiologists played in the COVID-19 crisis is well appreciated, different aspects of their engagements on a national level have not been reported to date.

There are approximately 900 anesthesiologists in Israel working in non-private hospitals, caring for a national population of about 9 million people. Most Israeli anesthesiologists are registered in the Israeli Society of Anesthesiologists (ISA). Despite early assumptions according to which Israel will face thousands of COVID-19 mechanically ventilated patients in mid-April, the rapid transmission of the disease was contained, in part due to governmental orders of isolation, curfew, and social distancing [2]. The peak of the first "wave" of the pandemic spread occurred in mid-April, but even at that point, in contrast to earlier predictions, less than 200 COVID-19 patients were severely ill, of which less than 140 were mechanically ventilated. Shortly after that peak, transmission rate decreased as well as the number of COVID-19 patients and the pandemic was considered under control, until the second wave started in July. Nevertheless, the healthcare system was still making extensive preparations to cope with the original predictions at that point. One consequence was the abrupt decrease in elective surgical activity and anesthesia providers' availability. The magnitude of this decrease and its ramifications were not measured. Additionally, as in the rest of the world, once the COVID-19 pandemic expanded, an acute shortage in medical equipment, personal protective equipment (PPE), and other supplies was noticed [3, 4]. The ISA has published its recommendations for safe airway management of patients suspected to carry SARS-CoV-2, including the use of N95 masks and goggles / face shields, but the adherence to these recommendations in light of the national shortage of PPE remains unknown. Similarly, the magnitude of SARS-CoV-2 infection in anesthesia personnel is also unknown.

The present national cross-sectional study was thus set to evaluate various aspects of the COVID-19 pandemic in anesthesia departments, including anesthesiologists' level of involvement in leadership and management, implementation of safety considerations designed to minimize COVID-19 infection and spread among anesthesia personnel, effects on anesthesiologists' health and availability, as well as anesthesia departments' activity. More so, the perspectives of departmental chairs on the opportunities arising from the COVID-19 pandemic were evaluated.

Methods

This nationwide cross-sectional study was conducted by an online questionnaire distributed to all anesthesia department chairs in Israel ($N = 28$), on April 14th 2020. The questionnaire was only identifiable on a departmental level. Reminders were set to be sent 3 days after the initial distribution to non-responders. The Tel-Aviv Medical Center institutional review board considered this survey of healthcare providers exempt from ethical approval, and consent was assumed by response to the survey. Since only organizational and institutional policy issues were addressed in this quality assurance project, with no identifiable or private health information, ethics committee approval and informed consent were waived.

The questionnaire consisted of 23 multiple-choice questions, some of which had an additional free-text response option. No question was mandatory. The main topics addressed by the survey were anesthesiologists' level of involvement in the COVID-19 crisis management, use of different components of PPE, modifications to the anesthesia induction and airway management methods, ramifications of the crisis on anesthesiologists' health and availability, and perceived opportunities arising from the situation. A full copy of the survey is available as **Supplementary File 1**.

Data were analyzed and presented with descriptive statistics. Pearson's Chi-square test was used in a post-hoc sensitivity analysis to compare the responses between large (number of hospital beds > 500) and small (< 500 hospital beds) anesthesia departments. We used a convenience sample of all anesthesia departments in Israel. This manuscript adheres to the applicable STROBE guidelines for reporting of cross-sectional studies.

Results

The questionnaire was completed and submitted by all 28 anesthesia department representatives within 2 days, so no reminders were sent (response rate 100%). Average (standard deviation) completion time was 10 (7) minutes. One third (9/28, 32%) of anesthesia departments include the intensive care unit (ICU), and one half (14/28, 50%) are in large hospitals (> 500 beds).

Leadership role and responsibilities: In two thirds of hospitals (19/28, 68%), anesthesiologists were leading COVID-19 patients' treatment, either by themselves or in collaboration with intensive care and internal medicine physicians. There was no difference between hospitals in which the ICU is part of the anesthesia department (6/9, 67%) and those in which they are

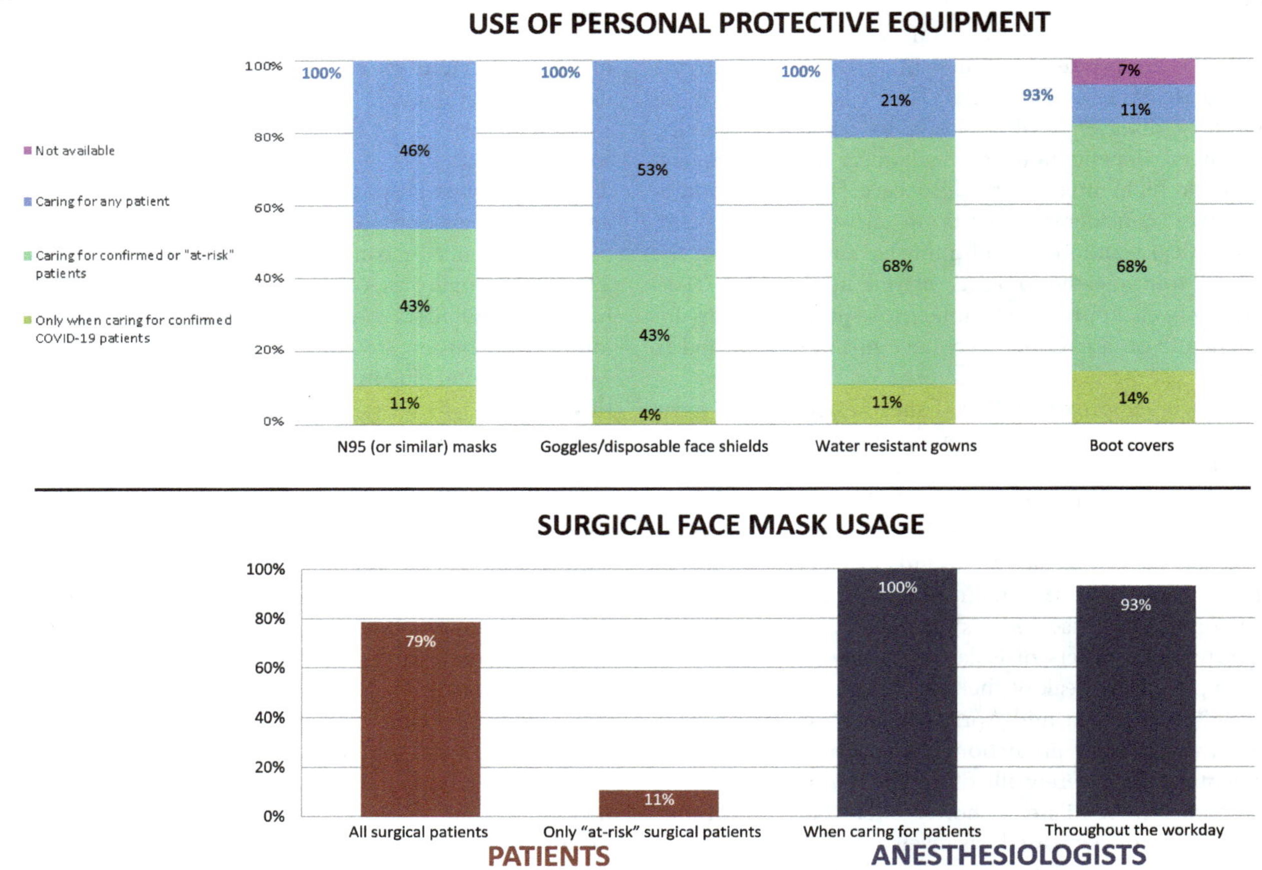

Fig. 1 Use of personal protective equipment. Upper panel – percentage of anesthesia departments using different components of protective equipment. Lower panel – usage of surgical face masks by patients and caregivers

managed independently (13/19, 68%). Other responsibilities of anesthesia departments included managing COVID-19 patients' airway (e.g., dedicated rapid response teams, 25/28), taking part in hospital crisis management and leadership (24/28), supervising the operating rooms (24/28), and clinical training and simulation to other disciplines in preparation to COVID-19 patients' treatment (19/28).

Anesthesia activity: As for elective surgical volume and anesthesia services, two thirds of departments reported a decrease of at least 40% in operating room activity (19/28, 68%), and 75% of departments reported cancellation of non-operating-room anesthesia cases.

Safety considerations (Fig. 1): Nearly all departments reported that anesthesiologists are wearing a surgical face mask constantly throughout the working day within the hospital (26/28, 93%), and in 79% of hospitals all patients arriving to the operating room also wear one. An aerosol protective mask (N95 or similar) is used in all hospitals when caring for confirmed COVID-19 patients, and in half of the departments when treating any patient arriving to the operating room (13/28, 46%). In most hospitals, one N95 mask is used throughout the day, and not replaced between cases ("re-use", 18/28, 64%). Goggles or face shields are used by all departments, either in all cases (15/28, 54%), or when caring for patients at-risk for SARS-CoV-2 infection. Similarly, water resistant gowns were used in all departments, either for all cases (6/28), for "at risk" cases (19/28), or only for confirmed COVID-19 cases (3/28). Boot covers were also commonly used (not available in only 2/28 centers). Ten departments reported using plastic covers on patients' heads to minimize potential aerosol exposure, and seven reported the use of aerosol boxes. Specific training for donning and doffing of PPE was performed in 86% of departments (24/28).

Two thirds of departments reported working in segregated shifts in order to minimize exposure and risk of transmission across caregivers. All but one hospital reported to have a dedicated operating room for COVID-19 cases (27/28, 96%), usually with a separate access than the other operating rooms (16/27, 59%), and with a dedicated area for donning and doffing of PPE (19/27, 70%). Eleven hospitals noted this operating room operates under negative pressure.

Airway management: When asked about specific components of airway management in COVID-19 patients, vast majority of departments reported that these intubations are performed by the most experienced provider (26/28, 93%), using rapid sequence induction (25/28, 89%), and after leaving only the minimal number of people necessary in the room (26/28, 93%). Video-laryngoscopes were the default device utilized according to 93% of respondents (26/28), and use of disposable airway equipment was reported by 75% of departments (21/28).

Anesthesia personnel considerations: One quarter of departments reported that at least 10% of their manpower was absent due to home isolation orders for suspected contact with a COVID-19 positive person at some point during the current crisis (7/28, 25%). Nevertheless, only one anesthesiologist throughout the country was reportedly sick with COVID-19, while the source of infection remains unknown.

Prospects arising from COVID-19 crisis (Table 1): Organizational processes related to anesthesia activity that were promoted by the pandemic as noted by anesthesia chairs included purchase of new required equipment (such as video-laryngoscopes and ultrasound machines), improvement in clinical care and training of caregivers, implementation of new technologies, execution of tele-medicine practices, and the launch of new research activities.

A sensitivity analysis evaluating differences between large and small hospitals (cut-off 500 beds) did not find any significant differences.

Discussion

This cross-sectional study collected data from all anesthesia departments in Israel, with a complete response rate. It was concluded within 2 days, and therefore well-represents the nationwide situation in the Israeli healthcare system in mid-April. Of note, hospital preparations for a large-scale pandemic aimed at coping with several thousands of mechanically ventilated COVID-19 patients were mostly completed at that point, while the actual number of ventilated patients across the country on April 16th was 140 [5].

The dramatic decrease in surgical and procedural volume requiring anesthesia services reported in all hospitals around the globe was also evident in Israel as noted in the present study. Two key factors contributed to this in Israel: First, national regulations that went into effect in mid-March mandated active decrease of elective medical and surgical activity in public hospitals [5]. Secondly, regulatory bodies mandated people to stay at home except for extreme circumstances, forbidding any kind of outdoor personal activity, thus decreasing the chance of acute injuries.

Table 1 perceived opportunities arising from the COVID19 crisis among Anesthesia department chairs in Israel ($n = 29$)

Perceived opportunities	Prevalence, %
Purchase of new equipment	96%
Training and improved clinical capabilities of caregivers	68%
Technological innovations implemented	68%
Transition to tele-medicine	57%
Research	36%

We found that anesthesia departments in Israel are highly engaged in COVID-19 crisis and in about two thirds of hospitals anesthesiologists led the way through the crisis. Anesthesiology chairs were the primary managers of different aspects of hospitals' preparation processes, staff anesthesiologists trained other physicians in ventilation modes, conducted simulations, and many were shifted away from the operating room to treat patients in the ICUs.

The nature of their job puts health workers overall, and anesthesiologists in particular, at increased risk of being infected with COVID-19. During the SARS outbreak In Toronto, Canada in 2003, one-third to one-half of all infections were in healthcare workers [6, 7]. An early report from Wuhan county in China found that as many as 29% of hospitalized patients with COVID-19 were healthcare professionals, that acquired SARS-CoV-2 infection while working in the hospital [8]. More so, once the disease becomes prevalent among healthcare workers, the workload on their healthy colleagues clearly increases. For reference, on the day of the present study survey closure, over 1400 Israeli healthcare professionals were under home isolation due to suspected unprotected contact with a positive SARS-CoV-2 person.

Protecting anesthesia teams has thus been the focus of hospital administrations across the country. One initiative was to train the staff in donning and doffing of PPE. A retrospective study evaluating risk factors for healthcare workers' acquisition of the original SARS infection in 2003 found that workers who did not undergo proper infection-control training had higher risk of transmission as a result of caring for SARS-positive patients [9]. Several national associations and international health organizations recommend specific training of PPE donning and doffing to facilitate healthcare workers' safety [10–13], but reports of actual adherence to these recommendations are scarce. A recent survey among Turkish anesthesiologists found that only one third of respondents (37%) underwent specific COVID-19 training [14]. In contrast, a review of the COVID-19 response in a tertiary hospital in Singapore reported thorough PPE training of all 180 anesthesia physicians by a small group of staff anesthesiologists [15]. Similarly, in Israel, as evident in the present study, the majority of anesthesiologists underwent such training.

Access to protective equipment, during high risk procedures or while being exposed to suspected or infected COVID-19 patients, is another critical measure to avoid infection with COVID-19. The local, national, and international shortage of PPE has led the most influencing agencies as the World Health Organization and the United States Center for Disease Control and Prevention to publish guidelines on potential extended use and re-use of some disposable protective items [11, 13, 16, 17]. Most of the published data about hospitals' and nations' preparedness report proper use of PPE, although much has also been published about improvised solutions to reduce aerosol exposure, presumably in low-resource situations where appropriate PPE is in shortage [18–20]. In Israel, following the Israeli Society of Anesthesiologists' recommendations, practically all anesthesia departments reported proper use of PPE when caring for confirmed or suspected COVID-19 patients, mostly in an extended use or re-use fashion. Many have also expanded the use of aerosol protection to all surgical cases.

Several national anesthesia societies have published recommendations on the proper modifications to anesthesia induction and airway management [10, 12, 21]. Aside of the use of aerosol-level PPE, these often include rapid-sequence inductions, use of video-laryngoscopes, leaving the minimal necessary number of people in the room, providing care by the most experienced provider, avoidance of mask ventilation and fiber-optic bronchoscopy unless specifically indicated, as well as avoidance of tubing disconnections. The Israeli Society of Anesthesiologists has published similar recommendations that were strictly followed with impressive compliance by Israeli anesthesiologists, presumably contributing to caregivers' safety and setting an example to other disciplines. Unsurprisingly, some of these practices were extended to be used when caring for "at risk" patients, and sometimes to all surgical patients. These practices are neither supported nor addressed by most official guidelines, leaving a gap that was filled by local initiatives. Taken together, proper use of PPE, its availability to anesthesiologists despite national shortage, and adherence to Israeli Society of Anesthesiologists' airway management regulations could, in part, explain the fact that out of about 900 anesthesiologists working in a non-private setting in Israel, only one was reported positive for SARS-CoV-2, the source of which remains unknown.

Finally, many departments were also able to find opportunities in the health crisis. Examples include innovative solutions to long-lasting gaps in information technologies, acquisition of long-needed medical equipment, and promotion of research projects.

The main limitation of our study originates from its design – an survey offering anesthesia department chairs to participate and report the situation, as well as perceived achievements and challenges, of the departments they manage. Although anonymous in nature, we cannot verify the objective accuracy of participants' answers, and some degree of reporting and recall biases cannot be ruled-out.

Conclusion

This cross-sectional study provides a glimpse on anesthesia departments' engagement in the COVID-19 crisis in Israel. It shows the inspiring role the anesthesia leadership took upon itself while keeping its members protected and safe, and despite the calamity and uncertainty found prospects for upgrading the profession. This encouraging message raises an opportunity to establish a more proper acknowledgement of the anesthesia profession and its importance, which used to suffer poor reputation and to lack public understanding of the various roles anesthesiologists are able to take in different setups [22].

Abbreviations

COVID-19: Coronavirus infectious disease 2019; ISA: Israeli society of anesthesiologists; PPE: Personal protective equipment; ICU: Intensive care unit

Acknowledgements

We thank the Israeli anesthesiologists who took the time to respond to the presented survey while running their anesthesia departments and caring for COVID19 as well as other patients.

Authors' contributions

IM and BC conceived the study. All authors contributed to survey design. BC, YB, and IM contributed to data analysis and interpretation. BC and YB drafted the manuscript. All authors have read, critically reviewed, and approved the final version of the manuscript.

Author details

[1]Division of Anesthesia, Intensive Care, and Pain Management, Tel-Aviv Medical Center, 6 Weizmann St., 6423906 Tel-Aviv, Israel. [2]Outcomes Research Consortium, Cleveland Clinic, Cleveland, OH, USA. [3]Division of Anesthesia, Operating Rooms, Pain, and Critical Care, Samson Assuta Ashdod University Hospital, Ben-Gurion University of the Negev, Ashdod, Israel.

References

1. Huang C, Wang Y, Li X, et al. Clinical features of patients infected with 2019 novel coronavirus in Wuhan, China. Lancet. 2020;395(10223):497–506. https://doi.org/10.1016/S0140-6736(20)30183-5.
2. The Novel Coronavirus, Ministry of Health. https://www.health.gov.il/English/Topics/Diseases/corona/Pages/default.aspx. Accessed April 26, 2020..
3. Artenstein AW. In Pursuit of PPE. N Engl J Medl. 2020:e46. https://doi.org/10.1056/nejmc2010025.
4. Ranney ML, Griffeth V, Jha AK. Critical supply shortages - the need for ventilators and personal protective equipment during the Covid-19 pandemic. N Engl J Med. 2020;382(18):e41. https://doi.org/10.1056/NEJMp2006141.
5. COVID-19 Press Releases, Ministry of Health. https://www.health.gov.il/English/Topics/Diseases/corona/Pages/press-release.aspx. Accessed April 26, 2020.
6. Booth CM. Clinical features and short-term outcomes of 144 patients with SARS in the greater Toronto area. JAMA. 2003;289(21):2801. https://doi.org/10.1001/jama.289.21.JOC30885.

7. Varia M, Wilson S, Sarwal S, et al. Investigation of a nosocomial outbreak of severe acute respiratory syndrome (SARS) in Toronto, Canada. CMAJ. 2003; 169(4):285–92 www.cmaj.ca. Accessed September 5, 2020.
8. Wang D, Hu B, Hu C, et al. Clinical characteristics of 138 hospitalized patients with 2019 novel coronavirus-infected pneumonia in Wuhan, China. JAMA. 2020;323(11):1061–9. https://doi.org/10.1001/jama.2020.1585.
9. Raboud J, Shigayeva A, McGeer A, et al. Risk factors for SARS transmission from patients requiring intubation: A multicentre investigation in Toronto, Canada. PLoS One. 2010;5(5). https://doi.org/10.1371/journal.pone.0010717.
10. Chen X, Liu Y, Gong Y, et al. Perioperative management of patients infected with the novel coronavirus: recommendation from the joint task force of the Chinese Society of Anesthesiology and the Chinese Association of Anesthesiologists. Anesthesiology. 2020;6:1307–16. https://doi.org/10.1097/ALN.0000000000003301.
11. Centers for Disease Control and Prevention (CDC). Coronavirus disease 2019 (COVID-19) - strategies for optimizing the supply of eye protection. Strateg Optim PPE Equip. 2020;2019:1–12 https://www.cdc.gov/coronavirus/2019-ncov/hcp/ppe-strategy/eye-protection.html.
12. Cook TM, El-Boghdadly K, McGuire B, McNarry AF, Patel A, Higgs A. Consensus guidelines for managing the airway in patients with COVID-19: guidelines from the difficult airway society, the Association of Anaesthetists the Intensive Care Society, the Faculty of Intensive Care Medicine and the Royal College of Anaesthetist. Anaesthesia. 2020;75:785–99. https://doi.org/10.1111/anae.15054.
13. World Health Organization (WHO). Rational use of personal protective equipment for coronavirus disease 2019 (COVID-19). World Heal Organ. 2020;(February):1–7..
14. Dost B, Koksal E, Terzi Ö, Bilgin S, Ustun YB, Arslan HN. Attitudes of anesthesiology specialists and residents toward patients infected with the novel coronavirus (COVID-19): a National Survey Study. Surg Infect. 2020; 21(X):1–7. https://doi.org/10.1089/sur.2020.097.
15. Wong J, Goh QY, Tan Z, et al. Preparing for a COVID-19 pandemic: a review of operating room outbreak response measures in a large tertiary hospital in Singapore. Can J Anesth. 2020. https://doi.org/10.1007/s12630-020-01620-9.
16. Public health O. *COVID-19 - What We Know So Far About Personal Protective Equipment Reuse.*; 2020. https://www.publichealthontario.ca/-/media/documents/ncov/covid-wwksf/what-we-know-reuse-of-personal-protective-equipment.pdf?la=fr. Accessed 14 May 2020.
17. Health EP. Considerations for acute personal protective equipment (PPE) shortages. Published 2020. https://www.gov.uk/government/publications/wuhan-novel-coronavirus-infection-prevention-and-control/managing-shortages-in-personal-protective-equipment-ppe. Accessed 14 May 2020.
18. Canelli R, Connor CW, Gonzalez M, Nozari A, Ortega R. Barrier enclosure during endotracheal intubation. N Engl J Med. 2020. https://doi.org/10.1056/nejmc2007589.
19. Matava CT, Julie Yu M, Simon DF. Clear plastic drapes may be effective at limiting aerosolization and droplet spray during extubation: implications for COVID-19. Can J Anesth Can d'anesthésie. 2020;67(7):902-4. https://doi.org/10.1007/s12630-020-01649-w.
20. Au Yong PS, Chen X. Reducing droplet spread during airway manipulation: lessons from the COVID-19 pandemic in Singapore. Br J Anaesth. 2020; 125(1):e176-8. https://doi.org/10.1016/j.bja.2020.04.007.
21. Şentürk M, El Tahan MR, Szegedi LL, et al. Thoracic anesthesia of patients with suspected or confirmed 2019 novel coronavirus infection: preliminary recommendations for airway management by the EACTA thoracic subspecialty committee. J Cardiothorac Vasc Anesth. 2020;000:1–13. https://doi.org/10.1053/j.jvca.2020.03.059.
22. Cohen B, Ogorek D, Oifa S, Cattan A, Matot I. Smart marketing may improve public understanding of the anesthesia profession. Isr J Health Policy Res. 2015;4(1):16. https://doi.org/10.1186/s13584-015-0011-1.

22

The oculocardiac reflex and depth of anesthesia measured by brain wave

Robert W. Arnold[1*], Aleah N. Bond[1], Melissa McCall[2] and Leif Lunoe[2]

Abstract

Background: The oculocardiac reflex (OCR), bradycardia that occurs during strabismus surgery is a type of trigemino-cardiac reflex (TCR) is blocked by anticholinergics and enhanced by opioids and dexmedetomidine. Two recent studies suggest that deeper inhalational anesthesia monitored by BIS protects against OCR; we wondered if our data correlated similarly.

Methods: In an ongoing, prospective study of OCR/TCR elicited by 10-s, 200 g square-wave traction on extraocular muscles (EOM) from 2009 to 2013, anesthetic depth was estimated in cohorts using either BIS or Narcotrend monitors. The depth of anesthesia was deliberately varied between first and second EOM tested.

Results: From 1992 through 2013, 2833 cases of OCR during strabismus surgery were monitored. Excluding re-operations and cases with anticholinergic, OCR from first EOM traction averaged − 20.2 ± 21.8% (S.D.) with a range from − 95 to + 25% in patients aged 0.2 to 90 (median 6.5) years. We did not find correlation between %OCR and brain wave for 97 patients with BIS monitoring and 91 with Narcotrend. With intra-patient controls between first and second muscle, the difference in brain wave did not correlate with difference in %OCR for BIS (r = 0.0002, 95% C. I -0.0002, 0.002, $p = 0.30$) or for Narcotrend ($r = -0.001$, 95% C. I -0.004, 0.001, $p = 0.32$). Secondary multi-variable analysis demonstrated significant association on %OCR particularly with BIS monitor, opioid, propofol and nitrous oxide concentration in the second EOM tensioned. Sevoflurane concentration correlated better with BIS monitor in second and third EOM tension. %OCR correlated with younger age ($p < 0.01$). OCR with rapid onset was more profound than those with gradual onset (difference in means 18, 95% C. I 10, 26%).

Conclusions: We were unable to confirm a direct correlation between brain wave monitor and OCR when using multifactorial anesthetic agents. The discrepency with other studies probably reflects direct impact of inhalational agent concentration and less deliberate quantification of EOM tension. We found no level of BIS or Entropy EEG monitoring that uniformly prevents OCR.

Keywords: Trigeminovagal reflex, Trigemino cardiac reflex, Bradycardia, Children, Squint

Background

The oculocardiac reflex (OCR) is a trigemino-vagal reflex associated with manipulations of the eye and orbit and specifically tension on the extraocular muscle during strabismus surgery [1]. The term Trigemino Cardiac Reflex (TCR) has efferent cardiac, respiratory and gastric vagal influence stimulated by any branch of the fifth cranial nerve [2, 3]. Of TCR and other vagal reflexes including diving response, the oculocardiac is not usually the most profound, however it has great intersubject variability occasionally producing profound bradydysrhythmias [1].

Anesthesiologists and ophthalmic surgeons make attempts to protect patients from the occasional profound oculocardiac reflex [4]. Gentle tension and release of tension by the ophthalmic surgeon limit or reverse the bradycardia [5, 6]. OCR can be inhibited by retrobulbar block and with anticholinergic medications [7], particularly when administered intravenous or intraglossally [8]. OCR is augmented by some opioids [9–11] and by dexmedetomidine [12, 13].

* Correspondence: eyedoc@alaska.net
[1]Alaska Children's EYE & Strabismus, 3500 Latouche St #280, Anchorage, Alaska 99508, USA

Yi, et all in 2008 reported that BIS values less than 50 in children undergoing strabismus surgery under sevoflurane anesthesia had less OCR [14]. Karaman, et al. in 2016 reported their experience suggesting that their cohort with lower BIS scores with nitrous oxide / desflurane general endotracheal anesthesia were associated with less bradycardia during deliberate, but non-quantified, extraocular muscle traction [15]. Was the reduction in OCR in these studies due to the inhalational agent concentration or the BIS score? Both anesthesia and surgeon have an influence on OCR. Depth of anesthesia is impacted by several components including inhalational agent concentration, nitrous oxide, opioids, propofol, sedatives, etc. OCR is also markedly influenced by the duration, form and amount of tension [5, 6, 16] on different extraocular muscles that were not controlled in former papers. We hypothesized that, over a range of anesthesia depths monitored by two different brain wave devices, we would find a correlation between specifically controlled oculocardiac reflex and lighter anesthesia.

Methods

From 1992 through 2013, patients undergoing strabismus or orbital surgery had deliberate, quantified extraocular muscle tension with prospective monitoring of electrocardiograph and anesthetic variables in an ongoing, HIPAA-compliant study with institutional review board approval from Providence Hospital (ClincalTrials.gov NCT03663413). This ongoing observational study complies with the Declaration of Helsinki and utilizes de-identified data; written informed consent has not been a requirement of the study. The intent of the study has been to monitor the oculocardiac reflex in community surgery centers with choice of agents up to the anesthesia teams. Since profound OCR is a relatively rare event, our ongoing prospective study using identical extraocular muscle stimulation provides a unique opportunity to observe large numbers of patients over time. This present report covers prospectively recorded anesthetic parameters in two cohorts representing different surgery centers and brain wave monitors, but identical strabismus rectus muscle stimulation to elicit oculocardiac reflex (Fig. 1). Patients were selected from all consecutive strabismus surgery patients of one surgeon (RWA) including ASA 1 and 2 patients some with developmental disabilities. There was no health or age related bias directing patients to either surgery center, however younger patients were more likely to receive pre-operative sedation- that may serve as a confounder with respect to age. Anesthesia staff was equally likely to increase or decrease anesthesia depth over the course off the surgery. The known confounder dexmedetomidine was not used in

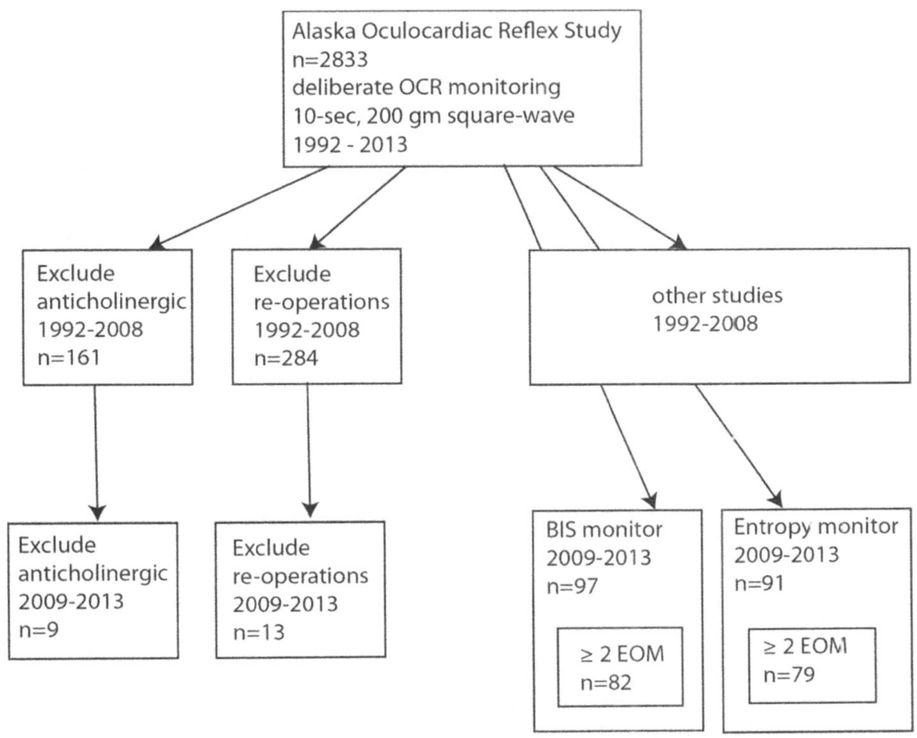

Fig. 1 Break down of patients recruited in the ongoing Alaska Oculocardiac Reflex Study. From 2009 through 2013, sequential patients in two different outpatient surgery centers were monitored with either BIS or Narcotrend brain wave monitors. Patients initially receiving anticholinergic medication or patients returning for re-operations were excluded

this study group [13]. Excluded were any patients given anticholinergic medication before OCR was measured and re-operations.

At the choice of the outpatient anesthesia team, some patients were given premedication: oral midazolam 0.5 mg/Kg. During induction, some patients were given IV fentanyl 1–2 mcg//Kg and/or propofol 3 mg/Kg. The children were induced with inhaled N2O and sevoflurane and then intravenous catheter inserted. No pre-operative, or induction anticholinergic was given. Most patients had laryngeal mask airway however some had general enotracheal. Few required rocuronium 0.5 mg/Kg. The anesthesiologist deliberately varied anesthetic agents, and specifically the inhalational agent concentration within customary levels to allow observation of the impact of lighter and deeper levels of anesthesia on the same patient.

From 2009 through 2013, each patient was monitored for electrocardiograph, end-tidal agent and CO2 concentration, and brain wave. Anesthetic depth was estimated using bispectral index (BIS) monitors (BIS XP, Aspect Medical Systems, Newton, Mass) in one center, and Narcotrend monitors (MonitorTechnik, Bad Bramstedt, Germany) in another surgical center. The monitors were applied to the forehead and temple according to manufacturer's instructions, and covered with adhesive, transluscent plastic drape after iodophore preparation. Additional monitoring included end-tidal agent concentration, CO2 monitoring and electrocardiograph. Oculocardiac reflex (OCR) was monitored during deliberate, 10-s, square wave tension on carefully isolated extraocular rectus muscles. Some cases involved surgery on just one extraocular muscle, while the majority of cases involved surgery on more than one muscle with time for heart rate to return to stable baseline between deliberate tension.

Oculocardiac reflex is reported as the maximum percent change in heart rate from stable, pre-tension ECG to the maximally different heart rate induced by the 10-s, deliberate extraocular muscle tension. Stability in brain wave monitor also preceded OCR monitoring. Although some define OCR as a 20% drop in heart rate [17], percent change better allows for comparison between children and adults with different resting heart rates. A negative percent represents bradycardia ((OCR heart rate – pre-heart rate)/pre-heart rate), whereas a positive percent oculocaridac could represent tachycardia. By this definition, more OCR (greater minus percent) implies more bradycardia and lower heart rate. We differentiated between oculocardiac with gradual onset from those with rapid onset- defined by at least 25% heart rate change in the first two seconds after extraocular muscle tension. For practical approach reasons, for uniformity, and because it produces the greatest OCR of the recti [18], inferior rectus muscles were most commonly tested. An example of rapid-onset, inferior rectus oculocardiac reflex can be observed at https://vimeo.com/robertarnold/oculocardiacreflex.

Statistical methods

Continuous data %OCR and brain wave monitor readings were analyzed with linear regression with calculations for coefficient of regression with 95% confidence intervals and Pearson product moment correlation with p values before and after adjustment for multiple comparisons. For cases with two muscles recorded of a given patient, the difference in %OCR from muscle 1 to muscle 2 was correlated to the difference in brain wave monitor reading at time of deliberate muscle tension. Linear regression was also employed comparing %OCR to age.

A multi-variable analysis then sought contributing related explanatory variables as might influence depth of anesthesia (midazolam, propofol, opioid, nitrous oxide, inhalational agent concentration). A p value less than 0.05 was considered significant. To address interaction, interaction terms were generated between pairs of explanatory variables with or without Robust standard errors and none of these contributed to additional significance.

A student's t-Test was employed to determine difference in means of cases showing rapid versus gradual onset OCR.

Sample size

For a correlation to detect an r of 0.3 or – 0.3 given power of 0.8 and alpha of 0.05, sample size would be 85.

For t-Test, given a power 0.8 and alpha 0.05, we estimate that we could detect a difference of 10% from a mean of – 20% OCR given S.D. of 18% with 51 samples.

Results

From 1992 through 2013, 2833 consecutive cases of OCR during strabismus surgery were monitored. Excluding 297 re-operations and 170 cases with anticholinergic, OCR from first EOM traction averaged – 20.2% (± 21.8% S.D., 95% C.I. -81, + 5%) with a range from – 95 to + 25% in patients aged 0.2 to 90.2 (median 6.5) years. No adverse cardiac event requiring rescusitation occured despite asystole occasionally longer then ten seconds. Release of tension was employed as the primary therapy for profound oculocardiac reflex. Some anethesiologists then employed intravenous anticholinergic before extraocular muscle manipulation resumed.

The number of patients with EEG monitoring (BIS 97 and Narcotrend 91) during strabismus surgery was 188 with a breakdown of their characteristics given in Table 1. Their initial OCR was – 19 ± 18% and the proportion of

Table 1 Demographics of cohorts

	BIS	Narcotrend
n	**97**	**91**
male/female	48/49	41/50
age minimum	1.3	0.5
age maximum	77	73
age mean	18 ± 23	17 ± 20
age median	5.7	6.5
Neuro disorder	5%	10%
opioid	52%	25%
rapid onset	16%	5%
midazolam	20%	5%
one EOM	9%	22%

Opioid and midazolam are the percent of patients receiving these drugs as a part of their anesthesia. Rapid onset are the percent pf patients with more than 25% drop in hear rate in the first two seconds. One EOM are the percent of cases with only one extraocular muscle operated. BIS and Narcotrend are the brain wave monitors used for each cohort

our patients with initial OCR greater than 10% was 56% while the proportion greater than 20% bradycardia was 43%. 98% of EOM traction was on the inferior rectus with 2% on the superior rectus. Table 2 shows the Pearson Product-moment correlation between %OCR and brain wave monitoring for BIS and Narcotrend for first, second and third EOM traction. The *p*-value is presented and adjusted for multiple comparisons. We did not detect a significant correlation under any of these conditions.

Table 2 also shows the difference in %OCR between first and second EOM correlated with the difference in

Table 2 Primary Outcome Variables: correlations between brainwave monitor (BIS and Narcotrend) and oculocardiac reflex (%OCR) for first, second and third extraocular muscle with 10-s, 200 g tension during strabismus surgery

	n	Pearson	*p*	*p'*
%OCR1				
BIS	97	− 0.12	0.24	0.43
Narcotrend	91	0.018	0.86	0.98
%OCR2				
BIS	82	−0.13	0.23	0.41
Narcotrend	79	−0.12	0.29	0.49
%OCR3				
BIS	54	−0.12	0.40	0.64
Narcotrend	39	0.08	0.62	0.86
ΔOCR				
ΔBIS	82	−0.12	0.30	0.51
ΔNarcotrend	79	−0.11	0.32	0.54

Pearson is the Product-Moment Correlation with p probability and p' adjusted for multiple comparisons. The lower table shows the correlations between the difference between OCR and monitor values with intra-subject control between first and second extraocular muscle tension in a given case

brain wave monitoring- our primary outcome variable with intra-subject control to test our hypothesis that deeper anesthesia monitored by brainwave would influence OCR. With deliberate change in agent percent and other anesthetic agents as directed by the anesthesiologist between first and second extraocular muscle tension in multiple-muscle cases, the average absolute difference readings between first and second reading at the time of oculocardiac measurement for BIS was 14.2 ± 16 units and for Entropy 16.3 ± 17 units. The interval between first EOM and second EOM in 134 cases was 16 ± 6 min while the interval between second and third EOM in the 74 cases was 8 ± 4 min. With BIS monitoring and the 82 cases with two-muscle comparison, no correlation between delta BIS and delta %OCR was found (r = 0.0002, 95% C. I -0.0002, 0.002, Pearson R (80) = − 0.12, *p* = 0.30). For the 79 two-muscle strabismus cases monitored with Narcotrend, no correlation between delta Narcotrend and delta %OCR was found (r = − 0.001, 95% C. I -0.004, 0.001, Pearson R (77) = − 0.11, *p* = 0.32).

Table 3 shows multi-variable analysis of potential determinates of %OCR including brain wave monitor, agent concentration, end tidal CO_2, and presence of pre-op midazolam, intravenous fentanyl and nitrous oxide for first, second and third EOM. Also, to facilitate comparison with other publications [17], OCR defined as 10% bradycardia and 20% bradycardia are analyzed. The oculocardiac reflex did not correlate with end-tidal carbon dioxide levels. No consistent pattern of interaction was noted except for second EOM and BIS monitor. Even then, for the 82 strabismus cases with %OCR2 correlated against BIS monitor, minimal correlation was noted ($r = -0.002$, 95% C.I. -0.006, 0.001, Pearson r (80) = − 0.133).

For this study group, we found that %OCR correlated with younger age (Fig. 2; $r = 0.002$, 95% C.I. 0.0005, 0.003, Pearson r (186) = 0.197, $p < 0.01$.) The linear regression formula is %OCR = 0.17 (age) -21.6%. OCR with rapid onset ($n = 21$, − 33 ± 18%) was more profound than in those with gradual onset (− 16 ± 18%; t-Test p < 0.01, difference in means 18, 95% C.I. 10, 26%).

Discussion

We deliberately monitored uniformly-generated oculocardiac reflex with brain wave monitoring in community surgery centers, then adjusted anesthetic parameters to allow patients to be internal controls for change in depth of anesthesia with two types of brain wave monitors. The 10-s, 200 g square-wave tension that generated the OCR for these 188 patients (− 19 ± 18%) which closely resembled the − 20 ± 22% from more than 2 decades of similar data collection. We employed continuous variables to increase the power of our observations. We

Table 3 Multi-variable linear regression Model

p Values		%OCR1	%OCR2	%OCR3		ΔOCR	OCR10%	OCR20%	Monitor1	Monitor2	Monitor3	
N2O	n=28	0.1	0.02	0.06		0.38	0.4	0.23	0.92	0.2	0.28	N2O
propofol	n=12	0.07	0.01	0.64		0.37	0.2	0.93	0.35	0.35	0.75	propofol
midazolam	n=19	0.75	0.77	0.11		0.09	0.63	0.81	0.03	0.28	0.96	midazolam
fentanyl	n=51	0.85	<0.01	0.68		0.01	0.43	0.89	0.66	<0.01	0.42	fentanyl
sevo		0.08	0.17	0.59			<0.01	0.19	0.18	0.02	<0.01	sevo
CO2		0.65	0.18	0.92			0.77	0.76	0.42	0.27	0.09	CO2
BIS		0.37	0.01	0.79	ΔBIS	***0.91***	0.6	0.94				BIS
		n=97	n=76	n=49		n=76	n=97	n=97	n=97	n=76	n=49	
N2O	n=15	0.65	0.26	0.92		0.07	0.62	0.34	0.11	0.79	0.68	N2O
propofol	n=23	0.44	0.69	0.67		0.24	0.31	0.7	0.62	0.89	0.37	propofol
midazolam	n=5	0.38	0.7	0.65		0.26	0.29	0.49	0.17	0.06	0.98	midazolam
fentanyl	n=23	0.95	0.72	0.35		0.19	0.87	0.86	0.76	0.44	0.48	fentanyl
sevo		0.07	0.75	0.19			0.02	0.2	0.55	0.05	0.52	sevo
CO2		0.81	0.24	0.75			0.79	0.19	0.91	0.75	0.46	CO2
Narcotrend		0.73	0.47	0.89	ΔNarco	***0.84***	0.42	0.33				Narcotrend
		n=91	n=58	n=25		n=58	n=91	n=91	n=91	n=58	n=25	

The significance (*p* value) for various anesthetic paramaters on oculocardiac reflex utilizing the brain wave monitors BIS (top seven rows) and Narcotrend (bottom seven rows.) First three columns represent separate analyses for percent oculocardiac reflex with the first extraocular muscle (EOM; 98% inferior rectus), the second EOM and the third EOM in strabismus surgery cases. Next column ΔOCR represents the difference between %OCR1 and %OCR2 correlated with the difference in brain wave monitors (ΔBIS and ΔNarcotrend). Next two colums added for comparison with other authors who employ ordinally defined oculocardiac reflex OCR10% and OCR20% as proportion with 10% bradycardia or 20% bradycardia. Final three columns determine impact of anesthetic variables on the readings from the BIS and Narcotrend monitors for first EOM, second EOM and third EOM observations. Far right and left columns highlight covariates nitrous oxide concentration (N2O), induction propofol, premedication oral midazolam, induction fentanyl, endtidal sevoflurane concentration (sevo), end-tidal carbon dioxide (CO2) and brain wave monitor reading. Below each column in the number of patients in that cohort

were unable to find a significant correlation between OCR and brain wave monitor levels alone, and we are not sure whether our observations of lack of brain wave correlation would impact other forms of trigemino cardiac reflex (TCR). This differs from the two other direct investigations on this subject and a systematic review of OCR/TCR that controlled other anesthetic conditions varying only inhalational agent concentration within pre-defined BIS monitor readings.

In the first publication on OCR and BIS, Yi, et al. [14] had three cohorts of 28 children varying sevoflurane to achieve BIS levels of 40–49, 50–59 and 60–69. They employed pre-op IM atropine and thiopentone in all patients. The surgeon was not masked to BIS and agent concentration and did not quatify EOM tension or duration, however tension was apparently gentle such that their initial ordinal definition of OCR had to be switched from 20% down to only 10% bradycardia. They reported more lateral rectus muscles tensioned than medial rectus and stopped traction if their defined 10% OCR was observed. The incidence of 10% OCR was 11% for deep cohort, 32% for mid cohort and 71% for the light anesthesia cohort.

In the other recent study on BIS and OCR, Karaman et al. also found less oculocardiac reflex in a study arm with lower BIS [15] Their prospective study used general endotracheal anesthesia with fentanyl, no anticholinergic and maintenance with 50% nitrous oxide and desflurane so the deep group of 31 children had BIS < 50 while the light group of 28 children had BIS ≥50. OCR, ordinally defined as 20% heart rate drop or arrythmia was 25% in the deep group, but 64% in the light group. Extraocular tension was deliberate but not quantified and a difference between medial rectus and lateral rectus was only noted in the light anesthesia group.

A systematic review of Trigemino-Cardiac Reflex (TCR) found a weak 1.2 fold increase with lighter anesthesia, but a 4.5 fold pooled risk of asystole when light anesthesia is compared to deeper anesthesia [19].

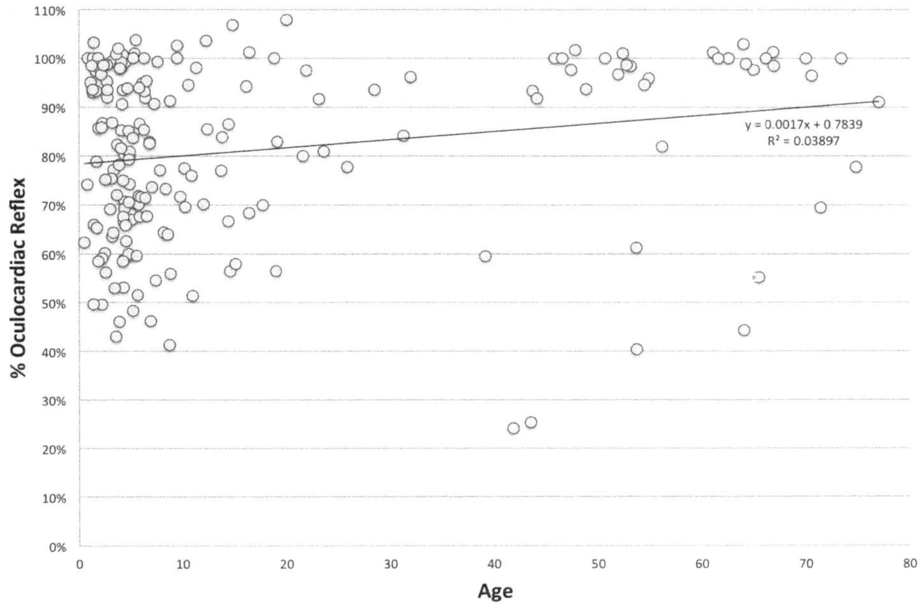

Fig. 2 Influence of age on percent oculocardiac reflex. *N* = 188

As a secondary outcome, we employed multi-variable analysis with respect to the continuous variable %OCR, additional anesthetic agents had a significant effect, noted more with BIS monitoring than with Narcotrend and more so with the second EOM than the initial EOM. This may be due to residual impact of midazolam pre-medication and the induction agents fentanyl and propofol. Compared to the studies by Yi [14] and Karaman [15], we had several additional pharmacologic confounders than just varied inhalational sevoflurane or desflurane. We suspect the levels of those agents, more so than the actual BIS reading itself, can impact OCR defined as a small percent change in heart rate, when the surgeon's extraocular tension is not uniformly controled. The amount and duration of EOM tension have a major impact on OCR [5, 6].

Both BIS and Narcotrend measure EEG activity, but employ different algorithms to derive a value [20]. Similar to others [21], we noted differences in the ability of Narcotrend compared with BIS to detect correlations that impacted OCR. Though our study was not intended to determine superiority of one brain wave monitor over the other, we did not have uniform correlation between brain wave and sevo concentraion but observed slightly better correlation between BIS and agent concentration than with Narcotrend (Table 2).

Under our current anesthetic conditions, the percent oculocardiac reflex correlated with age such that younger patients had a slightly greater heart rate change. This differs from our earlier findings also reported as percent OCR [22], perhaps due to different anesthetics and/or to pre-operative sedation that was more often employed in younger patients [5]. In prior studies, halothane and flurane were used with nitrous oxide, whereas most current cases employ sevoflurane. Midazolam, fentanyl or other agents (dexmedetomidine) are currently used pre-operatively mainly in children. In our experience, opioids and dexmedetomidine augment oculocardiac reflex; the latter was not employed in this study group [12]. We do not know whether opioids and dexmedetomidine augment other forms of TCR.

Approximately 11% of our cases are characterized by rapid onset- and these cases have substantially greater oculocardiac reflex.

Strengths of our study are the wide inclusion of strabismus patients from young children to adults, the strict control of extraocular muscle stimulation primarily on the inferior rectus muscles and our use of continuous variables for oculocardiac reflex and brain wave monitor readings. To enhance comparability with other historic studies, we also provide out data as if OCR was defined ordinally as 10% bradycardia, or 20% bradycardia. Given this, and the variety of anesthetic agents employed in community surgery centers, our study is genalizeable to a wide variety of patients. Weakness of our study include a non-uniform anesthetic protocol and more pre-operative sedation in younger patients; ideal conditions might involve double-blind randomization of the variable amount of one anesthetic component such as inhalational agent concentration unbeknown to anesthesiologist and to strabismus surgeon. We had sufficient numbers to have demonstrated a substantial correlation had there been one, but halved the cohort numbers employing two different types of monitors not intending to determine inferiority of one against the other.

Conclusions

Our observations, especially with BIS brain wave monitor, provide some more evidence that deeper anesthesia can provide some protection against the oculocardiac reflex. Further study is needed to fully delineate the relative roles of various anesthetic agents. Due to the high inter-subject variability of oculocardiac reflex, and our case-by-case use of a variety anesthetic agents, we observed some cases of profound oculocardiac reflex despite BIS and Narcotrend monitor readings indicating deep anesthesia.

Abbreviations

ASA: Amercian Society of Anesthesiologists; BIS: Bispectal index; C.I.: Confidence interval; CO2: Carbon dioxide; ECG: Electrocardiograph; EEG: Electroencephalogram; EOM: Extraocular muscle; HIPAA: Health Insurance portability and accountability" act"; IRB: Institutional review board; N2O: Nitrous oxide; OCR: Oculocardic reflex; S.D.: Standard deviation; TCR: Trigemino Cardiac Reflex

Acknowledgements

None.

Author' contributions

RWA, the corresponding author contributed to design, obtaining IRB, collecting data, writing and re-analysis. ANB contributed to data processing, writing and each edit. MM contributed to data collection and editing. LL contributed to data collection, design, and editing. All authors read and approved the final manuscript.

Authors' information

MM and LL are pediatric anesthesiologists. ANB is an anesthesiology resident at Wake Forest. RWA is a pediatric ophthalmologists.

Author details

[1]Alaska Children's EYE & Strabismus, 3500 Latouche St #280, Anchorage, Alaska 99508, USA. [2]Providence Anesthesia Group, Anchorage, Alaska, USA.

References

1. Arnold RW. The human heart rate response profiles to five vagal maneuvers. Yale J Biol Med. 1999;72(4):237–44.
2. Meuwly C, Golanov E, Chowdhury T, Erne P, Schaller B. Trigeminal cardiac reflex: new thinking model about the definition based on a literature review. Medicine (Baltimore). 2015;94(5):e484.
3. Schaller B, Cornelius JF, Prabhakar H, Koerbel A, Gnanalingham K, Sandu N, Ottaviani G, Filis A, Buchfelder M. Trigemino-cardiac reflex examination G: the trigemino-cardiac reflex: an update of the current knowledge. J Neurosurg Anesthesiol. 2009;21(3):187–95.
4. Scheiermann P, Herzog F, Siebenhofer A, Strametz R, Weberschock T. Intravenous versus inhalational anesthesia for pediatric inpatient surgery - a systematic review and meta-analysis>. J Clin Anesth. 2018;49:19–25.
5. Machida CJ, Arnold RW. The effect of induced muscle tension and fatigue on the oculocardiac reflex. Binoc Vis and Strabismus Quart. 2003;18(2):81–6.
6. Ohashi T, Kase M, Yokoi M. Quantitative analysis of oculocardiac reflex by traction on human extraocular muscle. Invest Ophthalmol Vis Sci. 1986;27:1160–4.
7. Garcia Guasch MR, Lapena Bayo C, Garcia de Oteyza J, Martinez de Salinas AD, Chavarria F, Nalda Felipe MA: [Oculocardiac reflex in strabismus surgery. Comparative study between atropine and retrobulbar block]. Rev Esp Anestesiol Reanim 1985, 32(6):284–287.
8. Arnold RW, Farah RS, Monroe G. The attenuating effect of intraglossal atropine on the oculocardiac reflex. Binocul Vis Strabismus Q. 2002;17(4):313–8.
9. Garg R. Remifentanil-induced bradycardia or oculocardiac reflex during strabismus surgery? Acta Anaesthesiol Scand. 2009;53(4):548–9.
10. Chung CJ, Lee JM, Choi SR, Lee SC, Lee JH. Effect of remifentanil on oculocardiac reflex in paediatric strabismus surgery. Acta Anaesthesiol Scand. 2008;52(9):1273–7.
11. Arnold RW, Jensen PA, Kovtoun TA, Maurer SA, Schultz JA. The profound augmentation of the oculocardiac reflex by fast acting opioids. Binocul Vis Strabismus Q. 2004;19(4):215–22.
12. Bond AN, Beerle BJ, Arnold RW. Dexmedetomidine nasal sedation produces more Oculocardiac reflex during strabismus surgery. J Pediatr Ophthalmol Strabismus. 2016;53(5):318.
13. Arnold RW, Biggs RE, Beerle BJ. Intravenous dexmedetomidine augments the oculocardiac reflex. J AAPOS. 2018;22(3):211–213.e211.
14. Yi C, Jee D. Influence of the anaesthetic depth on the inhibition of the oculocardiac reflex during sevoflurane anaesthesia for paediatric strabismus surgery. Br J Anaesth. 2008;101(2):234–8.
15. Karaman T, Demir S, Dogru S, Sahin A, Tapar H, Karaman S, Kaya Z, Suren M, Arici S. The effect of anesthesia depth on the oculocardiac reflex in strabismus surgery. J Clin Monit Comput. 2016;30(6):889–93.
16. Grover V, Bhardwaj N, Shobana N, Grewal S. Oculocardiac reflex during retinal surgery using peribulbar block and nitrous narcotic anesthesia. Ophthalmic Surg Lasers. 1998;23(3):207–12.
17. Meuwly C, Chowdhury T, Sandu N, Golanov E, Erne P, Rosemann T, Schaller B. Definition and diagnosis of the Trigeminocardiac reflex: a grounded theory approach for an update. Front Neurol. 2017;8:533.
18. Stump M, Arnold R. Iris color alone does not predict susceptibility to the oculocardiac reflex in strabismus surgery. Binoc Vis Strabismus Q. 1999;14(2): 111–6.
19. Meuwly C, Chowdhury T, Sandu N, Reck M, Erne P, Schaller B. Anesthetic influence on occurrence and treatment of the trigemino-cardiac reflex: a systematic literature review. Medicine (Baltimore). 2015; 94(18):e807.
20. Schmidt GN, Bischoff P, Standl T, Lankenau G, Hilbert M, Schulte Am Esch J. Comparative evaluation of Narcotrend, Bispectral index, and classical electroencephalographic variables during induction, maintenance, and emergence of a propofol/remifentanil anesthesia. Anesth Analg. 2004;98(5):1346–53.
21. Kreuer S, Bruhn J, Larsen R, Bialas P, Wilhelm W. Comparability of Narcotrend index and bispectral index during propofol anaesthesia. Br J Anaesth. 2004;93(2):235–40.
22. Stump M, Arnold RW. Iris color alone does not predict susceptibility to the oculocardiac reflex in strabismus surgery. Binocul Vis Strabismus Q. 1999; 14(2):111–6.

Bioelectrical impedance analysis of body composition for the anesthetic induction dose of propofol in older patients

Ana M. Araújo[1*], Humberto S. Machado[1], Amílcar C. Falcão[2] and Patrício Soares-da-Silva[3]

Abstract

Background: Older people are currently the fastest growing segment of the worldwide population. The present study aimed to estimate propofol dose in older patients based on size descriptors measured by bioelectrical impedance analysis (BIA).

Methods: A cross sectional study in adult and older patients with body mass index equal to or lower than 35 kg/m^2 was carried out. BIA and Clinical Frail Scale scoring were performed during pre-operative evaluation. Propofol infusion was started at 2000 mg/h until loss of consciousness (LOC) which was defined by "loss of eye-lash reflex" and "loss of response to name calling". Total dose of propofol at LOC was recorded. Propofol plasma concentration was measured using gas chromatography/ion trap-mass spectrometry.

Results: Forty patients were enrolled in the study. Total propofol dose required to LOC was lower in Age ≥ 65 group and a higher plasma propofol concentration was measured in this group. 60% of old patients were classified as "apparently vulnerable" or "frail" and narrow phase angle values were associated with increasing vulnerability scores. In the Age ≥ 65 group, the correlation analysis showed that the relationship between propofol dose and total body weight (TBW) scaled by the corresponding phase angle value is stronger than the correlation between propofol dose and TBW or fat free mass (FFM).

Conclusions: This study demonstrates that weight-based reduction of propofol is suitable in older patients; however FFM was not seen to be more effective than TBW to predict the propofol induction dose in these patients. Guiding propofol induction dose according to baseline frailty score should also be considered to estimate individualized dosage profiles. Determination of phase angle value appears to be an easy and reliable tool to assess frailty in older patients.

Keywords: Propofol induction dose, Older patients, Phase angle, Frailty

Background

Older people are currently the fastest growing segment of the worldwide population, and older patients are increasingly submitted to a multiplicity of surgical procedures [1, 2]. Physiologic changes and cognitive dysfunction associated with age, the presence of multiple comorbidities, the use of multiple medications and frailty increase the risk of older patients to adverse postoperative outcomes [1]. As a result, older people present a larger variation in terms of morbidity and physiological characteristics, which affect the predictability of their response to medications [3]. Variation in frailty likely contributes to this heterogeneity but its effects on pharmacokinetics (PK) and pharmacodynamics (PD) are not yet well understood [3]. Consequently, chronological age is a weak contributing factor of pharmacological response. Age-related physiologic changes per se are not always clinically significant and should not result in the same dose regimen alterations for all chronological old patients [3]. Despite these considerations, current guidelines recommend lower doses of anesthetic agents for

* Correspondence: amfariaaraujo@gmail.com
[1]Serviço de Anestesiologia, Centro Hospitalar Universitário do Porto, Largo Prof. Abel Salazar, 4099-001 Porto, Portugal

all chronologically older patients [4–6]. For induction of general anesthesia with propofol, it is generally recommended to decrease propofol dose from 40 mg every 10 s (2–2.5 mg/kg) to 20 mg every 10 s (1–1.5 mg/kg) until induction onset [7].

Additionally, bolus dose recommendations for adult non-obese patients are generally made as a function of total body weight (TBW) [8]. Physiologic changes that occur with aging, such as a decrease in total body water, a decrease in lean body weight (LBW) and an increase in body fat, may possibly require the adjustment of propofol doses based on different weight scalars [5, 9]. Mitchell et al. [9] have advocated that LBW may be an alternative choice for drug dose calculation in older patients. Nevertheless, the adequacy of TBW or other size descriptors as predictors of the propofol dose at LOC has not been studied yet in older patients.

Bioelectrical impedance analysis (BIA) is a reference method for the assessment of body composition by measuring resistance and reactance [9, 10]. Resistance is associated with the quantity of water present in tissues, and reactance is the resistive effect created by the cell membranes and tissue interfaces [11]. Phase angle can be calculated from resistance and reactance [arc-tangent (Reactance/Resistance)*180°/π] and it characterizes the relative effects of fluid (resistance) and cellular membranes (reactance) of the body [11, 12]. Consequently, phase angle has been interpreted as a determining factor of body cell mass, cell membrane integrity, intra and extracellular water distribution and it has also been proposed as a biological sign of cell death [10, 13]. The phase angle varies with sex, age and body mass index (BMI) but the average value for a healthy individual is generally comprised between 6 and 9 degrees [14].

Phase angle evaluation has been suggested as a prognostic factor in a number of clinical disorders, namely, human immunodeficiency virus infection, liver cirrhosis, chronic obstructive pulmonary disease, hemodialysis, sepsis and lung, breast, colorectal and pancreatic cancer [10]. BIA derived phase angle has also been proposed as an objective measure to recognize frail patients [15]. More recently, Mullie et al. [12] concluded that phase angle is strongly associated with sarcopenia and frailty in older patients, and that it is a promising noninvasive device to assess frailty.

Given the physiologic changes in body composition associated with aging, we planned to determine the appropriate size descriptor, measured by bioelectrical impedance, to estimate propofol induction dose in older patients. We also proposed to assess changes in phase angle values in frail patients. We hypothesized that LBW would be a more appropriate dosing scalar to calculate propofol induction dose in older patients and that old frail patients would require lower doses of propofol during induction of general anesthesia.

Methods

This study was performed at Centro Hospitalar e Universitário do Porto, Porto, Portugal, after Hospital Review Board and Ethical Committee approvals (IRB: N/REF.[a] 2015.221(183-DEFI/165-CES) and it provides secondary analyses of data registered at clinicaltrials.gov under the reference NCT02713698 on 23 February 2016.

The main purpose of the research published in clinical trials consisted in the development of a population pharmacokinetic-pharmacodynamic model for propofol when used for induction and maintenance of general anesthesia. Secondarily, sectorial evaluations of the results focusing on the induction and maintenance phases of anesthesia have also been conducted. The first study, planned to assess the ability of body size descriptors to estimate propofol induction dose in obese patients, has already been published [16].

The proposed study is a cross sectional analytical study and it conformed to the requirements of STROBE (Strengthening the reporting of Observational studies in epidemiology) statement. The whole anesthetic procedure was standard except for additional body composition assessment with body composition monitor (BCM, Fresenius Medical Care, Germany) and arterial blood sample. Written informed consent was obtained from all subjects participating in the trial.

Patients

Adult patients (18–64 years), with ASA (American Society of Anesthesiology) physical status I to III and BMI equal to or lower than 35 kg/m^2 scheduled for elective nose, ear or general surgery and older patients (with 65 or more years), with ASA physical status I to III and BMI equal to or lower than 35 kg/m^2 scheduled for orthopedic or elective nose or ear surgery were included in the study.

Exclusion criteria included the presence of predictive criteria for difficult airway management, dementia, severe hepatic or renal insufficiency, significant hemodynamic instability prior to the surgery and a known allergy to propofol at the time of enrolment. Patients with a pacemaker and pregnant women were also excluded.

Analysis of body composition by bioelectrical impedance

BIA was performed by Body Composition Monitor (BCM, Fresenius Medical Care, Germany) during preoperative evaluation in accordance with the manufacturer's recommendations [17].

Phase angle values at 50 kHz were registered and standardized values (z-score) were calculated based on reference values generated in a healthy German population [18] according to sex, age and BMI.

The values of resistance and reactance obtained at 50 kHz were used to estimate fat free mass (FFM) or fat mass (FM) based on specific predictive equations [19]. The equation proposed by Kyle et al. [20] was used in adult patients and the equation proposed by Roubenoff et al. [21] was used in older patients for the assessment of FFM.

$$FFM\ (Kyle\ equation) = -4.104 + \frac{0,518 Height^2}{Resistance} + 0.231 \times TBW + 0.130 \times Reactance + 4.229 \times Sex$$

$$FFM\ (Roubenoff\ equation) = -5.741 + \frac{0,4551 Height^2}{Resistance} + 0.1405 \times TBW + 0.0573 \times Reactance + 6.2467 \times Sex$$

Frailty assessment tools

The 9-point Clinical Frailty Scale (CFS) [22] developed by Geriatric Medicine Research (Dalhousie University, Halifax, Canada) was applied to each patient during preoperative assessment. The CFS was assigned from 1 (very fit) to 9 (terminally ill).

Anesthetic procedure

All patients were brought to the operating room without premedication. In the operating room, continuous pulse oximetry, electrocardiography, invasive blood pressure and neuromuscular blockade were applied in all patients. The bispectral index (BIS) was monitored using a BIS VISTA™ Bilateral Monitoring System (Covidien, Colorado, US) with a bilateral sensor on the forehead of the patient.

Each subject received a standardized dose of fentanyl (2 µg/kg) or a target controlled infusion of remifentanil (pharmacokinetic model of Minto [23]) was set at 3 ng/mL before propofol infusion. Propofol infusion (using Orchestra™ Mobile stand, Fresenius Vial, Brézins, France) was started at 2000 mg/h (33.3 mg/min) until LOC, defined by "loss of eye-lash reflex" and "loss of response to name calling". Total dose of propofol at LOC was recorded in all patients. After LOC, rocuronium was administered, propofol infusion rate was guided by the BIS and volume-controlled ventilation was started in all patients. Ventilation parameters setting were: tidal volume 7 ml/kg, respiratory rate 12–14 cycles per minute to attain normocapnia and PEEP 5cmH_2O.

Quantification of propofol concentration

Arterial blood samples were collected after LOC and they were centrifuged (2862×g for 5 min) at the end of the surgery. Serum samples were then preserved at −80 °C until analysis.

Propofol concentration was determined by gas chromatography/ion trap-mass spectrometry (GC/IT-MS) using the method described by Campos et al. [24]. The concentration range for the calibration curve was defined according to the expected serum concentrations (0.25, 0.5, 1, 2, 4, 5 and 10 µg/mL).

Sample size

Literature shows a moderate relationship ($r^2 = 0.49$) between propofol induction dose and TBW in adult patients with normal BMI [8]. To the author's knowledge there is no previous study evaluating the relationship between TBW and propofol induction dose in older patients. As a result, sample size considerations were based on association analyses using the Pearson correlation test. To detect a correlation of at least 0.7 between propofol induction dose and TBW a sample of at least 13 subjects was calculated to provide 80% power and a 0.05 level of significance.

Statistical methodology

The Shapiro-Wilk test was used to test for the normality of data. Categorical variables are presented as frequency (%). Continuous data are presented as mean or median (coefficient of variation, CV %). For comparison between groups, the Student's t-test and the Mann-Whitney-Wilcoxon test were used for continuous variables. The Fisher's exact test was used for categorical variables.

Fisher's exact test was used to estimate the association between CFS and phase angle values: *p*-values, odds ratio (OR) and respective 95% confidence intervals were obtained.

The relation among propofol dose at LOC, body size descriptors and phase angle was determined by linear regression analysis.

Statistical analyses were performed using GraphPad Prism 8.2.0 software (GraphPad Prism, San Diego, California). A *p*-value < 0.05 was considered to be statistically significant.

Results

Twenty adult patients (Age < 65 group) and twenty older patients (Age ≥ 65 group) were enrolled for participation in the study from April 2016 to March 2017. Patient's demographics and comorbidity indexes are presented in Table 1.

Table 1 Patient demographic characteristics and comorbidity indexes

Variables	Age < 65 group	Age ≥ 65 group
Age (years)	42.85 (26)[a]	77.8 (11)[a]
Gender		
Female	14 (70)[b]	12 (60)[b]
Male	6 (30)[b]	8 (40)[b]
ASA		
I	7 (35)[b]	1 (5)[b]
II	12 (60)[b]	15 (75)[b]
III	1 (5)[b]	4 (20)[b]
Charlson Comorbidity index		
0–1	18 (90)[b]	13 (65)[b]
2–3	2 (10)[b]	6 (30)[b]
4–5	0	1 (5)[b]

ASA American society of anesthesiology
[a]Data are present as mean (CV %)
[b]Data are presented as frequency (%)

The body composition of each patient evaluated by BIA is demonstrated in Table 2. The mean percentage of FFM in Age < 65 and Age ≥ 65 groups is 33.5 and 30.2%, respectively. There is a good agreement between the LBW values obtained by the Janmahasatian equation (LBW_j) [25] and FFM values measured by the BCM in both groups (Fig. 1).

With respect to phase angle values, Fig. 2 shows that lower values were observed in Age ≥ 65 group in comparison with those observed in the Age < 65 group. Figure 2 also shows that in Age ≥ 65 group the median standardized phase angle value *(z-score)* was lower than expected from a reference healthy population with the same sex, age and BMI.

No relevant changes in heart rate, blood pressure and BIS values were observed following opioid administration.

Table 3 shows that the median absolute dose of propofol to LOC was lower in the Age ≥ 65 group ($p = 0.005$). Despite the lower propofol induction dose, the mean variation of MAP (mean arterial pressure) was higher in the Age ≥ 65 group ($p = 0.046$). In this group, 6 patients showed a variation of MAP values before and after propofol dose higher than 40%. These patients were treated with ephedrine and fluid boluses to return MAP to baseline levels. No changes in heart rate that have required intervention were observed during propofol induction. Table 3 also shows that mean propofol plasma concentration after induction of general anesthesia was higher in the Age ≥ 65 group.

Table 2 Body composition according to bioelectrical impedance analysis

Variables	Age < 65 group	Age ≥ 65 group	*p*-value
Body mass index (kg/m^2)	25.9 (15)	24.3 (14)	0.09
Total body weight (kg)	70.2 (21)	63.0 (18)	0.18
Fat free mass (kg)	49.0 (23)	41.9 (23)	0.04
Fat free mass (%)	70.0 (10)	66.2 (10)	0.09
Fat mass (kg)	21.1 (33)	21.1 (24)	0.97

Data are present as mean (CV%)

Clinical frailty scale scores are presented in Table 4. These scores are statistically significant different between groups ($p < 0.001$). Actually, in the Age ≥ 65 group, 60% of patients were classified as *apparently vulnerable* or *frail* and in the Age < 65 group all the patients were classified as *very fit, well* or *managing well.* Figure 3 shows that lower z-scores are associated with high vulnerability CFS scores. The patients with a CFS score equal to or higher than 4 have been 23 times more often classified with a z-score lower than zero than patients with a CFS score lower than 4 (OR 0.044; 95% confidence interval 0.0072 to 0.2630; $p = 0.0002$).

Regarding the regression analysis, Fig. 4 indicates that propofol dose was similarly related to TBW and FFM in both groups ($r^2 = 0.39$ vs 0.36 and $r^2 = 0.48$ vs 0.45). When the TBW is scaled by the corresponding phase angle values, Age ≥ 65 group shows a stronger relationship than that observed in the Age < 65 group ($r^2 = 0.63$ vs 0.23). Figure 4 also compares the propofol doses at LOC with those that would be obtained using a standard bolus approach. Accordingly, the use of a bolus dose of propofol based on TBW (1 mg•TBW) would result in inappropriately low doses in some patients of the Age ≥ 65 group (Fig. 4d). Conversely, the use of the standard dose (2 mg•TBW) would be adequate for the Age < 65 group (Fig. 4a).

Discussion

In this study, older patients required a lower propofol dose than adult patients to clinical LOC when propofol was administered at a fixed infusion rate. In the Age ≥ 65 group, the relationship between propofol dose and TBW scaled by the corresponding phase angle values is stronger than the correlation between propofol dose and TBW or FFM.

In the present study, LOC was defined clinically by "loss of eye-lash reflex" and "loss of response to name calling". BIS values were not used to guide propofol dose because of the previously reported delay between clinical recognition of LOC and the decrease in BIS values [26], which may lead to propofol overdosing. The same infusion rate of propofol was adopted in the Age < 65 and Age ≥ 65 groups because propofol infusion rate has a critical impact on the dose and time required to induction of general anesthesia [27–

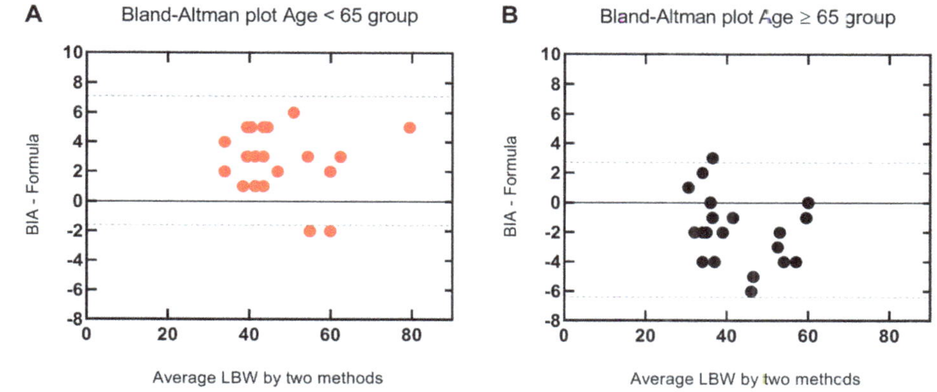

Fig. 1 Bland–Altman plots - Janmahasatian formula vs. body impedance analysis in Age < 65 group (**a**) and Age ≥ 65 group (**b**). The 95% limits of agreement are shown as dashed lines. BMI | Body mass index (kg/m^2)

29]. The use of different infusion rates appear alone to result in different dosing regimens and correlations levels. Additionally, a lower infusion rate (2000 mg/h) than that exposed in the recommendations (7200 mg/h) have been selected. According to Chan et al. [30] the use of slower infusion rates allowed more time to observe the specific clinical endpoint of LOC. It has also been published in several studies that the mean MAP variations were lower when slower propofol infusion rates (2000–3000 mg/h) were used [30–32].

For the fixed infusion rate adopted in the present study, propofol dose to LOC in adult patients was

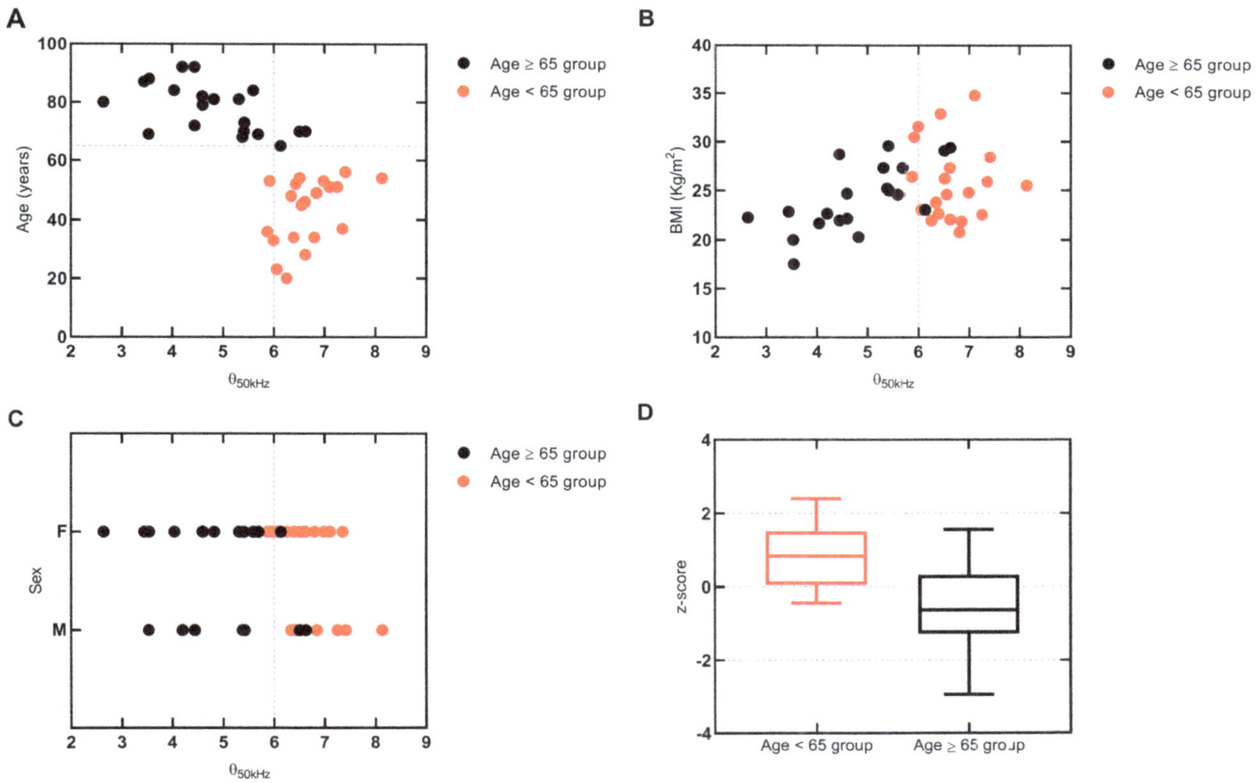

Fig. 2 Phase angle reference values. **a**, **b** and **c** represent the distribution of phase angle values according to age, BMI and sex. Vertical dashed lines represent lower phase angle reference value in healthy adult population. **d** shows the distribution of the standardized phase angle, *z score*, [*z score* = (observed phase angle-mean reference phase angle)/SD reference phase angle] for specific age, sex and BMI categories. BMI | Body mass index (kg/m^2). F | Female. M | Male. SD | Standard deviation

Table 3 Propofol dose until loss of consciousness

Variables	Age < 65 group	Age ≥ 65 group	*p*-value
Propofol (mg)	90 (40)[a]	68.5 (36)[a]	0.005
Propofol (mg/kg of TBW)	1.24 (30)[a]	1.09 (25)[a]	0.05
Time to LOC (min)	2.95 (1.18)[b]	2.17 (0.78)[b]	0.02
MAP variation[d] (mmHg)	19.62 (67)[c]	29.04 (54)[c]	0.05
Plasma [Propofol] (μg/mL)	3.96 (39)[c]	7.68 (34)[c]	< 0.001
Time after LOC[e] (min)	1.6 (1.3)[b]	1.5 (1)[b]	0.84
BIS[f]	49.5 (22)[a]	46 (27)[a]	0.88

LOC Loss of consciousness, *MAP* Mean arterial pressure, *TBW* Total body weight
[a]Data are presented as median (CV%)
[b]Data are presented as mean (SD)
[c]Data are presented as mean (CV%)
[d]Variation = [(MAP before propofol − MAP after propofol)/MAP before propofol]*100
[e]Time after LOC is the time when arterial blood sample was obtained after LOC
[f]Bispectral index value at the time of blood sample collection

similarly correlated with TBW and FFM, as also noticed by Ingrand et al. [8]. Similar considerations were herein observed in the results obtained for the Age ≥ 65 group (Fig. 4). These results are in accordance to the results of body composition evaluation by BIA providing that the expecting differences in FFM and FM associated with age [5] were not verified in the present study (Table 2).

By comparing the correlations obtained using TBW as a size descriptor (Table 3), it can also be seen that a lower dose per kg is required in older patients. This observation is in line with previous literature [7], whereby lower doses of propofol are recommended for older patients. However, the standard bolus dose (1 mg/kg based on TBW) may result in inappropriately low doses in some older patients (Fig. 4d).

The results obtained when TBW is scaled by the corresponding phase angle values showed a stronger correlation level in the Age ≥ 65 group (Fig. 4f). This correlation level was not verified in the Age < 65 group (Fig. 4c). Other authors have previously concluded that BIA derived phase angle can be associated with frailty and that phase angle values can be interpreted as a global marker of health in aging [15]. This fact was noted in the present study, namely on the association observed between standardized phase angle values and CFS scoring in the Age ≥ 65 group (Fig. 2). Therefore, the differences between the correlation levels obtained for the scalar TBW•θ in both groups appear to be related to the differences in the registered frail scores.

A small number of studies have previously assessed the effect of frailty as an independent PK predictor to determine thiopental [33] and propofol [34] dose. Additionally, it has been recommended that perioperative analgesia protocols should be individualized in frail patients [1, 3].

With respect to propofol plasma levels (Table 2), a higher value was found in older patients, thus corroborating the age-related decrease in volume of distribution and inter-compartmental clearance expected in these patients [5, 35]. Higher propofol plasma levels predispose older patients to cardiovascular side effects associated to propofol. In this study, the higher mean MAP variation was observed in the Age ≥ 65 group (Table 2). A slow induction has already been recommended for older patients in order to minimize post-induction hypotension [7]. Thus, when infusion rates higher than those adopted in this study are considered, increased MAP variations may be expected. Consequently, since low MAP and deep hypnosis is a predictor of excessive hospital length of stay and post-operative mortality [36], slow titration and monitoring of propofol action is judicious in this group of patients during induction of general anesthesia.

There are potential limitations associated to this study specifically the delay between clinical LOC and blood sample collection. Nevertheless, the average time was not significantly different between groups and the range of plasma concentrations measured ascertained the differences observed in propofol dose to LOC and hemodynamic side effects. Additionally, in this study, each patient received a standardized dose of fentanyl or remifentanil, according to the scheduled surgery. Notwithstanding the synergistic interaction between opioids and propofol for the suppression of purposeful movement to skin incision, the effect of opioids in the absence of a painful stimulus is limited [37]. It was shown by Milne et al. [38] that low target remifentanil concentrations (< 4 ng/mL) have low hypnotic potency and therefore a limited impact on propofol dose requirements when a painful stimuli is not applied. With respect to fentanyl, it has

Table 4 Clinical frailty scale

Age < 65 group	Clinical frailty scale		Age ≥ 65 group
	Item	Description	
2 (10)[a]	1	Very fit	0
11 (55)[a]	2	Well	2 (10)[a]
7 (35)[a]	3	Managing well	6 (30)[a]
0	4	Apparently vulnerable	7 (35)[a]
0	5	Mildly frail	4 (20)[a]
0	6	Moderately frail	1 (5)[a]
0	7	Severely frail	0
0	8	Very severely frail	0
0	9	Terminally ill	0

[a]Data are presented as frequency (%)

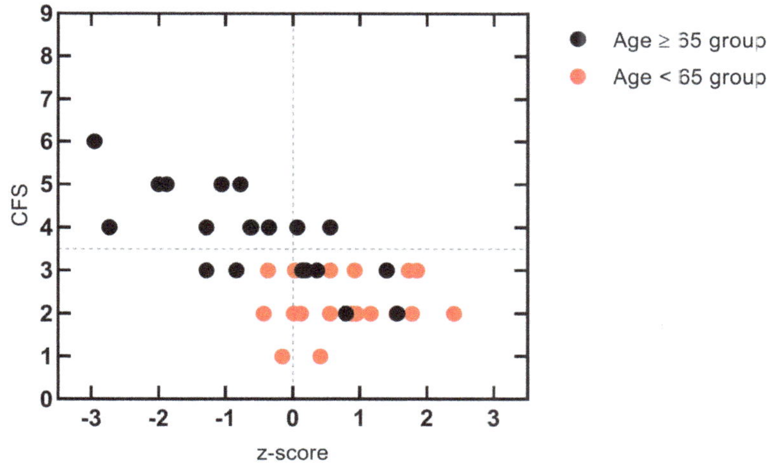

Fig. 3 Standardized phase angle *(z-score)* and clinical frail scale scores for each patient. CFS | Clinical frail scale

been concluded that the interaction between fentanyl and propofol for LOC is minor [39, 40].

Conclusion

For the fixed infusion rate of propofol (2000 mg/h) used in the present study, a lower dose of propofol based on TBW is suitable in older patients when compared to that required for adult patients. Nevertheless, the cumulative declines of physiologic systems and the baseline vulnerability to adverse outcomes specific of frail patients should also be measured to estimate individualized dosage profiles. Determination of phase angle appears to be

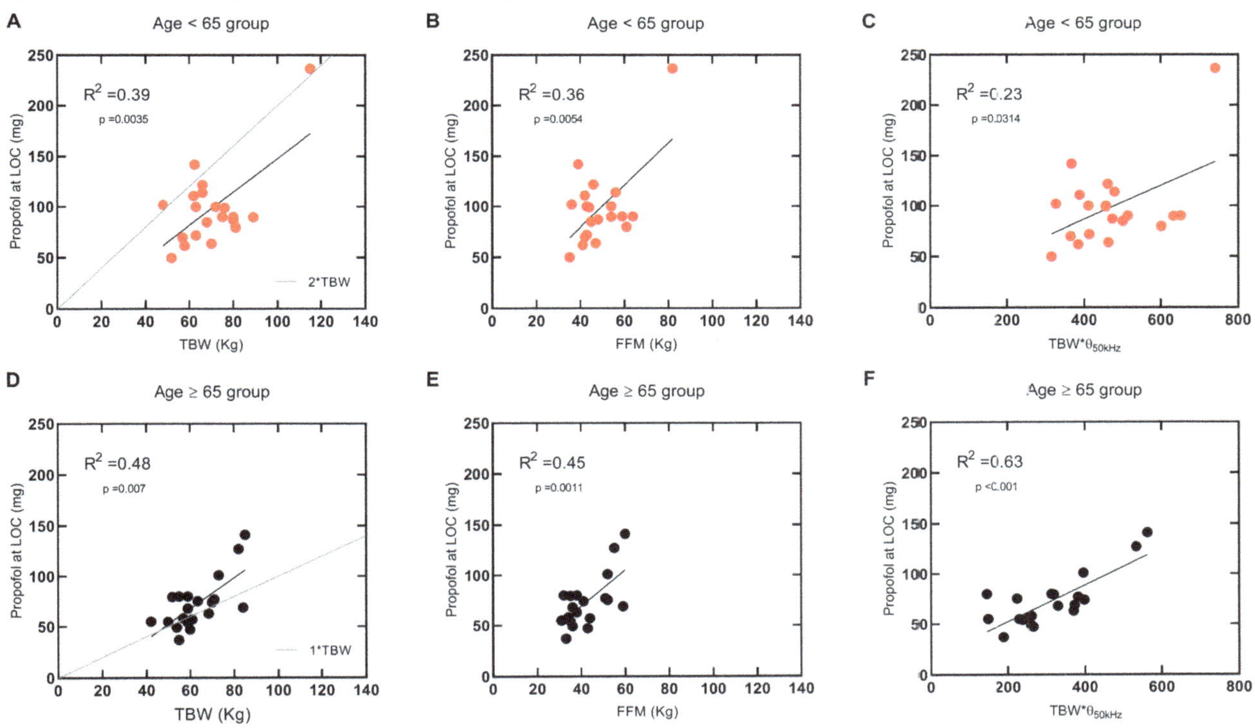

Fig. 4 Propofol dose at LOC. **a**, **b** and **c** show, respectively, the correlations of propofol induction dose with TBW, FFM and TBW•phase angle of Age < 65 group. **d**, **e** and **f** illustrate, respectively, the correlations of propofol induction dose with TBW, FFM and TBW•phase angle of Age ≥ 65 group. Grey line in **a** and **d** represents the function equivalent to the standard adult and older propofol dose (2 mg•TBW in **a** and 1mg•TBW in **d**), respectively. BMI | Body mass index. FFM | Fat free mass. LOC | Loss of consciousness. TBW | Total body weight

an easy and reliable tool to assess frailty in older patients. A multivariate analysis comparing adult and older healthy patients with adult and older frail patients is necessary to accurately determine the effect of frailty on propofol induction dose.

Abbreviations

ASA: American Society of Anesthesiology; BCM: Body composition monitor; BIA: Bioelectrical impedance analysis; BIS: Bispectral index; BMI: Body mass index; CFS: Clinical frailty scale; FFM: Fat free mass; FM: Fat mass; GC/IT-MS: Gas chromatography/ion trap-mass spectrometry; LBW: Lean body weight; LOC: Loss of consciousness; MAP: Mean arterial pressure; STROBE: Strengthening the reporting of Observational studies in epidemiology; TBW: Total body weight

Acknowledgments

The authors thank Toxicological Laboratory, Department of Biological Sciences, Faculty of Pharmacy, University of Porto for technical cooperation in propofol plasma dosing.

Authors' contributions

All authors designed the study, analyzed the data and contributed to manuscript preparation (drafting and revision). AA conducted the study protocol. All authors read and approved the final manuscript.

Author details

[1]Serviço de Anestesiologia, Centro Hospitalar Universitário do Porto, Largo Prof. Abel Salazar, 4099-001 Porto, Portugal. [2]Laboratory of Pharmacology, Faculty of Pharmacy, University of Coimbra, Pólo das Ciências da Saúde, Azinhaga de Santa Comba, 3000-548 Coimbra, Portugal. [3]Department of Biomedicine, Unit of Pharmacology and Therapeutics, Faculty of Medicine, University of Porto, Alameda Prof. Hernâni Monteiro, 4200-319 Porto, Portugal.

References

1. Griffiths R, Beech F, Brown A, Dhesi J, Foo I, Goodall J, Harrop-Griffiths W, Jameson J, Love N, Pappenheim K, et al. Peri-operative care of the elderly 2014: Association of Anaesthetists of Great Britain and Ireland. Anaesthesia. 2014;69(Suppl 1):81–98.
2. Amrock LG, Deiner S. The implication of frailty on preoperative risk assessment. Curr Opin Anaesthesiol. 2014;27(3):330–5.
3. McLachlan AJ, Bath S, Naganathan V, Hilmer SN, Le Couteur DG, Gibson SJ, Blyth FM. Clinical pharmacology of analgesic medicines in older people: impact of frailty and cognitive impairment. Br J Clin Pharmacol. 2011;71(3):351–64.
4. Rivera R, Antognini JF. Perioperative drug therapy in elderly patients. Anesthesiology. 2009;110(5):1176–81.
5. Akhtar S, Ramani R. Geriatric pharmacology. Anesthesiol Clin. 2015;33(3):457–69.
6. Klotz U. Pharmacokinetics and drug metabolism in the elderly. Drug Metab Rev. 2009;41(2):67–76.
7. Phillips AT, Deiner S, Mo Lin H, Andreopoulos E, Silverstein J, Levin MA. Propofol use in the elderly population: prevalence of overdose and association with 30-day mortality. Clin Ther. 2015;37(12):2676–85.
8. Ingrande J, Brodsky JB, Lemmens HJM. Lean body weight scalar for the anesthetic induction dose of propofol in morbidly obese subjects. Anesth Analg. 2011;113(1):57–62.
9. Mitchell SJ, Kirkpatrick CM, Le Couteur DG, Naganathan V, Sambrook PN, Seibel MJ, Blyth FM, Waite LM, Handelsman DJ, Cumming RG, et al. Estimation of lean body weight in older community-dwelling men. Br J Clin Pharmacol. 2010;69(2):118–27.
10. Gupta D, Lammersfeld CA, Vashi PG, King J, Dahlk SL, Grutsch JF, Lis CG. Bioelectrical impedance phase angle as a prognostic indicator in breast cancer. BMC Cancer. 2008;8:249.
11. Barbosa-Silva MC, Barros AJ. Bioelectrical impedance analysis in clinical practice: a new perspective on its use beyond body composition equations. Curr Opin Clin Nutr Metab Care. 2005;8(3):311–7.
12. Mullie L, Obrand A, Bendayan M, Trnkus A, Ouimet M-C, Moss E, Chen-Tournoux A, Rudski LG, Afilalo J. Phase angle as a biomarker for frailty and postoperative mortality: the BICS study. J Am Heart Assoc. 2018;7(17):e008721.
13. Stapel SN, Looijaard WGPM, Dekker IM, Girbes ARJ, Weijs PJM, Oudemans-van Straaten HM. Bioelectrical impedance analysis-derived phase angle at admission as a predictor of 90-day mortality in intensive care patients. Eur J Clin Nutr. 2018;72(7):1019–25.
14. Goswami PN, Munna K, Moinuddin. Bioelectrical impedance analysis: phase angle - an independent predictive health marker and its clinical applications. Berlin, Heidelberg: Springer Berlin Heidelberg; 2007. p. 321–4.
15. Wilhelm-Leen ER, Hall YN, Horwitz RI, Chertow GM. Phase angle, frailty and mortality in older adults. J Gen Intern Med. 2014;29(1):147–54.
16. Araujo AM, Machado HS, Falcao AC, Soares-da-Silva P. Reliability of body-weight scalars on the assessment of propofol induction dose in obese patients. Acta Anaesthesiol Scand. 2018;62(4):464–73.
17. BCM - Body Composition Monitor. http://www.bcm-fresenius.com/. Accessed Sept 2017.
18. Bosy-Westphal A, Danielzik S, Dorhofer RP, Later W, Wiese S, Muller MJ. Phase angle from bioelectrical impedance analysis: population reference values by age, sex, and body mass index. JPEN J Parenter Enteral Nutr. 2006;30(4):309–16.
19. Kyle UG, Bosaeus I, De Lorenzo AD, Deurenberg P, Elia M, Gomez JM, Heitmann BL, Kent-Smith L, Melchior JC, Pirlich M, et al. Bioelectrical impedance analysis--part I: review of principles and methods. Clin Nutr. 2004;23(5):1226–43.
20. Kyle UG, Genton L, Karsegard L, Slosman DO, Pichard C. Single prediction equation for bioelectrical impedance analysis in adults aged 20--94 years. Nutrition. 2001;17(3):248–53.
21. Roubenoff R, Baumgartner RN, Harris TB, Dallal GE, Hannan MT, Economos CD, Stauber PM, Wilson PW, Kiel DP. Application of bioelectrical impedance analysis to elderly populations. J Gerontol A Biol Sci Med Sci. 1997;52(3):M129–36.
22. Rockwood K, Song X, MacKnight C, Bergman H, Hogan DB, McDowell I, Mitnitski A. A global clinical measure of fitness and frailty in elderly people. CMAJ. 2005;173(5):489–95.
23. Minto CF, Schnider TW, Shafer SL. Pharmacokinetics and pharmacodynamics of remifentanil. II. Model application. Anesthesiology. 1997;86(1):24–33.
24. Campos SMJ, Antunes L, Branco PS, Ferreira LM, Pinho PG. Simultaneous quantification of propofol and its non-conjugated metabolites in several biological matrices using gas chromatography/ion trap – mass spectrometry method. J Anal Bioanal Tech. 2014;5(3):195.
25. Janmahasatian S, Duffull SB, Ash S, Ward LC, Byrne NM, Green B. Quantification of lean bodyweight. Clin Pharmacokinet. 2005;44(10):1051–65.
26. Iannuzzi M, Iannuzzi E, Rossi F, Berrino L, Chiefari M. Relationship between bispectral index, electroencephalographic state entropy and effect-site EC50 for propofol at different clinical endpoints. Br J Anaesth. 2005;94(4):492–5.
27. Kazama T, Ikeda K, Morita K, Kikura M, Ikeda T, Kurita T, Sato S. Investigation of effective anesthesia induction doses using a wide range of infusion rates with undiluted and diluted propofol. Anesthesiology. 2000;92(4):1017–28.
28. Doufas AG, Bakhshandeh M, Bjorksten AR, Shafer SL, Sessler DI. Induction speed is not a determinant of propofol pharmacodynamics. Anesthesiology. 2004;101(5):1112–21.
29. Struys M, Versichelen L, Thas O, Herregods L, Rolly G. Comparison of computer-controlled administration of propofol with two manually controlled infusion techniques. Anaesthesia. 1997;52(1):41–50.
30. Chan VW, Chung FF. Propofol infusion for induction and maintenance of anesthesia in elderly patients: recovery and hemodynamic profiles. J Clin Anesth. 1996;8(4):317–23.
31. Rather ZM, Rather MN, Afaq B, Farooq U, Ara Majid N. The effect of propofol when injected at different speeds for induction of general anesthesia: an observational study. Int J Clin Trials. 2018;5(2):7
32. Peacock JE, Lewis RP, Reilly CS, Nimmo WS. Effect of different rates of infusion of propofol for induction of anaesthesia in elderly patients. Br J Anaesth. 1990;65(3):346–52.
33. Hardman JG, Hopkins PM, Struys MMRF. Oxford textbook of anaesthesia. Oxford University Press; 2017.
34. Al-Rifai Z, Mulvey D. Principles of total intravenous anaesthesia: practical aspects of using total intravenous anaesthesia. BJA Educ. 2016;16(8):276–80.
35. Eleveld DJ, Colin P, Absalom AR, Struys MMRF. Pharmacokinetic-pharmacodynamic model for propofol for broad application in anaesthesia and sedation. Br J Anaesth. 2018;120(5):942–59.
36. Sessler DI, Sigl JC, Kelley SD, Chamoun NG, Manberg PJ, Saager L, Kurz A, Greenwald S. Hospital stay and mortality are increased in patients having a "triple low" of low blood pressure, low bispectral index, and low minimum alveolar concentration of volatile anesthesia. Anesthesiology. 2012;116(6):1195–203.

37. Vuyk J. TCI: supplementation and drug interactions. Anaesthesia. 1998; 53(Suppl 1):35–41.
38. Milne SE, Kenny GN, Schraag S. Propofol sparing effect of remifentanil using closed-loop anaesthesia. Br J Anaesth. 2003;90(5):623–9.
39. Smith C, McEwan AI, Jhaveri R, Wilkinson M, Goodman D, Smith LR, Canada AT, Glass PS. The interaction of fentanyl on the Cp50 of propofol for loss of consciousness and skin incision. Anesthesiology. 1994;81(4):820–8 discussion 826A.
40. Kazama T, Ikeda K, Morita K. Reduction by fentanyl of the Cp50 values of propofol and hemodynamic responses to various noxious stimuli. Anesthesiology. 1997;87(2):213–27.

24

Effects of awake caudal anesthesia on mean arterial blood pressure in very low birthweight infants

Frank Fideler[1*], Michael Walker[2] and Christian Grasshoff[1]

Abstract

Background: Intraoperative blood pressure is a relevant variable for postoperative outcome in infants undergoing surgical procedures. It is therefore important to know whether the type of anesthesia has an impact on intraoperative blood pressure management in very low birth weight infants. Here, we retrospectively analyzed intraoperative blood pressure in very low birthweight infants receiving either awake caudal anesthesia without sedation, or caudal block in combination with general anesthesia, both for open inguinal hernia repair.

Methods: Ethical approval was provided by the University of Tuebingen Ethical Committee on 05/29/2018 with the project number 403/2018BO2. Patient records of infants admitted by the neonatologist (median age at birth 31.1 ± 3.5 weeks, median weight at birth 1240 ± 521 g) which were scheduled for inguinal hernia repair were retrospectively evaluated for the course of mean arterial blood pressure and perioperative interventions to stabilize blood pressure. A total of 42 patients were included, 16 patients (11 boys, 5 girls) received awake caudal anesthesia, 26 patients (22 boys, 4 girls) a combination of general anesthesia and caudal block.

Results: Approximately 3% of the measured mean arterial blood pressure values in the caudal anesthesia group were below a critical margin of 35 mmHg, in contrast to 47% in the combined anesthesia group ($p < 0.001$). Patients in the latter group showed a significantly larger drop of mean arterial blood pressure below 35 mmHg (4.7 ± 2.7 mmHg vs. 1.9 ± 1.6 mmHg; $p < 0.005$) and a significantly longer time of mean arterial blood pressure below 35 mmHg (25.6 ± 26.0 min vs. 0.9 ± 2.3 min; $p < 0.001$), although they received more volume and vasopressor boluses for stabilization (27 ± 14.8 ml vs. 10 ± 4.1 ml; $p < 0.01$ and 0.15 ± 0.06 ml vs. 0 ml of cafedrine/theoadrenaline; $p < 0.001$).

Conclusions: The study indicates that the use of caudal block as stand alone procedure for inguinal hernia repair in very low birthweight infants might be advantageous in preventing critical blood pressure drops compared to a combination of caudal block with general anesthesia.

* Correspondence: frank.fideler@med.uni-tuebingen.de
[1]Departmnt of Anesthesiology and Intensive Care Medicine, University Hospital Tuebingen, Tübingen, Germany

Background

The outcome relevance of adequate blood pressure in pediatric surgery has been lately emphasized by several authors [1, 2]. For example, McCann et al. have reported a case series with pediatric patients suffering from infantile postoperative encephalopathy after the occurrence of intraoperative hypotension [3]. This raises the question whether the type of anesthesia has an impact on the need for active intraoperative blood pressure management. To keep blood pressure stable Marhofer et al. promoted the use of caudal and epidural anesthesia under sedation as one possibility to minimize the use of general anesthetic drugs [4]. The authors argued that by the use of regional techniques an avoidance of opioids during the perioperative period might help to reduce cardiorespiratory depression and improve gut function. However, to date there is little evidence supporting the concept that cardiocirculatory parameters in neonates are less impaired during caudal anesthesia compared with general anesthesia. So far, Ing et al. have demonstrated that spinal anesthesia performed in healthy infants undergoing pyloromyotomy results in reduced intraoperative blood pressure changes from baseline compared to general anesthesia [5]. Regarding caudal anesthesia, we already know from previous studies that arterial blood pressure is not altered by caudal anesthesia in children receiving general anesthesia [6], a finding that was supported by a prospective study in neonates by Deng et al. [7].

Thus, to determine whether the use of caudal block as a stand alone method may be advantageous in preventing critical blood pressure drops in the care of very low birthweight infants, we performed a retrospective analysis comparing patients with either awake caudal anesthesia without sedation (CA), or with a caudal block in combination with general anesthesia (GA + CA).

Methods

Ethical approval for this study was provided by the University of Tuebingen Ethical Committee on 05/29/2018 with the project number 403/2018BO2 (Chairperson Prof D. Luft). Anesthesia in both groups was performed by two senior anesthetists with more than 5 years of experience in the care of very low birthweight infants. Both anesthesiologists provided anesthetics of both types. The decision regarding the technique used was made up to their clinical preference.

Patients' characteristics

Patient records of infants admitted by the neonatologist which were scheduled for inguinal hernia repair between 01/01/2012 and 05/22/2014 were retrospectively evaluated. All children with hernia repair during that period have been evaluated ($n = 52$). We included only children who underwent an isolated inguinal hernia repair and who had no concomitant diseases ($n = 42$). Patients with congenital organ disorders like cardiovascular disease that could affect mean arterial pressure were not included into the study.

Definition of target size

In order to define a critical margin of mean arterial blood pressure we refer to a study by Rhondali et al. who conducted a retrospective analysis to compare the data of cerebral blood flow (CBF) and brain oxygenation in 180 children younger than 6 months. The authors stated that the mean arterial pressure is a good proxy of cerebral perfusion as they found that the CBF decreased proportionally with cerebral perfusion pressure. They regarded a mean arterial pressure beyond 35 mmHg during anesthesia to be safe and sufficient [8]. Therefore, we defined the incidence of a mean arterial pressure below 35 mmHg as the primary target. Secondary target sizes were the extent of fall of mean arterial pressure below the limit of 35 mmHg as well as the cumulative time per patient below that limit.

Data handling

Vital parameters were automatically recorded by use of a patient data management system (IntelliSpace Critical Care and Anesthesia (ICCA); Version H.02.01.001, Philips®). Evaluation of the data was carried out manually. Statistical analysis was performed by GraphPadPrism® 5.02. The Shapiro-Wilk's test for normality was used to check for normal distribution. Normal distributed groups were compared with the 2-sample 2-sided t-test. Otherwise the Mann-Whitney-U Test was used.

Results

In this study a retrospective analysis was performed in very low birthweight neonates (birthweight 1000 – 1500 g) receiving inguinal hernia repair. Two groups were compared: neonates with awake caudal anesthesia without sedation (CA) and neonates with a caudal block in combination with general anesthesia (GA + CA). At our institution we left treating preterm neonates for inguinal hernia repair without caudal block over a decade, since we rated the well-known advantages of regional anesthesia as so convincing [9, 10]. Therefore, a third study arm (general anesthesia alone) was not created. Table 1 shows that baseline characteristics are well balanced between both groups of very low birthweight infants. Patients who received CA had a lower body weight at the time of the surgical procedure. However, the difference is tiny and we therefore did not adjust for any baseline characteristic in our analysis. Median post menstrual age at birth was 31.6 weeks (GA + CA) vs 30.1 (CA). Post menstrual age at the time of operation was 39.8 weeks (GA + CA) vs 37.8 (CA).

Table 1 Baseline characteristics of very low birthweight infants receiving open inguinal hernia repair. Sixteen patients (11 boys, 5 girls) received a caudal anesthesia as a stand-alone method, 26 patients (22 boys, 4 girls) a combination of a general anesthesia with a caudal anesthesia. The baseline characteristics are well balanced between both groups (Mann-Whitney-U test)

	GA + CA (n = 26)			CA (n = 16)			
	Median	25–75% percentile	Min - Max	Median	25–75% percentile	Min - Max	P
birthweight [g]	1390	778–1850	560–2450	1220	869–1593	570–2150	0.32
PMA at birth [weeks]	31.57	29.68–34.07	25.57–38.86	30.07	27.00–32.72	24.29–34.29	0.11
Weight at OR [g]	2990	2375–3400	2000–3600	2400	2149–3050	2000–3600	0.05
PMA at OR [weeks]	39.79	36.86–41.61	35.14–48.29	37.79	36.40–39.71	35.43–43.71	0.11
Duration of surgery [min]	25.5	19.5–49.0	14.0–66.0	29.5	19.75–40.0	8.0–66.0	0.9

PMA Post menstrual age, *OR* Operation

Sixteen patients (11 boys, 5 girls) received a CA, while 26 patients (22 boys, 4 girls) received a GA + CA.

Caudal anesthesia was performed in patients in a lateral decubitus position with left side down. The puncture site was preoperatively anesthetized with EMLA®. After implementation of an intravenous infusion and monitoring of vital parameters the patient was placed in a lateral decubitus position with left side down. An Epican® Paed25G was guided by a SonoSite® M-Turbo with linear probe (5–13 MHz) in long axis in-plane-technique and the needle tip advanced under direct visualization. After negative aspiration, local anesthetic (ropivacaine 0.375%; 1 ml/kg) was applied and its spread assessed by ultra sound (Fig. 1).

The patients received no further medication until the end of anesthesia.

General anesthesia was either induced by mask ventilation with sevoflurane or by intravenous injection of 2–4 mg/kg propofol. In 12 patients the trachea was intubated, and in 14 patients the airway was secured by use of a laryngeal mask (Ambu® AuraOnce™). In order to facilitate intubation of the trachea the muscle relaxant vecuronium (0.1 mg/kg) was applied. General anesthesia was maintained with sevoflurane (0.5–2.9 Vol% corresponding to 0.3–1 MAC), 13 patients received additionally remifentanil (0.1–0.3 μg/kg/min) (Fig. 2, Table 2) After induction of general anesthesia, a caudal block was applied as described above. In contrast to patients with CA, the local anesthetic was used in a concentration of 0.2% (1 ml/kg). This anesthetic practice followed in-house standard operating procedures and was not changed within the study period. As a result, all caudal blocks were successful and there were no complications or side effects registered.

Patients in both groups received an intravenous isotonic full electrolyte solution including 1 % glucose with an infusion rate of 10 ml/kg/h. Basic vital parameters like blood pressure, heart rate, oxygen saturation and body temperature were continuously monitored during the operation and automatically recorded.

In accordance with the American Heart Association (AHA) recommendations for blood pressure measurement in children, cuff bladder width was at least 40% of the arm circumference halfway between the olecranon and acromion. The cuff covered at least 80% of the arm circumference.

In Fig. 3 we plotted the individual courses of the patients' mean arterial blood pressure. According to Rhondali et al. we defined a mean arterial pressure above 35 mmHg to be safe in this population [8]. The mean recording period was 47.4 ± 24.3 min. As demonstrated in Fig. 3a, approximately half of the mean blood pressure values were below the defined critical threshold of 35 mmHg in the GA + CA group, whereas this was the case in only 3% in the CA group (Fig. 3b). 57.7% of the patients in the GA + CA group underran the critical margin of 35 mmHg compared to 18.8% in the CA group.

In the following step we quantified these episodes with a critical mean arterial blood pressure. As depicted in Fig. 4, both severity of MAP (Fig. 4a) (4.7 ± 2.7 mmHg vs 1.9 ± 1.6 mmHg) and mean cumulative time per patient of MAP below 35 mmHg (Fig. 4b) (25.6 ± 26.0 min vs 0.9 ± 2.3 min) were significantly higher in the GA + CA group.

Intraoperative interventions to stabilize blood pressure are summarized in Table 3. The application of full electrolyte solution (Jonosteril®) or a vasopressor (Akrinor®; cafedrine/theoadrenaline) was at the discretion of the anesthesiologist. In the GA + CA group 15 out of 26 patients (57.7%) received a volume bolus in contrast to 3 out of 16 patients (18.8%) in the CA group. The median cumulative amount of bolus volume applied to patients in this group was significantly lower (10 ± 4.1 ml vs. 27 ± 14.8 ml; $p = 0.0015$). In accordance with this, vasopressor application was less frequent in the caudal anesthesia group (0% versus 19%).

Discussion

In this retrospective study we evaluated the course of intraoperative blood pressure in very low birthweight infants who received either caudal anesthesia, as a stand alone method, or a combination of general anesthesia, and caudal anesthesia, both for inguinal hernia repair. Anesthesia in both groups was performed by senior anesthetists with more than 5 years experience in the

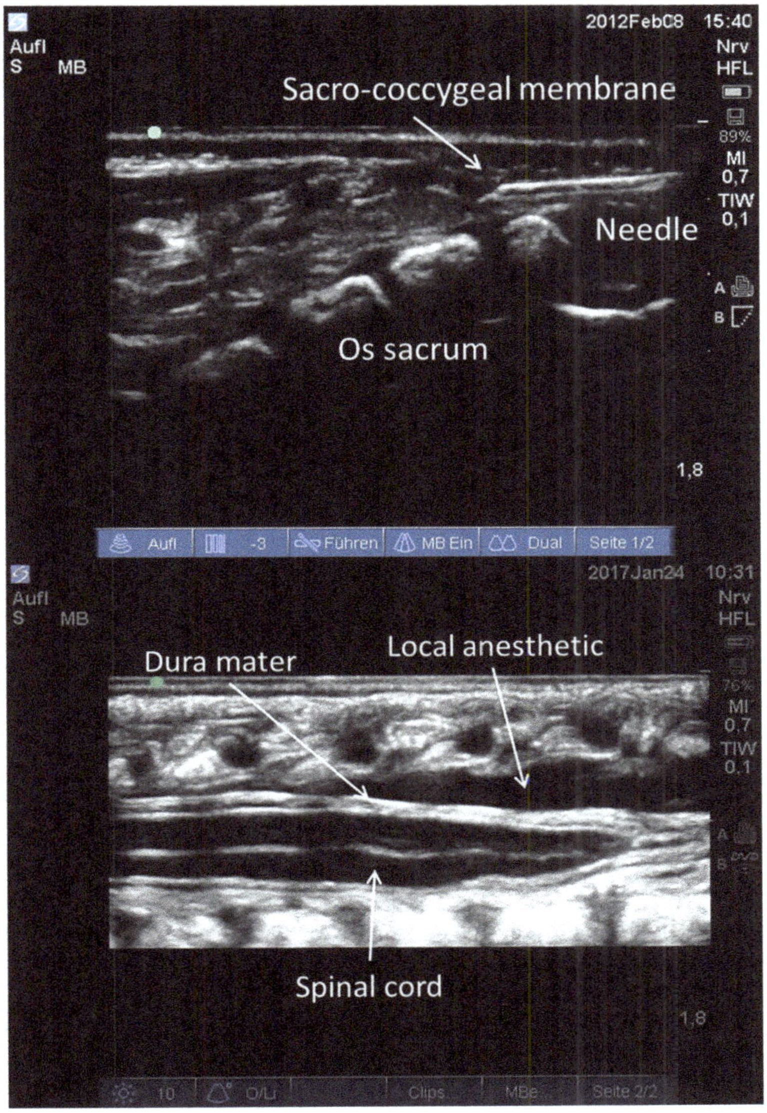

Fig. 1 Ultrasound images of the implementation of caudal anaesthesia in very low birth weight infants scheduled for open inguinal hernia repair. Caudal anaesthesia was implemented in infants placed in a lateral decubitus position with the left side down. Correct needle placement and distribution of the local anaesthetic was observed in all patients as visible on the ultrasound image and led to a surgically sufficient analgesia. Both pictures show a long axis view of the spinal canal. **a** Puncture with an Epican®Paed25G was performed in an in-plane technique by means of a SonoSite® M-Turbo with linear probe (5–13 MHz). **b** The ultrasound picture in in-plane technique demonstrates the spread of the local anaesthetic (ropivacaine 0.375%; 1 ml/kg)

care of very low birthweight infants. As reported in the results section we did not investigate the effects of general anesthesia as a stand alone method, although general anesthesia may still be used in many institutions for this type of surgery. In our opinion, the two study arms are justifiable since the aim of our study was to find out potential advantages of caudal anesthesia as a stand-alone method in preterm neonates. Furthermore, we know from literature that arterial blood pressure is not altered by caudal anesthesia in children receiving general anesthesia (Larousse et al. 2002), a finding that was supported by a prospective study in neonates by Deng et al. in 2008 [6, 7].

The most striking result is that the mean blood pressure was significantly lower in the GA + CA group although there were more pharmacological interventions like application of vasopressors or volume boluses. It is of even more importance that approximately 47% of the measured mean arterial blood pressure values in that group were below a critical margin of 35 mmHg, in contrast to only 3% in the CA group and that the cumulative time below 35 mmHg per patient was significantly

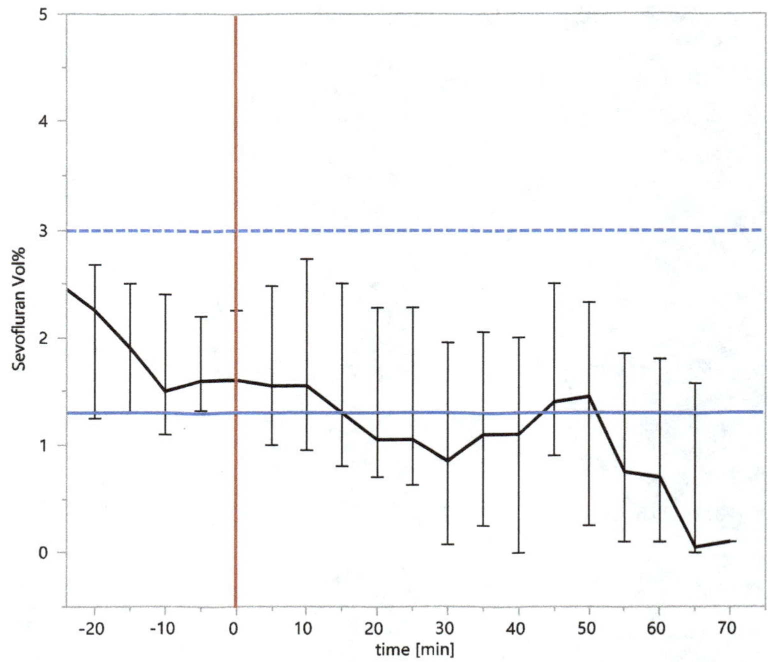

Fig. 2 Time course of the median sevoflurane concentration (median ± interquartile range) calculated from patients in the group of combined general- and caudal anesthesia. The time point "0 min" indicates the start of the surgical procedure and is marked by the vertical red line. The dashed blue line indicates a sevoflurane concentration of 3.0 vol% corresponding to 1 MAC. The blue line represents the median sevoflurane concentration of 1.3 vol% during the maintenance phase of general anesthesia

longer. A safe lower limit of blood pressure in infants is still a matter of debate. The incidence of hypotension in preterm neonates seems to be inversely related to gestational age and birth weight [11]. General anesthesia can contribute to hypotension, and thereby cause low cerebral perfusion [1, 8]. This seems to be less critical in preterm neonates who do not undergo surgical intervention since Alderliesten et al. described that a mean arterial blood pressure less than gestational age in weeks was not associated with lower neurodevelopmental outcome scores [11]. On the other hand McCann et al. reported on 6 infants who underwent elective surgery and developed postoperative encephalopathy, which had features most consistent with intraoperative cerebral hypoperfusion [3]. However, in a retrospective analysis in children younger than 6 months conducted by Rhondali et al., the authors compared data of two studies investigating the impact of sevoflurane anesthesia on cerebral blood flow by transcranial Doppler [12] and on brain oxygenation by NIRS [13]. The authors reported that in healthy infants scheduled for short procedures, the mean arterial pressure is a good surrogate parameter of cerebral perfusion. Even more Rhondali et al. stated that maintaining the mean arterial pressure above 35 mmHg during anesthesia is safe and sufficient [8], and we adopted this value as a lower threshold. It is important to mention that general anesthetics were administered at low concentrations, e.g. sevoflurane was dosed by approximately 0.5 MAC (median 1.3 vol%) during the maintenance phase of general anesthesia which is far less compared to sevoflurane concentrations reported in other studies (Fig. 2) [13, 14]. Even for sedation the application of either 8 vol% sevoflurane or up to 4 mg/kg propofol during the initiation of a caudal block were reported [15, 16]. Thus it can be estimated that with a less cautious use of general anesthetics even more episodes of low mean arterial pressure can be expected.

Table 2 The table summarizes the doses and ranges of anesthetic agents used in the group of combined general- and caudal anesthesia

Anesthetic agent	i.v. Induction (n)	Mask Induction (n)	maintenance of anesthesia (n)
Propofol [mg/kg]	2–4 (11)	–	–
Sevofluran [vol%]	–	0.6–7.3 (15)	0.5–2.9 [mean 1.3] (26)
Remifentanil [µg/kg/min]	–	–	0.1–0.3 (13)
Vecuronium [mg/kg]	0.1 (4)	–	–

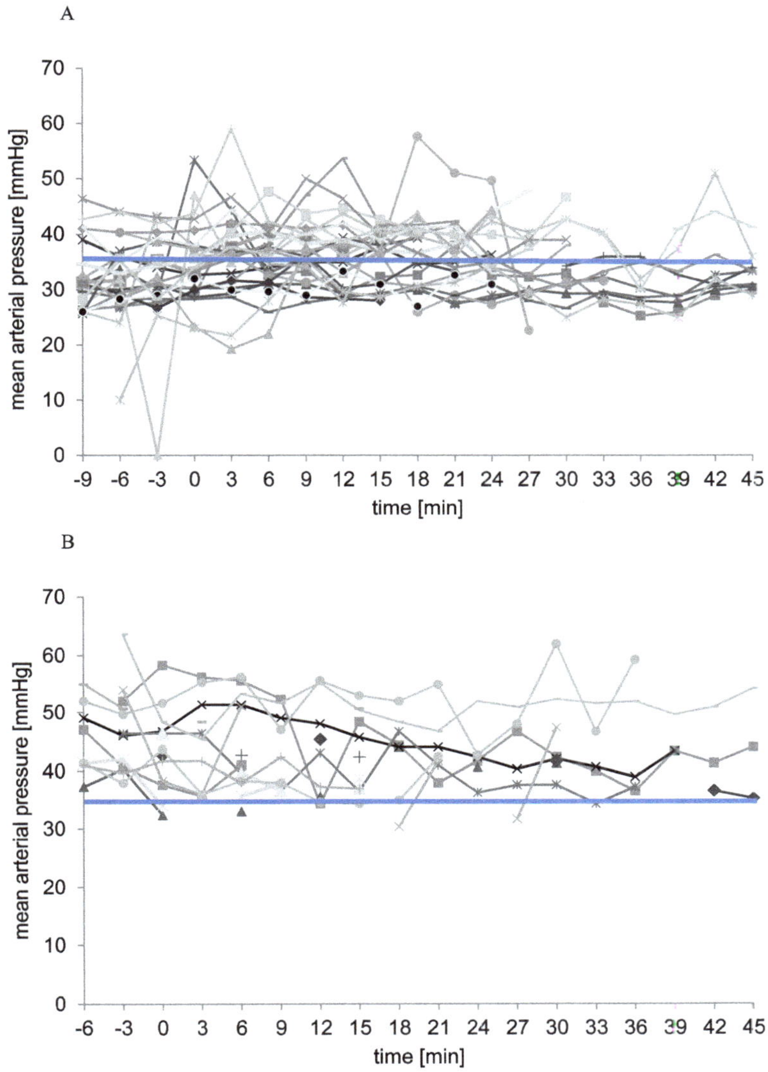

Fig. 3 The graph depicts the individual courses of mean arterial blood pressure in very low birth weight infants during open inguinal hernia repair. Each character represents a single patient. The surgical procedure started at the time point 0 min. For easier interpretation of the data a blue line was drawn at 35 mmHg, since this value marked the threshold that was defined to be safe according to Rhondali et al. [8] **a** The graph visualizes that in the group of combined general- and caudal anesthesia approximately half of the mean blood pressure values measured during inguinal hernia repair were below the critical threshold of 35 mmHg. **b** In contrast to the patients in the group of combined general- and caudal anesthesia only 3% of all mean blood pressure values measured in the caudal anesthesia group underran the critical margin of 35 mmHg

In very low birthweight infants we use caudal anesthesia rather than spinal anesthesia since the success rates are significantly higher [14, 15, 17, 18]. The quality of caudal blockade provided adequate surgical conditions in all cases although a lack of sufficient motor blockage was often considered to be disadvantageous [17, 19]. For this ropivacain 0,375% was used in the CA group without any side effects. In contrast to spinal anesthesia, the implementation of a caudal block is technically less difficult and became even more straightforward by use of ultrasound control since puncture and correct spread of the local anesthetic can be tracked visually, especially when the needle is visualized in long axis in a sagittal plane [20, 21]. Another advantage is the chance to identify anatomical anomalies like for example a terminal myelocystocele, a myelomeningocele or a tight filum terminale syndrome [22] before puncture.

The retrospective analysis suffers from some limitations like the limited number of patients being anesthetized by only two anesthetists or that an association of intraoperative hypotension to general anesthetics like remifentanil or sevoflurane cannot be derived. Likewise no sequelae could be recorded in this retrospective study. However, the anesthetists each had at least 5 years

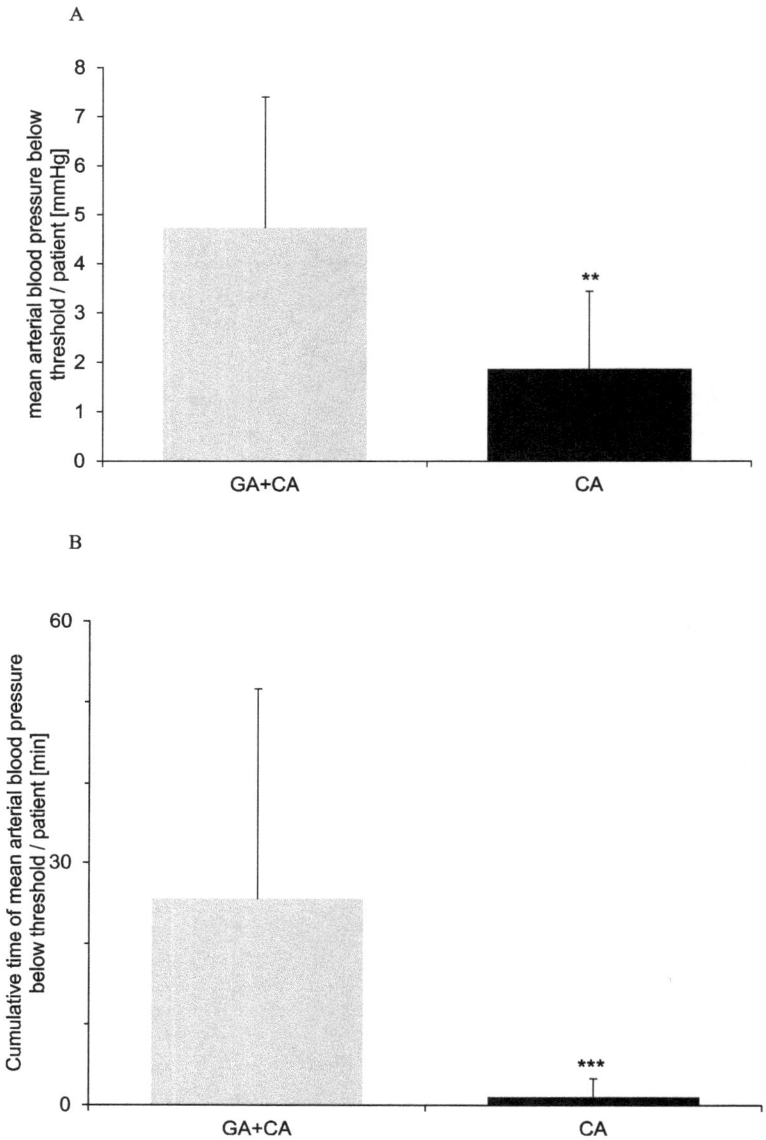

Fig. 4 Evaluation of potentially critical episodes (mean arterial blood pressure values below 35 mmHg) in both groups of very low birth weight infants receiving open inguinal hernia repair. **a** The figure demonstrates that the extent to which the critical limit of 35 mmHg was underran is significantly greater in the group of combined general- and caudal anesthesia (GA + CA) (**; $P < 0.01$). **b** Analysis of the mean cumulative time per patient with a mean arterial pressure value below 35 mmHg. Patients in the group of combined general- and caudal anesthesia (GA + CA) spent significantly longer time with mean arterial pressure below 35 mmHg compared to patients in the caudal anesthesia (CA) group (***; $P < 0.001$)

Table 3 depicts intraoperative interventions to raise blood pressure in very low birthweight children receiving open inguinal hernia repair. Full electrolyte solution boli (Jonosteril®) or vasopressor boli (Akrinor®; cafedrine/theoadrenaline) were administered at the discretion of the anaesthesiologist (Mann-Whitney-U test)

		GA + CA (n = 26)	CA (*n* = 16)	*P*
Fluid bolus	Patients n [%]	15 [57.7]	3 [18.8]	0.0046
	Average fluid bolus [ml/patient] [mean]	27 ± 14.8	10 ± 4.1	0.0015
Cafedrine / theoadrenaline	Patients n [%]	5 [19.2]	0 [0]	< 0.001
	Average vasopressor bolus [ml/patient] [mean]	0.15 ± 0.06	0	< 0.001

of experience in pediatric anesthesia and were aware of keeping the mean arterial pressure above 35 mmHg which was difficult in the group of combined general- and caudal anesthesia in spite of the use of volume boluses and vasopressors and resulted in significantly more episodes of critically low mean arterial blood pressure.

Conclusion

In summary this preliminary study provides support for the use of caudal block as a stand alone method for the care of very low birthweight infants as it shows advantages in preventing critical blood pressure drops compared to a combination of caudal block with general anesthesia.

Abbreviations

AHA: American heart association; CA: Awake caudal anesthesia without sedation; CBF: Cerebral blood flow; g: Gram; G: Gauge; G1%: Glucose 1%; GA + CA: General anesthesia with caudal block; ICCA: IntelliSpace Critical Care and Anesthesia information system; MAC: Minimum alveolar concentration; MAP: Mean arterial blood pressure; MHz: Megaherz; ml: Milliliter; mmHg: Millimeter mercury column; NIRS: Near-infrared spectroscopy; OR: Operation; PMA: Post menstrual age; vs: Versus

Acknowledgements

Not applicable.

Authors' contributions

FF helped with the planning of the study, the data collection, the compilation of statistics as well as the constitution of the manuscript. MW contributed to the data collection, evaluation of patient files and compilation of statistics. CG helped with the planning of the study, the compilation of statistics and the constitution of the manuscript. The authors read and approved the final manuscript.

Author details

[1]Departmnt of Anesthesiology and Intensive Care Medicine, University Hospital Tuebingen, Tübingen, Germany. [2]Clinic for Anesthesiology, Intensive, Emergency- and Pain-Therapy, Ludwigsburg, Germany.

References

1. Michelet D, Arslan O, Hilly J, Mangalsuren N, Brasher C, Grace R, et al. Intraoperative changes in blood pressure associated with cerebral desaturation in infants. Paediatr Anaesth. 2015;25(7):681–8.
2. Williams M, Lee JK. Intraoperative blood pressure and cerebral perfusion: strategies to clarify hemodynamic goals. Paediatr Anaesth. 2014;24(7):657–67.
3. McCann ME, Schouten AN, Dobija N, Munoz C, Stephenson L, Poussaint TY, et al. Infantile postoperative encephalopathy: perioperative factors as a cause for concern. Pediatrics. 2014;133(3):e751–7.
4. Marhofer P, Keplinger M, Klug W, Metzelder ML. Awake caudals and epidurals should be used more frequently in neonates and infants. Paediatr Anaesth. 2015;25(1):93–9.
5. Ing C, Sun LS, Friend AF, Kim M, Berman MF, Paganelli W, et al. Differences in intraoperative hemodynamics between spinal and general anesthesia in infants undergoing pyloromyotomy. Paediatr Anaesth. 2017;27(7):733–41.
6. Larousse E, Asehnoune K, Dartayet B, Albaladejo P, Dubousset AM, Gauthier F, et al. The hemodynamic effects of pediatric caudal anesthesia assessed by esophageal Doppler. Anesth Analg. 2002;94(5):1165–8 table of contents.
7. Deng M, Wang X, Wang L, Zheng S. The hemodynamic effects of newborn caudal anesthesia assessed by transthoracic echocardiography: a randomized, double-blind, controlled study. Paediatr Anaesth. 2008;18(11):1075–81.
8. Rhondali O, Andre C, Pouyau A, Mahr A, Juhel S, De Queiroz M, et al. Sevoflurane anesthesia and brain perfusion. Paediatr Anaesth. 2015;25(2):180–5.
9. Sanders RD, Ma D, Brooks P, Maze M. Balancing paediatric anaesthesia: preclinical insights into analgesia, hypnosis, neuroprotection, and neurotoxicity. Br J Anaesth. 2008;101(5):597–609.
10. Lonnqvist PA. Regional anaesthesia and analgesia in the neonate. Best Pract Res Clin Anaesthesiol. 2010;24(3):309–21.
11. Alderliesten T, Lemmers PM, van Haastert IC, de Vries LS, Bonestroo HJ, Baerts W, et al. Hypotension in preterm neonates: low blood pressure alone does not affect neurodevelopmental outcome. J Pediatr. 2014;164(5):986–91.
12. Rhondali O, Mahr A, Simonin-Lansiaux S, De Queiroz M, Rhzioual-Berrada K, Combet S, et al. Impact of sevoflurane anesthesia on cerebral blood flow in children younger than 2 years. Paediatr Anaesth. 2013;23(10):946–51.
13. Rhondali O, Juhel S, Mathews S, Cellier Q, Desgranges FP, Mahr A, et al. Impact of sevoflurane anesthesia on brain oxygenation in children younger than 2 years. Paediatr Anaesth. 2014;24(7):734–40.
14. Davidson AJ, Disma N, de Graaff JC, Withington DE, Dorris L, Bell G, et al. Neurodevelopmental outcome at 2 years of age after general anaesthesia and awake-regional anaesthesia in infancy (GAS): an international multicentre, randomised controlled trial. Lancet (London, England). 2016; 387(10015):239–50.
15. Brenner L, Kettner SC, Marhofer P, Latzke D, Willschke H, Kimberger O, et al. Caudal anaesthesia under sedation: a prospective analysis of 512 infants and children. Br J Anaesth. 2010;104(6):751–5.
16. Brenner L, Marhofer P, Kettner SC, Willschke H, Machata AM, Al-Zoraigi U, et al. Ultrasound assessment of cranial spread during caudal blockade in children: the effect of different volumes of local anaesthetics. Br J Anaesth. 2011;107(2):229–35.
17. Dalens B, Hasnaoui A. Caudal anesthesia in pediatric surgery: success rate and adverse effects in 750 consecutive patients. Anesth Analg. 1989;68(2):83–9.
18. Suresh S, Long J, Birmingham PK, De Oliveira GS Jr. Are caudal blocks for pain control safe in children? An analysis of 18,650 caudal blocks from the pediatric regional anesthesia network (PRAN) database. Anesth Analg. 2015; 120(1):151–6.
19. Hoelzle M, Weiss M, Dillier C, Gerber A. Comparison of awake spinal with awake caudal anesthesia in preterm and ex-preterm infants for herniotomy. Paediatr Anaesth. 2010;20(7):620–4.
20. Wang LZ, Hu XX, Zhang YF, Chang XY. A randomized comparison of caudal block by sacral hiatus injection under ultrasound guidance with traditional sacral canal injection in children. Paediatr Anaesth. 2013;23(5):395–400.
21. Ahiskalioglu A, Yayik AM, Ahiskalioglu EO, Ekinci M, Golboyu BE, Celik EC, et al. Ultrasound-guided versus conventional injection for caudal block in children: a prospective randomized clinical study. J Clin Anesth. 2018;44:91–6.
22. Unsinn KM, Geley T, Freund MC, Gassner I. US of the spinal cord in newborns: spectrum of normal findings, variants, congenital anomalies, and acquired diseases. Radiographics. 2000;20(4):923–38.

25

It's not you, it's the design - common problems with patient monitoring reported by anesthesiologists

David W. Tscholl[1*], Lucas Handschin[1], Julian Rössler[1], Mona Weiss[2], Donat R. Spahn[1] and Christoph B. Nöthiger[1]

Abstract

Background: Patient monitoring is critical for perioperative patient safety as anesthesiologists routinely make crucial therapeutic decisions from the information displayed on patient monitors. Previous research has shown that today's patient monitoring has room for improvement in areas such as information overload and alarm fatigue. The rationale of this study was to learn more about the problems anesthesiologists face in patient monitoring and to derive improvement suggestions for next-generation patient monitors.

Methods: We conducted a two-center qualitative/quantitative study. Initially, we interviewed 120 anesthesiologists (physicians and nurses) about the topic: common problems with patient monitoring in your daily work. Through deductive and inductive coding, we identified major topics and sub themes from the interviews. In a second step, a field survey, a separate group of 25 anesthesiologists rated their agree- or disagreement with central statements created for all identified major topics.

Results: We identified the following six main topics: 1. "Alarms," 2. "Artifacts," 3. "Software," 4. "Hardware," 5. "Human Factors," 6. "System Factors," and 17 sub themes. The central statements rated for the major topics were: 1. "problems with alarm settings complicate patient monitoring." (56% agreed) 2. "artifacts complicate the assessment of the situation." (64% agreed) 3. "information overload makes it difficult to get an overview quickly." (56% agreed) 4. "problems with cables complicate working with patient monitors." (92% agreed) 5. "factors related to human performance lead to critical information not being perceived." (88% agreed) 6. "Switching between monitors from different manufacturers is difficult." (88% agreed). The ratings of all statements differed significantly from neutral (all $p < 0.03$).

Conclusion: This study provides an overview of the problems anesthesiologists face in patient monitoring. Some of the issues, to our knowledge, were not previously identified as common problems in patient monitoring, e.g., hardware problems (e.g., cable entanglement and worn connectors), human factor aspects (e.g., fatigue and distractions), and systemic factor aspects (e.g., insufficient standardization between manufacturers). An ideal monitor should transfer the relevant patient monitoring information as efficiently as possible, prevent false positive alarms, and use technologies designed to improve the problems in patient monitoring.

Keywords: Patient monitoring, Signal processing, Qualitative research, Patient safety, Situation awareness

* Correspondence: david.tscholl@usz.ch
[1]Institute of Anesthesiology, University and University Hospital Zurich, Raemistrasse 100, 8091 Zurich, Switzerland

Introduction

The World Health Organization considers continuous patient monitoring during surgical interventions as "extremely important" for patient safety [1].

A patient monitor measures and displays the vital signs of a patient using various sensors and enables care providers to take corrective action if a patient's vital signs deviate from their normal range. Patient monitoring devices have gained significant relevance in our area of expertise. Anesthesiologists nearly always work directly with a patient monitor.

To perceive the data displayed on a patient monitor and to derive a mental model of the operating room situation, an exchange of information has to take place between the display of the patient monitor and the person interpreting the data shown there [2–8]. The patient monitor serves as the critical interface between the hardware and software components that measure physical quantities in the patient on the one hand and the sensorium and cognition of the human decision makers on the other hand. However, we know from previous research that current standard patient monitoring still has deficits regarding this information transmission. Today's monitors make use of numbers and curves to transfer vital sign information and display a multitude of individual numerical values and curve forms with very similar ranges of values, e.g., blood pressure, pulse rate and oxygen saturation can all three take a value of 95. Care providers must read all these numbers from the screen one after the other and afterwards cognitively integrate the data to derive meaning, before they can start to establish a complete picture of the patient situation [9–13]. Several research groups have developed innovative technologies, which, at least in theory, were able to communicate a situation overview to users in a faster and easier-to-understand fashion [14–18].

From previous research, we also learned that auditory and visual alarm displays represent a problem in patient monitoring. Alarms are set on the monitor to alert if a vital sign exits its normal range. They are often false positive, e.g., as a result of measurement artefacts, leading to alarm fatigue and potentially causing true positive alarms to go unnoticed because of induced insensitivity [19–24].

The rationale for this study was to learn more about the problems anesthesiologists consider common in their daily work with patient monitors. We hoped that these results would allow us to identify critical aspects for further development in future patient monitors.

Methods

The Ethics Committee of the Canton of Zurich, Zurich, Switzerland issued a declaration of no objection for this study (Business Administration System for Ethics Committees Req-2016-00103). Additionally, all participants signed an informed consent in which they agreed to the evaluation of their answers for medical research. We did not record audio or video.

Study design

In planning the study and conducting the analyses, we followed the "Consolidated Criteria for Reporting Qualitative Research" checklist and relevant guidelines for qualitative data analysis and reporting [25].

The study consisted of a qualitative and a quantitative part. First we conducted semi-structured interviews to identify major topics and subthemes from interviews of anesthesia professionals about common problems with patient monitors. Then, for the quantitative part, we derived a central statement for each major theme identified in the interviews and asked a separate group of anesthesiologists to rate their agree- or disagreement with these statements.

Study participants

The majority of the participants in this study were anesthesiologists from the anesthesia department of the University Hospital Zurich, a maximum care hospital with around 30,000 surgical procedures per year. One participant came from the anesthesia department of the Kantonsspital Winterthur, Switzerland, a teaching hospital with about 10,000 surgical procedures per year.

In both study steps, all participants were either attending or resident physicians, or nurse anesthetists. All staff physicians held an anesthesia board certification, and all nurse participants had completed their anesthesia sub specialization training. We recruited participants who responded to institutional e-mail invitations and additionally asked colleagues in person to participate according to their personal availability.

Most participants knew the data collectors personally before the study, as they worked in the same departments. We explained the background of the study, namely the development and evaluation of an avatar-based patient monitoring technology, in the invitation e-mails and, when approaching a participant directly, in person.

Part I: qualitative analysis of interview answers

Study setup and data collectors

The interviews were conducted at the end of data collection sessions conducted with the intend to develop a novel avatar-based visualization technology for patient monitoring (Visual Patient technology). The methodology and the results of other studies conducted for this project have been published [17, 18]. Before each interview, participants also completed a personal information survey, e.g., age, sex, previous experience with patient monitors.

Two doctors conducted the interviews. Physician one (CBN) was a senior physician at the Institute of Anesthesiology of the University Hospital Zurich with more than 20 years of clinical anesthesia experience. He works 100% clinically, has completed advanced Good Clinical Practice (GCP) courses, and has considerable experience in patient safety.

The second data collector (LH) was a junior doctor in the second year of his anesthesia residency. During this study, he worked in a 50% clinical and 50% research capacity at the University Hospital Zurich. He has completed entry-level GCP courses at the clinical trials center of the University of Zurich.

Description of the interview

We conducted the data collection sessions and interviews in the University Hospital Zurich. The question we asked the participants was: "What are the most common problems with patient monitoring in your daily work?"

The interviewers motivated the participants to answer the questions openly with anything that came to their minds. Otherwise, no prompts or instructions were given. There were no time limits.

As the subjects pared their thoughts, the interviewers typed notes into a Microsoft Word document (Microsoft Corp., Redmond, WA, USA) on an Aspire V15 Nitro laptop computer (ACER, Inc., Taipei, Taiwan).

The transcript was visible to participants during data entry and was provided at the end of the interview for comments and corrections if requested.

Analysis

Before the analysis, we translated the original answers from German to English and unified words of similar meaning to make it easier to count and code words into topics. The matched words were tangling = cable clutter; handling = operation. With the resulting English translation of the answers, we performed a word count (Additional file 1: Table S2) and created a tag cloud (Fig. 1) using Wordle.net. We omitted common English words like 'and' or 'the' in the word counts and the tag cloud.

Study author DWT, a senior physician, with previous experience in patient safety research, who had not conducted any of the interviews, coded the respondents' interview answers. Major topics and sub themes were derived from the interview transcripts by applying a two-step process consisting of deductive coding based on word count, followed by an inductive coding process based on the cognitive identification of topics that repeatedly came up in the answers but had not been identified with word counting.

We present and discuss these main topics and sub themes with examples in the results and in Table 2. Additionally, we provide a figure of the coding tree (Fig. 2). The complete dataset with unformatted original answers, the stepwise translation, and correction as well as the coding of the answers are provided in Additional file 1: Table S1.

For data management, we used the software Atlas TI 8.0 (Scientific Software Development GmbH, Berlin) and Microsoft Word.

Part II: quantitative analysis of statement ratings

For the second, quantitative part of this study, we conducted a field survey in which anesthesiologists rated their agree- or disagreement to the qualitative statements.

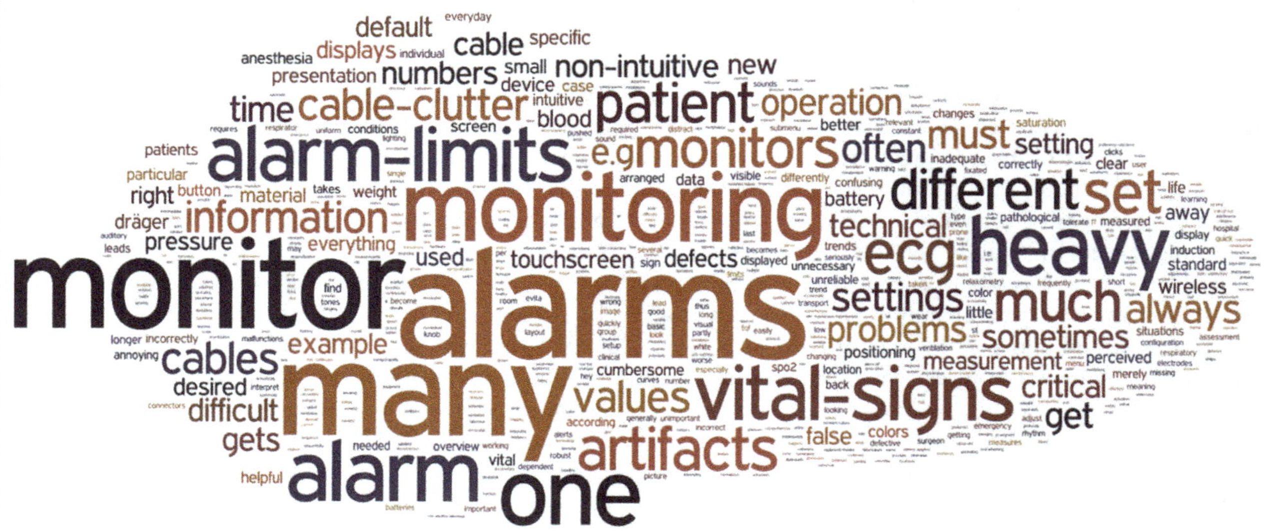

Fig. 1 A word cloud created from the participants' answers to visualize the most common topics. This word cloud was created with Wordle.net. All words were written in lowercase, and commonly occurring English words (e.g., the, is, and, to) were hidden

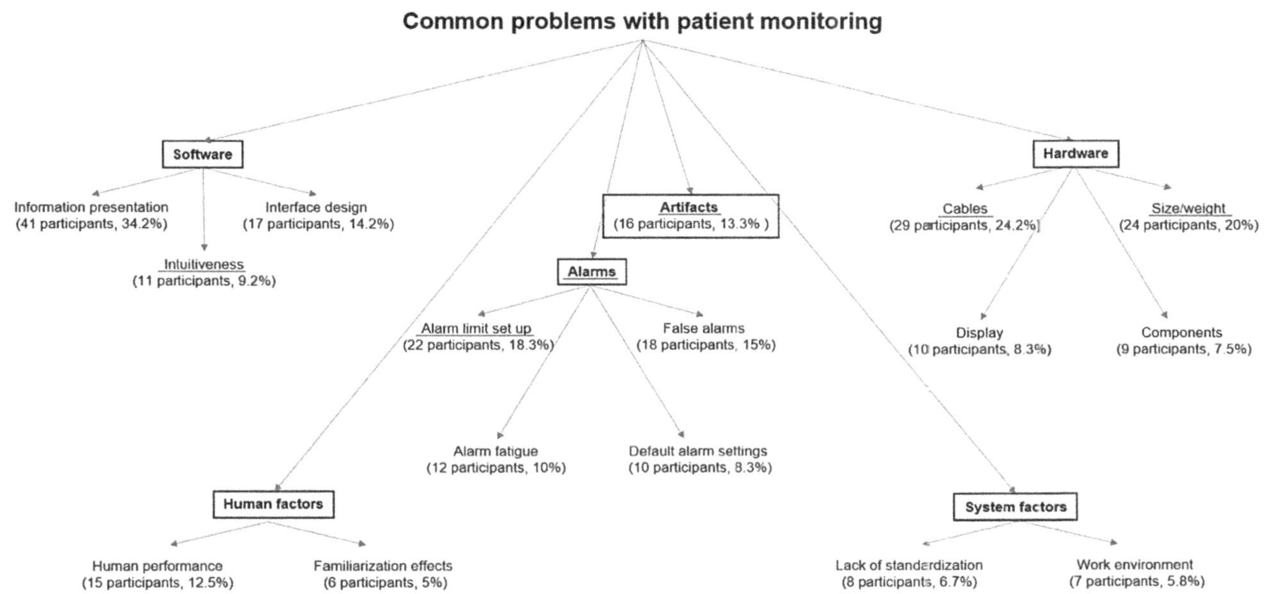

Fig. 2 The coding tree with major topics and sub themes, with participant numbers and percentages. We identified the terms underlined in blue by deductive coding based on word counting and the rest by inductive, free coding. We interviewed 120 individual anesthesia experts

Description of the field survey

In the field survey, we asked the participants to rate a total of six central statements based on the topics identified in the qualitative analysis of the interview responses. Specifically, we created a statement for each of the main theme common problems identified in the interviews. We tried to make these statements relevant for a better understanding of care providers' problems with patient monitoring.

The statements were evaluated by the participants on five-point Likert scales. The Likert scales consisted of five divisions: 1. "strongly disagree," 2. "disagree," 3. "neutral," 4. "agree," and 5. "strongly agree."

Statistical analysis

We present the results of the field survey for all six central statements as percentages and as medians with interquartile ranges (IQR). We used the Wilcoxon signed rank test to find out whether the sample medians were significantly different from the neutral rating option. We considered any difference from neutral as practically significant and considered p-values of < 0.05 as statistically significant.

Through the participants' ratings of the central statements, we tried to quantify the agree- or disagreement of the participants with the problems identified. Thereby, internal validity is given to the study.

Results

Study and participant characteristics

One hundred and thirty-seven anesthesia professionals participated in the study. For the qualitative part, we evaluated the responses given by 120 individual anesthesia experts. Twenty-five participants took part in the second quantitative part. Eight participants who participated in the interviews also participated in the follow-up study, resulting in a crossing-over between the interview participants and field survey participants of 6%.

The samples in both study steps were gender-, profession-, and experience balanced. Table 1 outlines the study and participant characteristics in full detail.

As we conducted this study at the University Hospital Zurich, all participants indicated to possess experience with patient monitors of the manufacturer Dräger (Drägerwerk AG & Co. KGaA. Lübeck, Germany), which were in use at the University Hospital Zurich at the time of the study. Additionally, about one of two participants had previous experience with monitors of Philips Healthcare (Koninklijke Philips N. V, Amsterdam, The Netherlands), and about one in six had previous experience with monitors of GE (General Electric Company, Boston, MA, USA).

Part I: qualitative analysis of interview answers

The word count revealed that the participants most frequently used the following words: alarm = 52, cable = 24, heavy = 20, alarm limits = 19, artifacts = 15, ECG (electrocardiogram) = 15, non-intuitive = 6.

Figure 1 shows the tag cloud created from the words people used in their answers.

Based on the word count and additional inductive, i.e., free coding, we identified the following six main topics with sub themes: 1. "Alarms" with sub themes "alarm

Table 1 Study details and demographic data of study participants. IQR = Interquartile range

	Part I: (participant Interview)	Part II: (field survey)
Duration of data collection in days	248 (April 12th 2016 – December 16th 2016)	16 (December 5th 2018 – December 21st 2018)
Total number of participants	120	25
Crossing over between parts I and II	8 participants (6%)	
Number of senior physicians (%)	36 (30%)	12 (50%)
Number of residents (%)	45 (37.5%)	12 (50%)
Number of nurse anesthetists (%)	39 (32.5%)	/
Number of female and male participants (%)	57 (47.5%) / 63 (52.5%)	12 (50%) / 12 (50%)
Median (IQR) anesthesia experience group of participants in years	5 to 10 (1 to 5 – more than 10)	6 (2–9.5)
Median (IQR) number of monitoring manufacturers whose products the participants had work experience with:	2 (1–3)	
Number of participants who had experience with the products of the three most common monitor manufacturers in this study:	Dräger (Drägerwerk AG & Co. KGaA. Lübeck, Germany): 120 (100%) Philips (Koninklijke Philips N. V, Amsterdam, The Netherlands): 55 (46%) GE (General Electric Company, Boston, MA, USA): 21 (17.5%)	

limit setup", "false alarms," "alarm fatigue," and "default settings," 2. "artifacts," 3. "software" with sub themes "information presentation," "interface design," and "intuitiveness," 4. "hardware" with "cables," "size/weight," "display," and "components," 5. "human factors" with sub themes "human performance" and "familiarization effects," and 6. "system factors" with sub themes "lack of standardization" and "work environment." We describe all major topics and sub themes with participant numbers, percentages, and examples in Table 2 and present the coding tree in Fig. 2.

Parent themes

1. **Alarms**

Alarms were a common major common problems topic. Twenty-two interviewees (18%) mentioned alarm limits and alarm configuration as problematic. Other themes included lack of standardization in alarm management, alarm limit settings, e.g., the requirement for different alarm thresholds for different phases of care or different patients.

False alarms were mentioned as problematic by 18 participants (15%). Participants criticized false positive alarms, i.e., a warning when all is ok, and too frequently reoccurring alarms. Twelve (10%) participants specifically used the term "alarm fatigue" and mentioned the danger of desensitization, which may cause a critical patient status to go unnoticed. Participants talked about the sound characteristics of the audio alarms and the problem of discerning which of two or more alerts is more important.

2. **Artifacts**

Artifacts were mentioned as problematic by 16 anesthesiologists (13%). The participants mentioned interactions in measurement such as electrocautery and the ECG or the oxygen saturation probe and patient movement, and the problems of distinguishing artifacts from real problems. One participant suggested that, similar to alarm fatigue, frequent artifacts can lead to ignoring of this sensor and, thereby, losing it for informed decision making. With problems caused by the empty invasive arterial blood pressure measurement sodium chloride infusion bag, another example of a frequently occurring artifact was named.

3. **Software**

Forty-three (34%) interviewees provided problems regarding the presentation of information. The participants complained that they consider the display of information in current monitoring confusing, e.g., the information is number-coded, and interpretation requires skills. The participants reported that they often feel overloaded with information. In addition, participants complained about a lack of standardization in the design and presentation of monitoring information

Table 2 The major topics and sub themes with participant counts, percentages and examples. $N = 120$

Major topics	Sub themes	Examples
Alarms	Alarm limit set up (22 participants, 18.3%)	Participant #14: Alarm-limits are set differently by different people - > either the monitor then alerts very quickly or not at all for long.
	False alarms (18 participants, 15%)	Participant #9: There are too many false alarms that have no relevance. The ideal would be: If there is no message displayed on the monitor, everything is fine.
	Alarm fatigue (12 participants, 10%)	Participant #48: Frequent false alarms lead to ignoring of alarms.
	Default settings (10 participants 8.3%)	Participant #71: Impractical default alarm-limits.
Artifacts	16 participants (13.3%)	Participant #12: SpO2 artifacts. Artifacts of the ECG caused by improper positioning of the electrodes.
		Participant #66: Cautery artifacts on the ECG.
		Participant #107: Distinguish artifacts from reality.
Software	Information presentation (41 participants, 34.2%)	Participant #49: Much visual and auditory information, the sense for the relevant gets lost.
		Participant #102: For a comprehensive state assessment, the gaze must travel across multiple monitors and numbers, which must then be interpreted.
	Interface design (17 participants, 14.2%)	Participant #47: Too many clicks needed to configure the monitor. Great tools hidden in submenus, so they are hard to find.
		Participant #71: In unfamiliar monitors, the patient is effectively worse off due as the vital-signs are perceived much worse and slower.
	Intuitiveness (11 participants, 9.2%)	Participant #23: The screen layout should be easily adjustable (intuitive as Apple products).
		Participant #98: Operation is non-intuitive.
Hardware	Cables (29 participants, 24.2%)	Participant #23: Wireless would be interesting. A wish: a single device on the patient, which measures all vital signs.
		Participant #106: Always cable-clutter.
		Participant #108: Cable disconnected / incorrect values measured.
	Size/weight (24 participants, 20%)	Participants #41: Sometimes difficult to transport, smaller transport monitors would be better.
		Participants #63: Not robust enough for the everyday run (much wear material).
		Participant #110: Patient monitoring is too heavy (kg).
	Display (10 participants, 8.3%)	Participant #36: Small display with reduced resolution. Touchscreen would probably be better or above all more intuitive.
		Participant #46: Numbers too small, not visible from a distance.
	Components (9 participants, 7.5%)	Participant #63: Not robust enough for the everyday run (much wear material).
		Participant #74: loose contacts...
		Participant #98: Unreliable battery life.
Human factors	Human performance (15 participants, 12.5%)	Participant #82: One pays too little attention to the monitor.
		Participant #82: Although a pathological value is on the monitor, the user does not recognize it because a number is not readily perceptible.
		Participant #95: Tired: One has to look several times until the information arrives.
	Familiarization effects (6 participants, 5%)	Participant #13: When changing the hospital or the monitor type, it takes a long time (up to many days) to get used to the new monitors.
System factors	Lack of standardization (8 participants, 6.7%)	Participant #23: Presentation / standard alarm-limits not uniform.
	Work environment (7 participants, 5.8%)	Participant #97: Lighting conditions and viewing angle to the monitor.
		Participant #114: A relatively large area with different displays that one must monitor continuously.
Comments/ Suggestions	26 participants (21%)	Participant #54: Measured values for non-continuous data collection (e.g., blood pressure) should disappear after a specific time (e.g., 3 or 5 min).
		Participant #116: In emergency situations, one must get a quick and safe overview, which is not always possible with the current monitoring.

between different manufacturers and hospitals. Eighteen participants (14%) mentioned software interface design aspects, e.g., a lack of intuitiveness in interface designs and the importance of customizability.

4. **Hardware**

Of the 120 total participants, 29 (24%) mentioned problems with cables. On one hand, problems with the technical aspects of cables, e.g., unplugged cables, bent or worn out plugs, ECG electrodes coming off with certain patient conditions, e.g., wet skin or a special patient positioning. On the other hand, the answers included examples of situations in which working with cables is most bothersome, e.g., when changing the patient's position or transferring a patient. Participants mentioned the large amount of individual cables, the length of the cables and constant entanglements as problematic and wished for a wireless solution.

Twenty-four (20%) participants addressed weight and industrial design issues of the monitoring devices, e.g., bulkiness. Ten (8%) participants complained about the technical characteristics of the displays. They wished for monitoring displays with these properties: "removable," "large format," "touchscreen," "high-resolution", "vibrant." Nine participants (8%) mentioned problems with individual components of the monitors. Mainly issues with battery life and built quality of parts, e.g., connectors.

5. **Human factors**

The human factors main topic included human performance and habituation effects, which were named by 15 (13%) and six subjects (5%), respectively. The human factors aspects included problems of interpretation of vital data in a numerical and wave-form presentation and problems with information overload caused by our limited and fatigue sensitive working memory. Participants described habituation effects as substantial and considered switching between different monitoring manufacturers difficult.

6. **System factors**

The anesthesiologists complained about insufficient standardization in monitoring - in both, the hospital and the global healthcare context. Unfavorably mounted monitors, poor operating room lighting conditions, the requirement for a large number of individual monitors, e.g. respirator, patient monitor, syringe pumps, to capture the situation were all mentioned as problematic. A few participants mentioned the poor transport capability of monitors as bothersome.

Comments/suggestions

Twenty-six participants (21%) provided ideas that did not fit into any of the major topics outlined above. These included aspects relevant for safety design, e.g., the wish of an anesthesiologist that trend images should always be visible and slow changes over time should be made recognizable for the care provider, or that the alarm off button should only mute the alarm for which it is pressed. Alarm tones should be made more explicit. One participant mentioned that despite all monitoring, we should never forget to look at the patient and the monitors: "Treat the patient, not the monitor."

Part II: quantitative analysis of statements rated in an online survey

Figure 3 shows the results of the ratings of the six central statements derived from the qualitative analysis (study part I). The sample medians of all six statements statistically significantly differed from neutral.

Discussion

In this qualitative and quantitative study, we analyzed the responses that 120 individual anesthesia experts gave in semi-structured interviews to an open-ended interview question asking them what problems commonly occur in their daily work with patient monitors. We then extracted central statements from the interviews and validated them in a quantitative approach through confirmation by a new group of 25 anesthesia professionals. All six statements were significantly agreed on, which by quantitative confirmation of the agreement with the central statements, increases the validity of the results. Although alarm fatigue [19–22], information overload [23], and measurement artifacts [24], had already been identified as problematic, this study confirms that these issues are still regarded as problematic by anesthesiologists in 2018 and, additionally, there still seems to be considerable need for improvement also in previously less-known areas of ubiquitously used patient monitors. As a descriptive example, in Fig. 4, we provide a photo, which illustrates the problem of "too many alarms" and the users' response to it. In our monitors, the most worn out button is the "all alarms off" button.

Through the evaluation of problems with current monitors, we found answers to the fascinating question: "What properties would an ideal patient monitor have?" The answer to this question could be particularly interesting for virtual and augmented reality head mounted devices of the future, as the desirable characteristics could be tested and implement there easily because it would merely be virtual and not physical, as todays patient monitors.

Based on the responses, an ideal patient monitor would be a high-quality built, lightweight and compact,

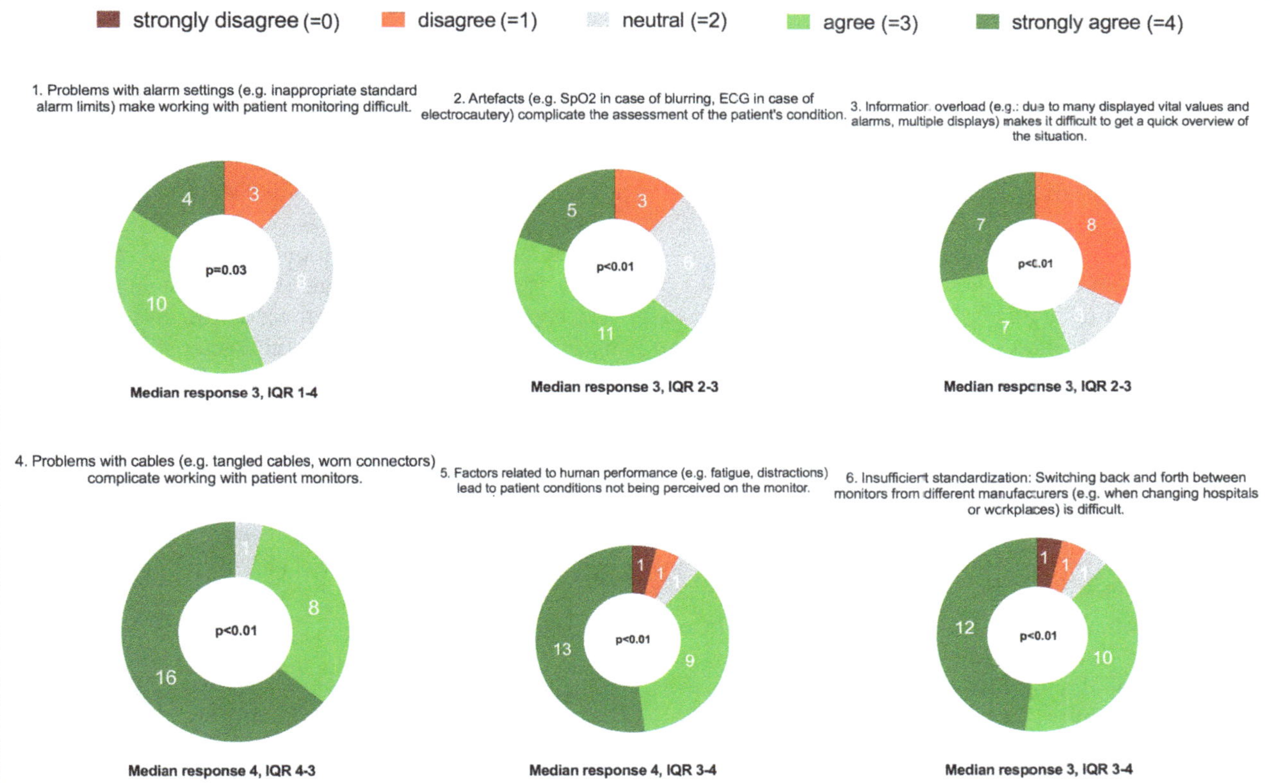

Fig. 3 Presentation of the results of the field survey as donut charts with the number of participants who chose a particular category. We used the Wilcoxon signed rank test to evaluate whether the sample medians were significantly different from neutral. IQR = interquartile range. 0 = strongly disagree, 1 = disagree, 2 = neutral, 3 = agree, 4 = strongly agree. $N = 25$

but still robust device, with a large, high resolution, non-reflecting touchscreen display. It would feature intuitive controls and large, vibrant and colorful, easy to understand visual display of the patient's situation presenting integrated information from all sensors. It would be resistant to artifacts and only issue an alarm in case of a true positive event. Data transmission, maybe even sensing, would be wireless and immediate. This system would do without cables. Work ergonomics would be excellent, and an international standardization for the appearance of monitoring data would be in effect. The hardware and software components, e.g., display, sensors, cables, interface design, and information presentation of an ideal monitor would make it easy for users to preserve both mental and physical energy, and, thereby, be able to maintain their alertness and performance longer and easier than with today's state-of-the-art.

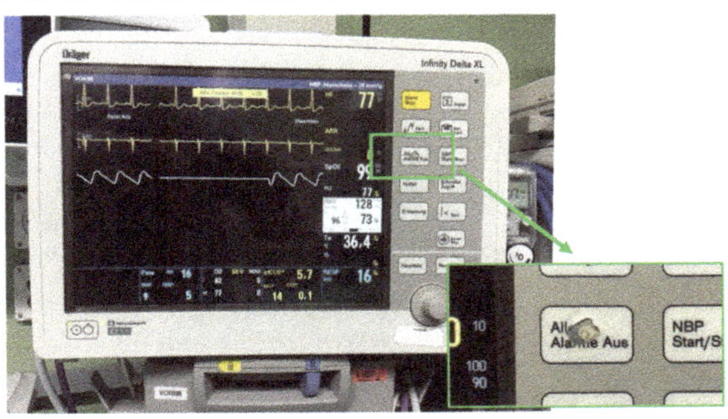

Fig. 4 The fact that too many alarms are a common problem is illustrated by the fact that the most worn button on our patient monitors is the "all alarms off" button

In our quantitative analysis 88% of the anesthesiologists agreed to the central statement that factors related to human performance (e.g. fatigue, distractions) can lead to important information being overlooked. It is well known that preserving mental and physical energy of care providers is safety critical, because fatigue (physical, alarm- and other kinds of fatigue) causes errors, which may ultimately lead to patient harm [26–29].

These aspects are important for the heterogenous group of patient monitoring users in healthcare, for example, non-experts, trainees, intensivists, emergency care providers, general ward nurses, paramedics, and tele monitoring, and consumer health users.

There is still much room left for improvement in patient monitoring systems and, based on this study and previous research, we claim that standardization [30], easy understanding [3, 9, 10, 17, 18], and fatigue prevention [31–37] should be sought after to reduce the risk of accidents to happen and improve patient safety and operator well-being in the perioperative area. Policy makers and creators of patient monitors should feel encouraged to satisfy these needs.

Limitations

The first part of the study has the inherent limitations of interview-based qualitative research. The qualitative analysis gives a complete, detailed description. There is no attempt to assign frequencies to the features identified in the data. Rare phenomena receive the same attention as more common phenomena. The main drawback of a qualitative analysis is that its results cannot be transferred to broader populations with the same certainty as quantitative results. This is because the research results are not checked to see if they are statistically significant or random. [38]

However, initially using a qualitative approach in our study context has yielded many benefits. We were able to identify everyday problems that caregivers have with traditional patient monitoring systems and develop a deeper understanding of the causes of these problems. The results contribute to a better understanding of patient monitoring and provide clues for its further improvement. In the first part of the study, our goal was to explore the full range of problems in patient monitoring without weighing these issues quantitatively. Since the participants in this study were asked to describe the problems, they felt were relevant, the analysis likely truly identified problems that the participants experience when working with patient monitoring and, furthermore, we were able to improve the validity of the central statements through their quantitative rating [39, 40].

Finally, this study was conducted in a small area of Central Europe in an environment with a high standard of care. The work values and thus the user perceived problems may vary in different parts of the world.

Conclusions

To our knowledge, this study is the first to provide a global overview of the problems anesthesiologists commonly experience when working with patient monitors in real-life patient care. This study confirmed findings of previous research that anesthetists are inconvenienced by inadequate alarms, artifacts, and information overload. Some of the new aspects discovered by this study included the findings that anesthesiologists feel bothered by problems related to monitoring cables and that they considered human factor and systemic factor aspects as relevant in patient monitoring. Human factor aspects included fatigue and distraction, which participants indicated may cause patient monitoring information to not be perceived and systemic factor aspects, which included difficulties in switching back and forth between monitors of different manufacturers. Furthermore, this study enabled us to draft a hypothetical prototype of an ideal monitor. An ideal monitor should have an alarm system that reduces false positive alarms to a minimum, works with as few cables as possible and transfer relevant information easily and quickly and, thereby, make it easier for participants to preserve both mental and physical energy, and maintain their alertness and performance longer and easier. These characteristics of a patient monitor would help keep patient safety and user satisfaction high. Further research should focus on the development of new monitoring technologies to provide the necessary information to care providers as quickly and efficiently as possible. Such developments should undergo extensive testing in realistic simulators before being carefully applied in real patients.

Additional file

Additional file 1: Table S1. The complete dataset, language translation and encoding of participants' answers to the question "What are the most common problems with patient monitoring in your daily work?" Columns two and three are presented in their original form to allow traceability and may, therefore, contain typos and syntax errors. In column four, "Adjusted English translation," the Google translation (Alphabet Inc., Mountainview, CA, USA) was adjusted by hand for meaning and syntax using Grammarly (Grammarly Inc., San Francisco, CA, USA). In column 4, we matched words with comparable meaning to facilitate word counting and coding. The matched words were tangling = cable-clutter; not intuitive = non-intuitive; use, handling = operation, parameters = vital-signs; weight, heavy = heavy weight. **Table S2.** The results of the word count with all words that have occurred more than five times. The dark gray shading displays the topics identified by the word count. Irrespective of singular or plural, uppercase or lowercase, the word count of these words was: alarm = 52, cable = 24, heavy = 20, alarm limits = 19, artifacts = 15, ECG = 15, non-intuitive = 6. ECG = electrocardiogram. (DOCX 94 kb)

Abbreviations

ECG: Electrocardiogram; GCP: Good Clinical Practice; IQR: Interquartile Range

Acknowledgements

The authors are thankful to the study participants for their time and effort.

Authors' contributions

DWT, LH, JR, MW, DRS and CBN helped to design the study. DWT, LH, JR and CBN helped to collect the data. DWT, LH and JR helped to analyse the data. DWT, LH, JR, MW, DRS and CBN helped to write the article and reviewed and approved the final version.

Author details

[1]Institute of Anesthesiology, University and University Hospital Zurich, Raemistrasse 100, 8091 Zurich, Switzerland. [2]Department of Management, School of Business and Economics, Free University of Berlin, Garystrasse 21, 14195 Berlin, Germany.

References

1. World Alliance for Patient Safety. WHO guidelines for safe surgery. Geneva: Switzerland World Health Organization; 2008.
2. Helmreich RL. On error management: lessons from aviation. BMJ. 2000;320: 781–5.
3. Endsley MR. Toward a theory of situation awareness in dynamic systems human factors. Hum Factors. 1995;37:32–64.
4. Fioratou E, Flin R, Glavin R, Patey R. Beyond monitoring: distributed situation awareness in anaesthesia. Br J Anaesth. 2010;105:83–90.
5. Gaba DM, Howard SK, Small SD. Situation awareness in anesthesiology. Hum Factors. 1995;37:20–31.
6. Schulz CM, Endsley MR, Kochs EF, Gelb AW, Wagner KJ. Situation awareness in anesthesia: concept and research. Anesthesiology. 2013;118:729–42.
7. Schulz CM, Burden A, Posner KL, et al. Frequency and type of situational awareness errors contributing to death and brain damage: a closed claims analysis. Anesthesiology. 2017;127(2):326-37.
8. Schulz CM, Krautheim V, Hackemann A, Kreuzer M, Kochs EF, Wagner KJ. Situation awareness errors in anesthesia and critical care in 200 cases of a critical incident reporting system. BMC Anesthesiol. 2015;16:4.
9. Drews FA, Westenskow DR. The right picture is worth a thousand numbers: data displays in anesthesia. Hum Factors. 2006;48:59–71.
10. Endsley MR, Jones DG. Designing for situation awareness: an approach to user-centered design. 2nd ed. Boca Raton: CRC Press, Inc.; 2011.
11. Ford S, Birmingham E, King A, Lim J, Ansermino JM. At-a-glance monitoring: covert observations of anesthesiologists in the operating room. Anesth Analg. 2010;111:653–8.
12. Loeb RG. Monitor surveillance and vigilance of anesthesia residents. Anesthesiology. 1994;80:527–33.
13. Degani, A, Jorgensen, CC, Iverson D, Shafto M, Olson L. On organization of information: approach and early work. Moffett Field: NASA Ames Research Center; 2009.
14. Drews FA, Doig A. Evaluation of a Configural vital signs display for intensive care unit nurses. Hum Factors. 2014;56(3):569–80.
15. Agutter J, Drews F, Syroid N, Westenskow D, Albert R, Strayer D, Bermudez J, Weinger MB. Evaluation of graphic cardiovascular display in a high-fidelity simulator. Anesth Analg. 2003 Nov;97(5):1403–13.
16. Wachter SB, Johnson K, Albert R, Syroid N, Drews F, Westenskow D. The evaluation of a pulmonary display to detect adverse respiratory events using high resolution human simulator. J Am Med Inform Assoc. 2006;13(6):635–42.
17. Tscholl DW, Handschin L, Neubauer P, Weiss M, Seifert B, Spahn DR, Noethiger CB. Using an animated patient avatar to improve perception of vital sign information by anaesthesia professionals. Br J Anaesth. 2018 Sep;121(3):662–71.
18. Tscholl DW, Weiss M, Handschin L, Spahn DR, Nöthiger CB. User perceptions of avatar-based patient monitoring: a mixed qualitative and quantitative study. BMC Anesthesiol. 2018;18(1):188.
19. Srinivasa E, Mankoo J, Kerr C. An evidence-based approach to reducing cardiac telemetry alarm fatigue. Worldviews Evid-Based Nurs. 2017 Aug;14(4):265–73.
20. Ruskin KJ, Hueske-Kraus D. Alarm fatigue: impacts on patient safety. Curr Opin Anaesthesiol. 2015 Dec;28(6):685–90.
21. Cvach M. Monitor alarm fatigue: an integrative review. Biomed Instrum Technol. 2012 Jul-Aug;46(4):268–77.
22. Schmid F, Goepfert MS, Kuhnt D, Eichhorn V, Diedrichs S, Reichenspurner H, et al. The wolf is crying in the operating room: patient monitor and anesthesia workstation alarming patterns during cardiac surgery. Anesth Analg. 2011;112(1):78–83.
23. McFarlane DC, Doig AK, Agutter JA, Mercurio JL, Mittu R, Brewer LM, Syroid ND. Defeating information overload in health surveillance using a metacognitive aid innovation from military combat systems. J Defense Modeling Simulation. 2017;14(4):371–88.
24. Hoorweg AJ, Pasma W, van Wolfswinkel L, de Graaff JC. Incidence of artifacts and deviating values in research data obtained from an anesthesia information management system in children. Anesthesiology. 2018 Feb; 128(2):293–304.
25. Tong A, Sainsbury P, Craig J. Consolidated criteria for reporting qualitative research (COREQ): a 32-item checklist for interviews and focus groups. Int J Qual Health Care. 2007;19:349–57.
26. Caplan RA, Vistica MF, Posner KL, Cheney FW. Adverse anesthetic outcomes arising from gas delivery equipment: a closed claims analysis. Anesthesiology. 1997;87:741–8.
27. Way LW, Stewart L, Gantert W, et al. Causes and prevention of laparoscopic bile duct injuries: analysis of 252 cases from a human factors and cognitive psychology perspective. Ann Surg. 2003;237:450–9.
28. Reason J. Human error: models and management. BMJ. 2000;320:768–70.
29. Reason J. Safety in the operating theatre - Part 2: human error and organisational failure. Qual Saf Health Care. 2005 Feb;14(1):56-60.
30. Davies MA, Tales H. Enhancing patient safety through a standardized model of physiologic monitoring. Healthc Q. 2005;8 Spec No:49–52.
31. Prottengeier J, Petzoldt M, Jess N, et al. The effect of a standardised source of divided attention in airway management: a randomised, crossover, interventional manikin study. Eur J Anaesthesiol. 2016;33:195–203.
32. McKinley J, Dempster M, Gormley GJ. 'Sorry, I meant the patient's left side': impact of distraction on left–right discrimination. Med Educ. 2015;49:427–35.
33. Haynes AB, Weiser TG, Berry WR, Lipsitz SR, Breizat AH, Dellinger EP, Herbosa T, Joseph S, Kibatala PL, Lapitan MC, Merry AF, Moorthy K, Reznick RK, Taylor B, Gawande AA. Safe surgery saves lives study group. A surgical safety checklist to reduce morbidity and mortality in a global population. N Engl J Med. 2009;360:491–9.
34. Drews FA, Musters A, Markham B, Samore MH. Error-producing conditions in the intensive care unit. In: Proceedings of the human factors and ergonomics society 51st annual meeting; 2007. p. 702–6.
35. Wallace DJ, Angu DC, Barnato AE, Kramer AA, Kahn JM. Nighttime intensivist staffing and mortality among critically ill patients. N Engl J Med. 2012;366: 2093–101.
36. Lockley SW, Cronin JW, Evans EE, et al. Effect of reducing Interns' weekly work hours on sleep and attentional failures. N Engl J Med. 2004;351:1829–37.
37. Dawson D, Reid K. Fatigue, alcohol and performance impairment. Nature. 1997;388:235.
38. Atieno O. An analysis of the strengths and limitation of qualitative and quantitative research paradigms. Problems of education in the 21st century, vol. 13; 2009. p. 13–38.
39. Brown C, Hofer T, Johal A, Thomson R, Nicholl J, Franklin BD, Lilford RJ. An epistemology of patient safety research: a framework for study design and interpretation. Part 2. Study design. Qual Saf Health Care. 2008;17:163–9.
40. Brown C, Hofer T, Johal A, Thomson R, Nicholl J, Franklin BD, Lilford RJ. An epistemology of patient safety research: a framework for study design and interpretation. Part 3. End points and measurement. Qual Saf Health Care. 2008;17:170–7.

26

A case of an unexpected posterior mediastinal functional paraganglioma

Zhuqing Yang[1], Qinye Shi[1] and Fangping Bao[1,2*]

Abstract

Background: Paraganglioma can be found in a wide range of locations. However, paraganglioma in the posterior mediastinum is rare. An unexpected paraganglioma located in the posterior mediastinum was found during surgery. The anesthesia management of this patient was challenging.

Case presentation: A 65-year-old male with a posterior mediastinal tumor was scheduled for thoracoscopic mediastinal tumor resection. Severe hemodynamic changes during the operation and postoperative pathological diagnosis showed that the patient had a rare case of posterior mediastinal functional paraganglioma, which was not found before the operation. Although the patient did not experience side effects after surgery, he did experience a dangerous surgical process.

Conclusions: The correct diagnosis of paraganglioma, intensive preoperative screening, adequate preoperative preparation, and accurate intraoperative anesthesia management could provide better anesthesia for paraganglioma patients.

Keywords: Mediastinal tumor, Paraganglioma, Pheochromocytoma

Background

Pheochromocytoma and paraganglioma (PPGL) are a rare class of neuroendocrine tumors that originate from tumors of the adrenal medulla and extra-adrenal sympathetic chain. If the tumor is located in the adrenal gland, it is referred to as pheochromocytoma (PCC), and if it is found outside the gland, it is called paraganglioma (PGL). PCC tumors account for about 80–85% of all PPGLs and synthesize and secrete catecholamines, causing a series of clinical symptoms. PGL accounts for 15–20% of all PPGLs but typically does not produce catecholamines [1, 2]. PGL can be found in a wide range of locations, such as the chest, abdomen, pelvis, and the head and neck. However, PGL is rare in the posterior mediastinum.

In March 2018, a PGL located in the posterior mediastinum was treated in our hospital. This was an unexpected neuroendocrine tumor as we did not diagnose the patient before surgery. Therefore, the patient was operated without receiving adequate preoperative preparation. The patient experienced dramatic fluctuations in hemodynamics during the surgery. The symptoms were treated, and the patient did not experience side effects after surgery. However, he did experience a dangerous surgical process. Therefore, we share this rare disease aiming to inform on how to choose appropriate perioperative management for such patients.

Case presentation

A 65-year-old male was admitted to our hospital for "a mediastinal tumor with cough for more than two

* Correspondence: baofp@zju.edu.cn
[1]Department of Anesthesiology, the Fourth Affiliated Hospital of Zhejiang University School of Medicine, N1 Shangcheng Road, Yiwu, Zhejiang Province, China
[2]Department of Anethesiology, the First Affiliated Hospital of Zhejiang University School of Medicine, 79 Qingchun Road, Hangzhou, Zhejiang Province, China

months" on March 22, 2018. Two months prior, the patient fell during mountain climbing, resulting in a painful left chest. He was conscious when he was injured and started coughing. He went to the local hospital emergency department, and a chest CT showed a "left posterior mediastinum mass". The patient received conservative treatment for the pain. As the patient kept experiencing symptoms, such as coughing and feeling uncomfortable, he came to our hospital for further treatment. The patient had a 4-year history of hypertension, for which he took 20 mg/day of sustained-release nifedipine. This was enough to keep his blood pressure stable within the normal range. He had no family history and no history of diabetes, surgery, or smoking and drinking. He is 162 cm in height and weighed 49.3 kg. His physical examination revealed heavy breathing sounds, but no other abnormalities were found. His blood pressure was 138/81 mmHg, heart rate 88 beats/min, respiratory rate 21 beats/min, and temperature 36 °C. His laboratory tests, such as CRP, blood routine, liver and kidney function, tumor markers, and blood gas analysis were all within the normal range. His fasting blood glucose was 7 mmol/l. His chest enhanced CT suggested: 1. Left posterior mediastinal mass, and therefore a neurogenic tumor was considered; 2. Chronic bronchitis, emphysema, multiple pulmonary bullae in the apex of both lungs; 3. Little inflammation in the lower right lung (Fig. 1). No obvious abnormality was found on his ECG, nor by abdominal and cardiac ultrasound. The pulmonary function examination displayed "Mildly restrictive pulmonary ventilation dysfunction". Given these characteristics, our initial diagnosis was: "left posterior mediastinum tumor; chronic bronchitis; hypertension". The patient continued to use nifedipine after admission, and his blood pressure was well-controlled.

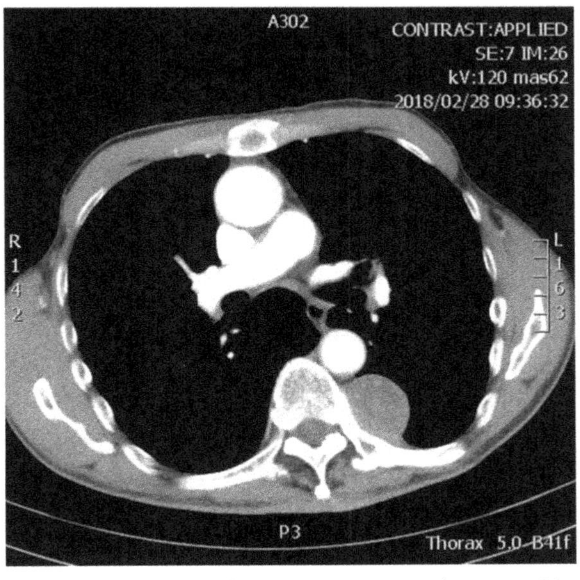

Fig. 1 Chest CT. The size of tumor was approximately 4.1 cm × 3.2 cm in the left spinal column, and the enhanced scan showed uniform enhancement

On March 28, 2018, the patient underwent thoracoscopic mediastinal tumor resection under general anesthesia. When he arrived in the operation room, the invasive arterial blood pressure (ABP), electrocardiogram (ECG), oxygen saturation (SPO_2), heart rate (HR), and respiratory rate (RR) were measured for baseline values and were continued to be monitored throughout the surgery. The baseline ABP was 147/78 mmHg, HR was 85 beats per min (bpm), and the SPO_2 was 98%. Intravenous anesthesia was induced and he was intubated successfully. During the operation, intravenous anesthesia, combined with inhalation anesthesia, was used. The patient was placed in the right lateral position for thoracoscopic surgery. The ABP (115–140/64-80 mmHg) and HR (80-89 bpm) were stable but suddenly increased during the exploration of the tumor. His ABP sharply increased to 214/81 mmHg, HR increased to 110 bpm, and the SPO_2 was steady at 97%. Deeper anesthesia and urapidil (10 mg) iv were used to attempt to control the hypertension, but this was ineffective. The anesthesiologist suspected that the tumor was secreting catecholamines. Nicardipine was given as a continuous infusion at 2 ~ 10 μg/(kg.min) to control the blood pressure. Esmolol 0.5 mg/kg was repeatedly administered to control the heart rate, and 500 ml colloid solution was given to expand the blood volume. When the patient's blood pressure returned to 140/63 mmHg, and the heart rate dropped to 95 bpm, Nicardipine and Esmolol were discontinued while the tumor was completely removed. After tumor resection, the patient showed circulatory fluctuations again, with the ABP decreasing between 101 and 110/59–80 mmHg and the HR between 95 and 104 bpm. After reducing the depth of the anesthesia, the patient's blood pressure still showed a decreasing trend (ABP 74/45 mmHg, HR 97 bpm, SPO_2 96%). The liquid infusion rate was increased, and 0.03 ~ 0.15 μg/(kg.min) norepinephrine was given to maintain the blood pressure at 100–110/60–70 mmHg. During the whole operation (3 h), a total of 2600 ml liquid was injected into the patient, of which 500 ml was colloidal liquid. Surgical bleeding was 300 ml, and the urine volume was 300 ml. Considering the intraoperative hemodynamic fluctuations, the patient was transferred to the ICU for intensive care after surgery. The vasoactive agents were continuously decreased under surveillance. Four hours after the operation, the patient's hemodynamics returned to a stable state, and the endotracheal tube was successfully removed. The patient was transferred back to the ward on the first day after surgery. The drainage tube was removed on the third day after the operation, and he was discharged after ten days.

Postoperative immunohistochemistry results showed that the tumor was positive for CgA, CD56, NSE, and SYN (Fig. 2), and negative for CK (AE1/AE3), MelanA, ki-67, and s-100. The mass was diagnosed as PGL by postoperative immunohistochemical tests (neuroendocrine markers (CgA, CD56, SYN) were positive) and by a chest enhanced CT scan (uniform enhancement of the tumor).

The patient was followed up in the outpatient clinic for over a year and did not present with recurrences or metastasis of the tumor, and his blood pressure and heart rate remained stable at 135/77 mmHg and 76 bpm with o.p. sustained-release nifedipine.

Discussion and conclusions

In this case report, we describe an unexpected PGL found during surgery when the patient experienced hemodynamic surges. Severe hemodynamic surges during surgery and the postoperative pathological diagnosis showed that the patient had a rare case of posterior mediastinal functional PGL. This was not detected before the operation, resulting in the patient experiencing a dangerous surgical process.

Clinically, PPGL (PCC and PGL) are incidental adrenal tumors. About 5% of adrenal incidentalomas are PPGLs [3–5]. Due to its secretion of catecholamines, PPGL often presents clinical symptoms such as paroxysmal or persistent hypertension, palpitations, headache, sweating, and hyperglycemia [2, 3]. Between 0.2 and 0.6% of hypertension in patients is caused by PPGL [3]. However, some PPGLs are clinically silent, which makes the diagnosis more difficult [2, 6, 7]. PGL is a neuroendocrine tumor derived from the paraganglia of the sympathetic and parasympathetic nervous systems. They are most commonly found in the head, neck, chest, abdomen, and pelvis, while PGL located in the mediastinum are rare. PGL in rare anatomical locations may cause confusion and diagnostic errors [8]. The patient described here had hypertension, which was well-controlled, without headache, sweating, cold extremities, or other symptoms. For this patient, the lack of symptoms and rare PGL location resulted in missing the diagnosis of PGL. Therefore, the patient did not receive sufficient preoperative preparation, which caused the hemodynamic surges during the surgery.

The primary method for the qualitative diagnosis of PPGL is the detection of hormones and their metabolites [3, 7, 9]. Determination of catecholamine metabolites can improve the sensitivity of the PPGL diagnosis. In addition, PGL/PCC have the highest rate of germline susceptibility, which is at almost 40% [10–12]. Thus

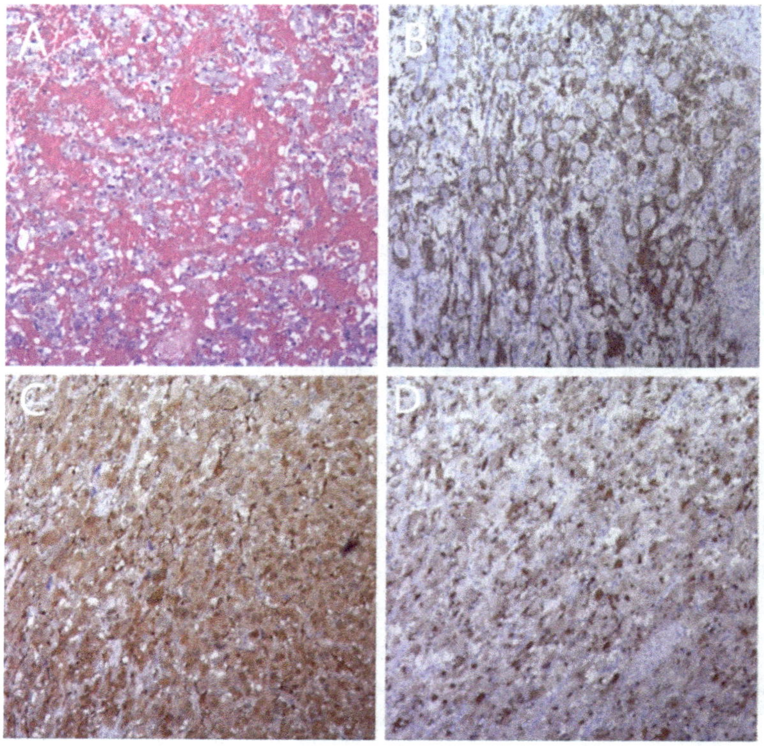

Fig. 2 Pathology diagnosed the posterior mediastinum tumor as PGL. **a** Postoperative pathology showed a patchy distribution of tumor cells with blue-purple cytoplasm and abundant interstitial blood sinuses. **b** CD56(+); **c** CgA(+); **d** SYN(+)

genetic testing, combined with clinical manifestations, biochemical, and imaging assessments, can help to understand tumor secretion, tumor malignancy, and develop treatment and follow-up plans for PPGL [12, 13]. For this missed diagnosis, tests for hormones and their metabolites or genetics were not performed.

A previously reported on a patient with bilateral asymptomatic adrenal masses, which were diagnosed as nonfunctional tumors based on the negative laboratory tests (hormones and their metabolites) [14]. Without sufficient preoperative preparation, a hypertensive crisis occurred during the right adrenal resection. Her pathology revealed a pheochromocytoma. Our patient was similar to this case, a silent PGL with severe hemodynamic fluctuations during the operation. Preoperative preparation such as α-adrenergic blockade should be considered in all PGL patients, even if the patient is clinically silent.

PPGL patients' anesthesia management is very challenging. First, preoperative preparation should be adequate, such as the use of αblockers and augmentation of blood volume [15, 16]. Second, hemodynamic monitoring during the surgery is essential. Monitoring ABP, CVP, the cardiac output (CO), systemic vascular resistance (SVR), and stroke volume variation (SVV) (with the Flotrac/Vigileo system) can provide precise guidance to fluid management. With the guidance of hemodynamic monitoring, adequate fluid therapy and appropriate vasoactive medications can reduce cardiopulmonary complications [17]. Third, appropriate and reasonable use of vasoactive drugs to control perioperative blood pressure fluctuations. Hypertension induced by catecholamine secretion can be treated with the following drugs such as sodium nitroprusside, urapidil, nicardipine, phentolamine, esmolol. Administration of volume expanders and antihypotensive drugs noradrenaline, phenylephrine, vasopressin, or dopamine would be critical in treating hypotension after tumor removal [18]. Fourth, attention should be focused on the clinical manifestations and complications associated with a sudden increase or decrease in catecholamine levels after operation [19]. When encountered intraoperatively with undetected catecholamine secreting PPGL, we should immediately perform adequate hemodynamic monitoring, prepare appropriate vasoactive agents, and give an appropriate amount of fluid treatment.

Fortunately, the patient's hemodynamic fluctuations were treated promptly, and there were no other life-threatening severe complications. Moreover, what we can learn from this case: (1) The clinical manifestations of PGL patients are diverse, of which 50–80% are often asymptomatic [20, 21]. Patients with a potential mediastinal tumor should be identified from PGL, especially tumors near the vertebral column. Early recognition is essential to manage PGL patients properly. (2) Less hemodynamic monitoring of this patient. We only monitored ABP at that time, and CVP could not be performed as the patient was in a lateral position, and the Flotrac/Vigileo system was not available. As considering the cardiopulmonary complications of over fluid therapies, the fluid dilatation might be insufficient for less hemodynamic monitoring during the operation. This may lead to serious hypotension after the removal of the tumor. (3) Short-acting vasoactive drugs are preferred and recommended to control hypertension, such as sodium nitroprusside, urapidil, and phentolamine. In our first attempt, urapidil was ineffective for reducing hypertension. Sodium nitroprusside and phentolamine were not given priority, because we did not prepare them in advance. Nicardipine, which successfully reduced the blood pressure during the removal of the tumor, can reduce brain and kidney damage, but may lead to serious hypotension after tumor removal as it has a long duration of action. Better drug choices might be more conducive to the patient's blood pressure management. (4) When facing an unexpected PGL with hemodynamic surges, promptly terminating the operation should be considered. If the hemodynamic surges appear at the entrance of the operation room, anesthesia induction time, changing of position, or during the operation but cannot be controlled, it should be communicated to the surgeons to cancel the surgery. In this case, hemodynamic parameters were stable until the separation of the tumor and could be controlled with vasoactive drugs and, therefore, the surgery continued.

Studies have shown that PGL have the potential to become malignant and are not sensitive to chemotherapy and radiation [3, 22]. Therefore, patients with PGL should be followed up for life after surgical treatment [23]. We followed up this patient for over one year after the operation and found no tumor recurrence or metastasis, and will continue to follow up. The patient's hypertension has remained stable using the same dose of nifedipine. His hypertension did not recover after the PGL tumor excision, which might confirm that the tumor was a silent PGL.

Conclusions

In this case report, we discuss a rare posterior mediastinal tumor, which was a functional PGL that was missed before surgery. Our experiences should alert all surgeons and anesthesiologists, to pay attention to the differential diagnosis of PGL, strengthen preoperative screening, and improve intraoperative anesthesia management to provide better anesthesia for such patients.

Abbreviations

PPGL: Pheochromocytoma and paraganglioma; PGL: Paraganglioma; PCC: Pheochromocytoma;; ABP: Arterial blood pressure;

ECG: Electrocardiogram; SPO_2: Oxygen saturation; HR: Heart rate; RR: Respiratory rate; bpm: Beats per min; ICU: Intensive care unit; CVP: Central venouspressure; CO: Cardiac output; SVR: Systemic vascular resistance; SVV: Stroke volume variation

Acknowledgements
Not applicable.

Authors' contributions
QS collected the data of the patient. ZY contributed to writting the manuscript.FB contributed to performing of anesthesiaand revising the manuscript. All authors read and approved the final manuscript.

References

1. Gunawardane PTK, Grossman A. Phaeochromocytoma and paraganglioma. Adv Exp Med Biol. 2017;956:239–59.
2. Neumann HPH, Longo DL, Young WF, Eng C. Pheochromocytoma and Paraganglioma. N Engl J Med. 2019;381:552–65.
3. Lenders JW, Duh QY, Eisenhofer G, Gimenez-Roqueplo AP, Grebe SK, Murad MH, et al. Pheochromocytoma and paraganglioma: an endcrine society clinical practice guideline. J Clin Endocrinol Metab. 2014;99(6):1915–42.
4. Bülow B, Ahrén B. Swedish Research Council Study Group of Endocrine Abdominal Tumours Adrenal incidentaloma experience of a standardized diagnostic programme in the Swedish prospective study. J Intern Med. 2002;252:239–46.
5. Kasperlik-Zaluska AA, Roslonowska E, Slowinska-Srzednicka J, OTTO M, Cichocki A, Cwikla J, et al. 1,111 patients with adrenal incidentalomas observed at a single endocrinological center: incidence of chromaffin tumors. Ann N Y Acad Sci. 2006;1073:38–46.
6. Motta-Ramirez GA, Remer EM, Herts BR, Gill IS, Hamrahian AH. Comparison of CT findings in symptomatic and incidentally discovered pheochromocytomas. Am J Roentgenol. 2005;185:684–8.
7. Lenders JW, Pacak K, Walther MM, Walther M, et al. Biochemical diagnosis of pheochromocytoma: which test is best? JAMA. 2002;287(11):1427–34.
8. Asa SL, Ezzat S, Mete O. The diagnosis and clinical significance of Paragangliomas in unusual locations. J Clin Med. 2018;77(9):280.
9. Nerli RB, Musale A, Ghagane SC, Hiremath MB, Dixit NS, et al. Adrenal hemorrhagic pseudocyst-A case report of a rare presentation of pheochromocytoma. Urol Case Rep. 2018;21:5–7.
10. Castro-Vega LJ, Letouzé E, Burnichon N, Buffet A, Disderot P-H, Khalifa E, et al. Multi-omics analysis defines core genomic alterations in pheochromocytomas and paragangliomas. Nat Commun. 2015;6:6044.
11. Jochmanova I, Pacak K. Genomic landscape of pheochromocytoma and paraganglioma.Trends. Cancer. 2018;4:6–9.
12. Kantorovich V, Pacak K. New insights on the pathogenesis of paraganglioma and pheochromocytoma. F1000Res. 2018:1–7. https://doi.org/10.12688/f1000research.14568.1.
13. Buffet A, Ben Aim L, Leboulleux S, Drui D, Vezzosi D, Libé R, et al. Positive impact of genetic test on the management and outcome of patients with Paraganglioma and/or Pheochromocytoma. J Clin Endocrinol Metab. 2019;104:1109–18.
14. El-Doueihi RZ, Salti I, Maroun-Aouad M, El Hajj A. Bilateral biochemically silent pheochromocytoma, not silent after all. Urol Case Rep. 2019;24: 100876.
15. Ohara N, Kaneko M, Yaguchi Y, Ishiguro H, Ishizaki F, Maruyama R, et al. A case of normotensive incidentally discovered adrenal pheochromocytoma. Clin Case Rep. 2018;6:2303–8.
16. Lenders JW, Eisenhofer G, Mannelli M, Pacak K. Phaeochromocytoma. Lancet. 2005;366:665–75.
17. Groeben H, Walz MK, Nottebaum BJ, Alesina PF, Greenwald A, Schumann R, et al. International multicentre review of perioperative management and outcome for catecholamine-producing tumours. Br J Surg. 2020;107(2): e170–8.
18. Ramachandran R, Rewar V. Current perioperative management of pheochromocytomas. Indian J Urol. 2017;33:19–25.
19. Mamilla D, Araque K, Brofferio A, Gonzales M, Sullivan J, Nilubol N, et al. Postoperative Management in Patients with Pheochromocytoma and Paraganglioma. Cancers. 2019;11:936.
20. Wald O, Shapira OM, Murar A. Paraganglioma of the mediastinum: challenges in diagnosis and surgical management. J Cardiothorac Surg. 2010;5:19.
21. Suzawa K, Yamamoto H, Ichimura K, Toyooka S, Miyoshi S. Asymptomatic but functional paraganglioma of the posterior mediastinum. Ann Thorac Surg. 2014;97(3):1077–80.
22. Stenman A, Zedenius J, Juhlin CC. The Value of Histological Algorithms to Predict the Malignancy Potential of Pheochromocytomas and Abdominal Paragangliomas-A Meta-Analysis and Systematic Review of the Literature. Cancers (Basel). 2019;11:3–12.
23. Alrezk R, Suarez A, Tena I, Pacak K. Update of Pheochromocytoma Syndromes: Genetics, Biochemical Evaluation, and Imaging. Front Endocrinol (Lausanne). 2018;9:515.

Clinical outcomes and anesthetic management of pregnancies with placenta previa and suspicion for placenta accreta undergoing intraoperative abdominal aortic balloon occlusion during cesarean section

Peng Li[1†], Xia Liu[2†], Xiangkui Li[1], Xinchuan Wei[1] and Juan Liao[3*]

Abstract

Background: This retrospective study aimed to compare the clinical outcomes of parturients with placenta previa (PP) and placenta accreta (PA) according to their severity, when they were managed with intraoperative abdominal aortic balloon occlusion (IAABO) during cesarean section.

Methods: We retrospectively examined 57 cases of PP and suspicion for PA in which IAABO was performed during cesarean section between April 2014 and June 2016. Based on preoperative examination and clinical risk factors, patients were divided into the low suspicion PA group and the high suspicion PA group. We compared the demographic characteristics, methods of anesthesia, intra- and postoperative parameters, and maternal and neonatal outcomes.

Results: The two groups showed similar demographic characteristics and intraoperative outcomes. Four women underwent cesarean hysterectomy. Eight neonates were admitted to the neonatal intensive care unit and three did not survive. Neonatal Apgar scores were significantly higher in the low suspicion PA group. Eight patients experienced postoperative femoral artery thrombosis and one patient complicated hematoma in the front wall of the common femoral artery. Patients who received neuraxial anesthesia showed significantly lower intraoperative blood loss, lower intraoperative, postoperative and total blood transfusion and shorter surgery than patients who received general anesthesia.

Conclusions: Our data suggested that the severity of aberrant placental position does not affect intraoperative blood loss during a cesarean section while the IAABO is performed. We propose that neuraxial anesthesia is preferred for conducting these surgeries without contraindications.

Keywords: Placenta previa, Placenta accreta, Cesarean section, Intraoperative abdominal aortic balloon occlusion, Anesthetic management

* Correspondence: 109497731@qq.com
†Peng Li and Xia Liu contributed equally to this study and shared first authorship
[3]Department of Stomatology, Sichuan Academy of Medical Sciences & Sichuan Provincial People's Hospital, Chengdu, Sichuan, China

Background

Placenta accreta spectrum, composed of placenta accreta, increta, and percreta, can result in severe hemorrhage, and lead to significant maternal morbidity and mortality rates [1, 2]. In fact, the term "accreta" was viewed as a common term for the above three conditions. Risk factors for abnormally invasive placentation include placenta previa with or without previous uterine surgery, prior myomectomy, prior cesarean delivery, Asherman's syndrome, submucous leiomyomata and maternal age older than 35 years [3]. The rates of PP and PA are increasing due to the rising incidence of cesarean section [3, 4]. Careful management of the anesthetic protocol is critical for women with placenta previa who have a history of cesarean section or abnormally invasive placentation [5].

IAABO has been extensively used in major pelvic surgical procedures and is effective in reducing intraoperative hemorrhage [6]. Moreover, this intravascular interventional therapy has been shown to effectively reduce intraoperative hemorrhage in patients with placenta accreta [7, 8]. Therefore, this technique is performed in our hospital to control severe intraoperative hemorrhages in patients with PP and suspicion for PA. However, not much is known about the best anesthetic protocol to choose when dealing with this situation. Therefore, this retrospective study was performed to compare the clinical outcomes of parturients with placenta previa and placenta accreta according to their severity, when they were managed with IAABO during cesarean section. In addition, we also evaluated the influence of the anesthesia method on postoperative clinical outcomes in this population.

Methods

Subjects

This retrospective study included 57 pregnancies between April 2014 and June 2016 at the Sichuan Provincial People's Hospital (Chengdu, China). This study was approved by the Ethics Committees of the Sichuan Academy of Medical Sciences and Sichuan Provincial People's Hospital and consent was waived.

We included patients with placenta previa and suspicion for placenta accreta who opted for IAABO during their cesarean section. Whether to perform the IAABO on patients was actually depended on the surgeons' synthetic judgment and patients' will. The aortic catheterization was performed on patients by interventional radiology preoperatively who were diagnosed with PP and suspected of having placenta accreta. Before the surgeon made an incision in the serous membrane of the uterus, according to the surgeon's request, sterilizing saline was injected into the balloon to control bleeding. The volume of the sterilizing saline was based on the situation of preoperative intervention, which demonstrated a satisfactory outcome of interfering with blood flow. After the placenta was extracted without active bleeding, the balloon was deflated by drawing saline out slowly. The duration of IAABO was less than 60 min at one time. If the surgeons wanted to occlude blood flow again, there should be at least 10-15 min periods of intermittence to restore blood flow. The catheters were usually extracted by the radiologists when the pregnancies' vital signs were stable after surgery.

The subjects in our study were divided into a low suspicion PA group and a high suspicion PA group conducted by two specialistic obstetricians on the basis of preoperative diagnosis by ultrasound or MRI (magnetic resonance imaging) and clinical risk factors [9]. High suspicion PA group comprised cases meeting the following criteria: (1) high suspicion for PA according to ultrasonography or MRI imaging findings including deficiency of retroplacental sonolucent zone; segmental retroplacental myometrial thinning < 1 mm; multiple vascular lacunae presenting a 'moth hole' appearance [10]; (2) pernicious placenta previa defined as PP with anterior placenta overlying a previous scar. In addition, low suspicion PA group included cases: (1) low-suspicion ultrasound for PA and anterior placenta without history of caesarean surgery; (2) PP without ultrasound signs for PA but with one previous caesarean section [9].

The following information was recorded: age, parity, gestational age, history of surgical abortion, previous cesarean section, type of anesthesia, intraoperative blood loss, blood transfusion, neonatal Apgar scores, duration of surgery and postoperative complications. After data collection, subjects were further stratified into a neuraxial anesthesia group or a general anesthesia group.

Statistical Analysis

Statistical analysis was carried out using SPSS Statistics 24.0 (IBM, Chicago, IL, USA). Data were presented as mean ± SD or median (range). Intergroup differences were assessed for significance using Student's *t*, Kruskal-Wallis, chi-squared or Fisher exact tests, as appropriate. $P < 0.05$ was considered statistically significant.

Results

As listed in Fig. 1, a total of 3840 pregnant women underwent cesarean section between April 2014 and June 2016 in our hospital. After excluding cases whose preoperative diagnosis was not PP and suspicion for PA and without use of IAABO, we included 65 pregnant women meeting the inclusion criteria. Also, there were 8 patients without detailed recording. Thus, our study totally included 57 subjects for analysis. In our study, we finally made sure 32 pregnancies diagnosed with PA. The incidence of PA was found to be 0.83% (32/3840) of all pregnancies contemporarily. During the same period, the rate of utilization of the technique of IAABO was

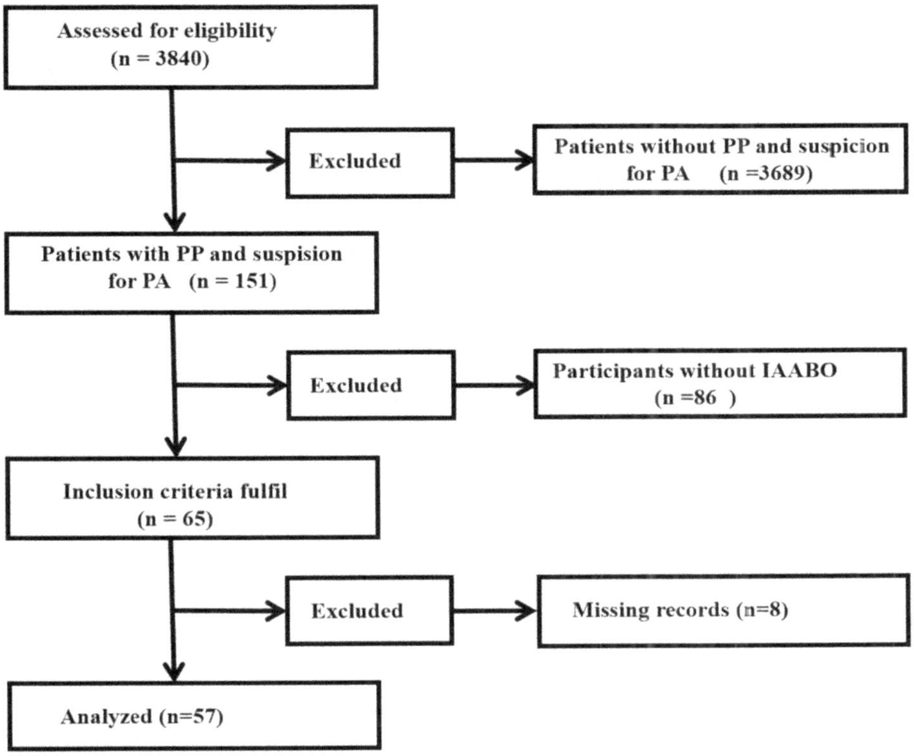

Fig. 1 Flow chart of the trial

43% (65/151) among the patients diagnosed with placenta previa and suspicion for placenta accreta.

A total of 57 pregnant patients were included in this study, of whom 27(47.3%) were older than 35 years. The sites of placenta attached to the uterus were anterior wall (n = 32,56%), posterior wall (n = 20, 35%) and lateral wall(n = 5, 9%). Across all deliveries, gestational age was 248 ± 20.8 days and 48 (84.2%) required emergency surgery. Reports on previous history revealed that the median and range of surgical abortion for all patients was 2 (0–6) with 3 (0–7) for uterine surgery (Table 1). Patients were divided into low suspicion or high suspicion for PA groups based on preoperative examination and clinical risk factors. Although the high suspicion PA group was more of the history of surgical abortion, cesarean section or uterine surgery than the low suspicion PA group, there was no difference of statistics.

Post-surgery data showed neonatal Apgar scores were higher in the low suspicion PA group compared to scores reported for the high suspicion PA group. Eight (17.0%) neonates from the high suspicion PA group were admitted to the neonatal intensive care unit, compared

Table 1 Baseline characteristics for patients with abnormal placenta position

Characteristic	Total (n = 57)	Low suspicion group (n = 10)	High suspicion group (n = 47)	P
Preoperative comorbidity	14 (24.6%)	5 (50.0%)	9 (19.1%)	0.098
Preoperative hemoglobin	107 ± 13.7	104 ± 12.4	107 ± 14.0	0.457
Emergency surgery	48 (84.2%)	9 (90.0%)	39 (83.0%)	0.940
Gestational age (days)	248 ± 20.8	243 ± 19.6	249 ± 21.0	0.353
Patient age (years)	36 ± 7.9	37 ± 8.9	36 ± 7.7	0.749
Parity	4 (1–8)	2.5 (2–8)	4 (1–8)	0.169
Previous surgical abortions	2 (0–6)	1 (0–6)	2 (0–6)	0.121
Previous cesarean sections	1 (0–2)	0 (0–1)	1 (0–2)	0.073
previous uterine surgeries	3 (0–7)	1 (0–7)	3 (0–7)	0.064

Values are n (%), mean ± SD or median (range)

to none of the neonates from the low suspicion PA group. In the high suspicion PA group, there were three twin pregnancies, one of which resulted in the death of both babies after the family refused admission to the NICU (neonatal intensive care unit) and left the hospital against medical advice. One patient from the low suspicion PA group and 6 (12.8%) from the high suspicion PA group were moved into the ICU (intensive care unit). Four patients were admitted to ICU as a result of the greater intraoperative blood loss (≥2000 ml) and other 3 patients mainly were respectively on account of postoperative loss of consciousness, twin pregnancy combined with severe preeclampsia preoperatively and paroxysmal supraventricular tachycardia operatively. These differences in rates of admission to the neonatal or standard intensive care units were not statistically significant (Table 2).

After abdominal aortic balloon occlusion during cesarean section, we found no significant differences in intraoperative blood loss, intraoperative blood transfusion, duration of surgery and postoperative hospital stay between the two groups. Because of bleeding during periods of intermittence of IAABO, the intrauterine balloon tamponade was used in 2 (20%) patients in the low suspicion PA group and 1 (2.1%) in the high suspicion PA group. Besides, the patients performed uterine artery embolization were 1 (10%) and 8 (17.0%) in each group respectively. Though there were no statistical difference with regard to clotting variables postoperatively between two groups, the intervention of the

Table 2 Maternal and neonatal intra- and postoperative outcomes for low and high suspicion for PA patients

Outcome	Low suspicion group (*n* = 10)	High suspicion group (*n* = 47)	*P* [a]
Intraoperative data			
Intraoperative blood loss (ml)	500 (200–800)	500 (200–3500)	0.784
Intraoperative blood transfusion (U)	0 (0–2)	0 (0–14)	0.818
Duration of surgery (min)	62 ± 10.0	79 ± 44.4	0.239
Intrauterine balloon tamponade	2 (20%)	1 (2.1%)	0.076
Uterine artery embolization	1 (10%)	8 (17.0%)	1.000
Hysterectomy	0	4 (8.5%)	1.000
Postoperative complications			
Femoral artery thrombosis	0	8 (17.0%)	1.000
Anesthesia-related complications	0	1 (2.1%)	1.000
Operation-related complications	1 (10%)	2 (4.3%)	1.000
Postoperative data			
Postoperative hospital stay (day)	5.5 ± 1.4	5.2 ± 2.7	0.745
Hemoglobin on postoperative day 1	106 ± 12.7	98 ± 15.1	0.139
Admission to ICU	1 (10%)	6 (12.8%)	1.000
Postoperative diagnosis with PA	2 (20%)	30 (64%)	0.016
Placenta accreta	1	14	
Placenta increta	1	10	
Placenta percreta	0	6	
Postoperative clotting variables			
Platelets(10^9/L)	166 (95–333)	171 (71–328)	0.826
INR	0.92 (0.81–1.12)	0.93 (0.79–1.28)	0.842
PT(s)	10.8 (10.5–13.5)	10.5 (9.2–12.4)	0.122
Neonatal data			
Neonate Apgar score			
1 min	10 ± 0.0	8.9 ± 2.0	0.001
5 min	10 ± 0.0	9.5 ± 1.0	0.003
10 min	10 ± 0.0	9.7 ± 0.7	0.004
Weight (g)	2751 ± 491.6	2958 ± 470.2	0.237
Admission to NICU	0	8 (17.0%)	0.327

Values are n (%), mean ± SD or median (range) or median (range)

balloon block led to femoral artery thrombosis in 8 (17.0%) and local hematoma of the common femoral artery in 1 (4.3%) from the high suspicion PA group. Six patients underwent arteriotomy of the femoral artery plus embolectomy and two patients used low molecular heparin for anticoagulation. The patient complicated local hematoma refused further examination and the pain in her leg was obviously relieved in the postoperative day 3.

It is worth noting that 4 (8.5%) patients from the high suspicion PA group, but no one from the low suspicion PA group, underwent hysterectomy because of hemorrhaging and difficulties related to placenta dissection during surgery. The placentas of another 53 patients were dissected by hand or surgical instruments as much as possible without leaving placenta in situ. One patient in the high suspicion PA group also experienced anesthesia-related complications. The patient suffered postoperative nausea, vomiting, pain and diminished consciousness and then treated by mechanical ventilation for 2 days.

Postoperative operation-related complications were observed in three patients. A uterine artery embolization was performed on one patient in the low suspicion PA group in order to stop bleeding after the gauze was removed from the vagina. One subject from the high suspicion PA group experienced a pelvic hematoma, disturbance of blood coagulation and was treated with an abdominal laparotomy and received 1.5 units plasma transfusion. Another high suspicion for PA patient underwent cystourethroscopy for the evacuation of a cystic hematoma and was subsequently diagnosed with placenta percreta. Operative blood loss was 3500 ml and the patient received operative blood transfusion containing 10 units red blood cells, 4 units fresh frozen plasma and 10 units of cryoprecipitate. The patient remained in the hospital for 14 days, of which 3 were spent postoperatively in the intensive care unit without ventilation. No maternal mortality was reported. Placenta accreta was definitively diagnosed postoperatively based on pathology examination or surgeons' classification when separating the placenta. Based on postoperative diagnosis, the low suspicion PA group actually contained 2 (20%) patients with placenta accreta, compared to 30 (64%) patients in the high suspicion PA group (Table 2).

To determine the effect of anesthesia on maternal and neonatal outcomes, patients were stratified based on whether they received neuraxial anesthesia ($n = 43$) or general anesthesia ($n = 14$). Thirteen (30.2%) patients underwent the subarachnoid anesthesia (L3–4) with injection 0.5% bupivacaine 2 ml. Another 30 patients with spinal-epidural anesthesia (L3–4) were injected the same local anesthetic without additional supplementary for analgesia. The induction drugs for general anesthesia mostly were propofol (2–2.5 mg.kg^{-1}), remifentanil (1.0 μg.kg^{-1}) and succinylcholine (1–1.5 mg.kg^{-1}) or rocuronium (0.6 mg.kg^{-1}). The anesthesia was maintained with remifentanil (0.2–0.25 μg.kg^{-1} min^{-1}), propofol (4–6 mg.kg^{-1} h^{-1}) and sevenflurane less than 1 MAC (minimum alveolar concentration). After the baby was took out, sufentanil (0.3–0.4 μg.kg^{-1}) and midazolam (0.03–0.05 mg.kg^{-1}) were injected to deepen anesthesia. The neuraxial anesthesia group comprised 8 patients from the low suspicion PA group and 35 from the high suspicion PA group; general anesthesia, 2 and 12. One patient firstly received regional anesthesia and then was switched to general anesthesia by anesthesiology team for the following concerns: history of thalassemia and severe preeclampsia, extended time of surgery, twin pregnancy, massive hemorrhage and hemodynamic instability. The two anesthesia groups showed significant differences in intraoperative blood loss, intraoperative blood transfusion, postoperative blood transfusion, total blood transfusion and duration of surgery (Table 3). The general anesthesia group tended to suffer greater blood loss and require more transfusion, longer surgery and more venous puncture.

Discussion

Anesthetic management plays a significant role in ensuring the safety of patients with placenta previa and/or accreta. Factors contributing to the abnormally invasive placenta should be identified prior to medical intervention. Anesthetists should then take these risk factors into account and collaborate with other healthcare professionals to aid in planning the most appropriate anesthesia plan.

A review of 62 placenta accreta cases found that 73% of patients had at least one previous cesarean delivery, and 45% were older than 35 years [11]. Our study found a higher proportion of patients who were older than 35 years (47.3%), which could explain the increased ratio of surgical abortion (82.5%). The incidence of cesarean hysterectomy in our study (7%) was much lower than the range of 48–100% in previous studies [12–15]. As some studies demonstrated, IAABO might be helpful in decreasing the likelihood of hysterectomy [7, 16–18]. We did not observe any maternal mortalities, in contrast, a previous study reported maternal deaths in the absence of interventional operation [5]. Further research is required to determine whether the technique of IAABO could consistently reduce the rate of maternal mortalities. Some researchers may be afraid that the radiation originated from preoperative intervention may cause fetal damage. However, the International Commission on Radiological Protection (ICRP) suggested that the fetal teratogenic risk does not increase when the radiation dose is less than 100 mGy [19]. Besides, the article reported fetal radiation exposure doses resulting from the technique of IAABO were 4.9 ± 2.9 mGy [20]. Three

Table 3 Comparison of clinical data between pregnancies involving neuraxial or general anesthesia

	Neuraxial anesthesia ($n = 43$)	General anesthesia ($n = 14$)	P [a]
Baseline characteristics			
Gestational age (days)	250 ± 18.4	252 ± 18.1	0.583
Patient age (years)	35 ± 7.8	38 ± 7.7	0.246
Emergency surgery	36 (83.7%)	12 (85.7%)	1.000
Preoperative comorbidity	9 (20.9%)	5 (35.7%)	0.271
CVC	1 (2.3%)	3 (21.4%)	0.042
Arterial catheterization	3 (7.0%)	4 (28.6%)	0.054
Intraoperative data			
Use of vasoactive agents	7 (16.3%)	2 (14.3%)	1.000
Intraoperative blood loss (ml)	500 (200–2000)	700 (300–3500)	0.017
Intraoperative blood infusion (U)	0 (0–4)	1.5 (0–14)	0.018
Duration of surgery (min)	65.7 ± 16.4	107.5 ± 70.4	0.046
Postoperative data			
Postoperative blood infusion (U)	0 (0–4)	0 (0–15.5)	0.001
Total blood infusion (U)	0 (0–6)	2.625 (0–29.5)	0.009
Maternal admission to ICU	3 (7.0%)	4 (28.6%)	0.054
Postoperative hospital stay (days)	4.9 ± 1.5	6.6 ± 4.2	0.146
Anesthesia-related complications	0	1 (7.1%)	0.246
Postoperative diagnosis with PA	23 (53.5%)	9 (64.3%)	0.479
Placenta accreta	13	2	
Placenta increta	8	3	
Placenta percreta	2	4	
Neonatal data			
Neonatal Apgar scores			
1 min	9.2 ± 1.75	8.9 ± 2.3	0.539
5 min	9.6 ± 0.9	9.5 ± 1.2	0.554
10 min	9.7 ± 0.7	9.7 ± 0.8	0.834
Neonatal admission to ICU	5 (11.6%)	3 (21.4%)	0.391

Values are n (%), mean ± SD or median (range)

other articles compared IAABO and bilateral internal iliac artery balloon occlusion in terms of the radiation dose and concluded that the former resulted in a lower fetal radiation dose [21–23]. Therefore, just like articles claimed the prophylactic use of abdominal aortic balloon occlusion in patients with placenta accreta is safe and effective [7, 8, 24].

Our study found no significant differences between the low and high suspicion PA groups in intraoperative blood loss and transfusion, postoperative hospitalization or rate of admittance to the ICU. These results suggest that the severity of aberrant placental position do not compromise the ability of IAABO to control severe hemorrhage. For example, we found an estimated median blood loss of 500 ml for the low and high suspicion PA groups, and this loss ranged from 200 to 3500 ml across the two groups. This was much lower than for patients who did not undergo such catheterization in previous studies [4, 24]. This variation in blood loss may be related to the technique of IAABO [16, 24]. When the 57 pregnancies diagnosed with PP and suspicion for PA based on preoperative examination (ultrasound or MRI) and clinical risk factors, the decision of using IAABO conducted by a multidisciplinary team (anesthesiologist, obstetrician, interventional radiologist and neonatologist). However, we should note that our study actually contained 32 patients with placenta accreta (accreta 15, increta 11, percreta 6) based on postoperative diagnosis. In fact, there were other 25 patients finally diagnosed with PP but with IAABO. Based on preoperative examinations (ultrasound, MRI) and clinical signs, 56.1% (32/57) of the patients suspicion for PA were identified correctly. Though there was still lack of definitive preoperative diagnostic tool, we should be well prepared for patients suspected of PA (even in low suspicion patients) because of high risk for massive bleeding. Meanwhile, we should pay more caution for its intervention-related complications. Altogether 8 (14.0%) of the patients in our study suffered from femoral artery thrombosis and some of them required femoral artery embolectomy. This catheterization-related complication may be due to the length of occlusion. According to literature, the best safety outcomes for IAABO occur when total occlusion time is less than 60 min [25]. Since the IAABO time was not included in medical records, we could not examine the effect of occlusion time on postoperative thrombosis in our study. Future studies should pay more attention to this. However, we could suppose that the occlusion time was shorter in the low suspicion PA. Moreover, Patients with the risk of femoral artery thrombosis was lower in the low suspicion PA group than the high suspicion PA group based on duration of surgery (62 ± 10.0 vs 79 ± 44.4), which needed to further investigation.

In this retrospective study, neuraxial anesthesia was used in 8 (80%) of the low suspicion PA pregnancies and 35 (74.5%) of the high suspicion PA ones, while only 2 (20%) patients of the low suspicion PA group and 12 (25.5%) of the high suspicion PA group performed general anesthesia. Final diagnosis with placenta accreta included totally 32 cases (accreta 15, increta 11, percreta 6), of whom 23 (71.9%) patients performed neuraxial anesthesia. The above results suggested that neuraxial anesthesia was used more often than general anesthesia for intraoperative aortic balloon occlusion intervention during a cesarean section. In contrast, one study found that general anesthesia was preferred during treatment of placenta previa, in order to avoid the risk of bleeding [5]. Another study indicated that general anesthesia was used almost exclusively for women strongly suspected of having placenta accreta, while spinal anesthesia was used in nearly two-thirds of cases with placenta previa without suspicion of placenta accreta [26]. These differences in anesthetic protocols may be attributed to the fact that we enrolled only patients who underwent intraoperative - abdominal aortic balloon occlusion during a cesarean section.

As argued by Guasch, general anesthesia was a risk factor for transfusion [27]. In our study, we also found more perioperative blood loss, transfusion and duration of surgery in the general anesthesia group than that in the neuraxial anesthesia group. However, in this retrospective study, the parturients' underlying conditions cannot be guaranteed to be absolutely consistent. The more blood loss and transfusion in the general anesthesia group could not completely exclude the influence of parturients' coagulation disorders. Besides, there was one patient whose anesthetic method was switched from neuraxial anesthesia to general anesthesia due to massive hemorrhage intraoperatively. Thus, the general anesthesia group could be biased towards a potentially high risk of bleeding, which could be the limitation of this study.

The anesthesia methods for pregnant women with placenta previa (PP) and suspicion for placenta accreta (PA) were determined by many factors. For example, the will of patients', preoperative comorbidities, coagulation conditions, duration of surgery, fetal condition, the risk for massive hemorrhage were all taken into account by a multidisciplinary team (anesthesiologist, obstetrician, interventional radiologist and neonatologist). There are some important risk factors for general anesthesia including coagulation disorders, massive bleeding in the third trimester, sever hemodynamic instability, fetal distress and severe pre-eclampsia [27]. However, faced with patients with placenta previa and suspicion for placenta accreta undergoing IAABO, neuraxial anesthesia may be preferable in our center excepting contraindications (coagulation disorders, infection of insertion point, sever lumbar spinal stenosis, hypovolemic shock and so on). This conclusion can be consistent with some previous studies, which concluded that neuraxial anesthesia is now employed more frequently for pregnancies with placenta accreta [12, 28]. The benefit of neuraxial anesthesia may include: (1) improvement of postoperative analgesia by PCEA (patient-controlled epidural analgesia);(2) related to less blood loss than general anesthesia at the time of hysterectomy [29]; (3) offered as an adjuvant to prevent thrombosis in high-risk patients [30]; and associated with lower incidence of postoperative thrombosis [31]; (4) minimization of the risk of failed intubation, ventilation and aspiration [32].

Only a small percentage of patients received arterial lines (12.3%) or central venous catheters (7%), which are lower than percentages reported in other studies [5, 26, 33]. We suspect the lower rate of invasive puncture is due to the expected decrease in bleeding after IAABO, but these patients should nevertheless be closely monitored.

In conclusion, the management of patients diagnosed with placenta previa and suspicion for placenta accreta requires a multidisciplinary approach. The anesthesiologist, obstetrician and interventional radiologist should formulate a plan to safely handle a massive hemorrhage that may occur during surgery. Prophylactic use of an abdominal aorta balloon catheterization may reduce the rate of cesarean hysterectomy and maternal mortality but needs further evidenced-based research to validate. Due to the potential advantages of neuraxial anesthesia, we prefer for this type of anesthesia in the absence of contraindications during abdominal aorta balloon catheterization intervention when treating patients diagnosed as placenta previa and suspicion for placenta accreta. Clinicians should, however, be aware of complications arising from the intraoperative abdominal aortic balloon occlusion.

Abbreviations

PP: Placenta previa; PA: Placenta accreta; IAABO: Intraoperative abdominal aortic balloon occlusion; NICU: Neonatal intensive care unit; ICU: Intensive care unit; INR: International normalized ratio; PT: Prothrombin time; CVC: Central venipuncture catheterization

Acknowledgements

Not applicable.

Authors' contributions

Authors' Contributions JL: Designed and analyzed the data. PL: Collected, analyzed the data, and revised the manuscript. XL: Collected, analyzed the data, and wrote the manuscript. XKL: Analyzed the data and revised the manuscript. XCW: Revised the manuscript. All authors read and approved the final manuscript.

Author details

[1]Department of anesthesiology, Sichuan Academy of Medical Sciences & Sichuan Provincial People's Hospital, Chengdu, Sichuan, China. [2]North Sichuan Medical College, Nanchong, Sichuan, China. [3]Department of Stomatology, Sichuan Academy of Medical Sciences & Sichuan Provincial People's Hospital, Chengdu, Sichuan, China.

References

1. Berg CJ, Atrash HK, Koonin LM, Tucker M. Pregnancy-related mortality in the United States, 1987-1990. Obstet Gynecol. 1996;88(2):161–7.
2. Hayes E, Ayida G, Crocker A. The morbidly adherent placenta: diagnosis and management options. Curr Opin Obstet Gynecol. 2011;23(6):448–53.
3. Committee on Adolescent Health Care. ACOG Committee Opinion no. 599: Committee on Adoscent Health Care: Adolescent confidentiality andelectronic health records. Obstet Gynecol. 2014;123(5):1148–50.
4. Wu Q, Liu Z, Zhao X, Liu C, Wang Y, Chu Q, Wang X, Chen Z. Outcome of pregnancies after balloon occlusion of the Infrarenal abdominal aorta during caesarean in 230 patients with placenta Praevia Accreta. Cardiovasc Intervent Radiol. 2016;39(11):1573–9.
5. Kocaoglu N, Gunusen I, Karaman S, Ergenoglu AM, Firat V. Management of anesthesia for cesarean section in parturients with placenta previa with/without placenta accreta: a retrospective study. Ginekol Pol. 2012;83(2):99–103.
6. Martinelli T, Thony F, Declety P, Sengel C, Broux C, Tonetti J, Payen JF, Ferretti G. Intra-aortic balloon occlusion to salvage patients with life-threatening hemorrhagic shocks from pelvic fractures. J Trauma. 2010; 68(4):942–8.
7. Chen L, Wang X, Wang H, Li Q, Shan N, Qi H. Clinical evaluation of prophylactic abdominal aortic balloon occlusion in patients with placenta accreta: a systematic review and meta-analysis. BMC Pregnancy Childbirth. 2019;19(1):30.
8. Shahin Y, Pang CL. Endovascular interventional modalities for haemorrhage control in abnormal placental implantation deliveries: a systematic review and meta-analysis. Eur Radiol. 2018;28(7):2713–26.
9. Weiniger CF, Elram T, Ginosar Y, Mankuta D, Weissman C, Ezra Y. Anaesthetic management of placenta accreta: use of a pre-operative high and low suspicion classification. Anaesthesia. 2005;60(11):1079–84.
10. Wang Y, Gao Y, Zhao YY, Chong YW, Chen YS. Ultrasonographic diagnosis of severe placental invasion. J Obstet Gynaecol Res. 2018;44(3):448–55.
11. Miller DA, Chollet JA, Goodwin TM. Clinical risk factors for placenta previa-placenta accreta. Am J Obstet Gynecol. 1997;177(1):210–4.
12. Lilker SJ, Meyer RA, Downey KN, Macarthur AJ. Anesthetic considerations for placenta accreta. Int J Obstet Anesth. 2011;20(4):288–92.
13. Roethlisberger M, Womastek I, Posch M, Husslein P, Pateisky N, Lehner R. Early postpartum hysterectomy: incidence and risk factors. Acta Obstet Gynecol Scand. 2010;89(8):1040–4.
14. Shellhaas CS, Gilbert S, Landon MB, Varner MW, Leveno KJ, Hauth JC, Spong CY, Caritis SN, Wapner RJ, Sorokin Y, Miodovnik M, O'Sullivan MJ, Sibai BM, Langer O, Gabbe SG. The frequency and complication rates of hysterectomy accompanying cesarean delivery. Obstet Gynecol. 2009;114(2 Pt 1):224–9.
15. Taylor NJ, Russell R. Anaesthesia for abnormally invasive placenta: a single-institution case series. Int J Obstet Anesth. 2017;30:10–5.
16. Luo F, Xie L, Xie P, Liu S, Zhu Y. Intraoperative aortic balloon occlusion in patients with placenta previa and/or placenta accreta: a retrospective study. Taiwan J Obstet Gynecol. 2017;56(2):147–52.
17. Masamoto H, Uehara H, Gibo M, Okubo E, Sakumoto K, Aoki Y. Elective use of aortic balloon occlusion in cesarean hysterectomy for placenta previa percreta. Gynecol Obstet Investig. 2009;67(2):92–5.
18. Panici PB, Anceschi M, Borgia ML, Bresadola L, Masselli G, Parasassi T, Perrone G, Brunelli R. Intraoperative aorta balloon occlusion: fertility preservation in patients with placenta previa accreta/increta. J Matern Fetal Neonatal Med. 2012;25(12):2512–6.
19. ICRP. The 2007 recommendations of the international commission on radiological protection. ICRP publication 103. Ann ICRP. 2007; 37:1–332.
20. Duan XH, Wang YL, Han XW, Chen ZM, Chu QJ, Wang L, Hai DD. Caesarean section combined with temporary aortic balloon occlusion followed by uterine artery embolisation for the management of placenta accreta. Clin Radiol. 2015;70(9):932–7.
21. Wang YL, Duan XH, Han XW, Wang L, Zhao XL, Chen ZM, Chu QJ, Zhang W. Comparison of temporary abdominal aortic occlusion with internal iliac artery occlusion for patients with placenta accreta - a non-randomised prospective study. Vasa. 2017;46(1):53–7.
22. Song P, Wu N. The application of temporary balloon occlusion technique in performing cesarean section for patients with pernicious placenta previa. J Int Radiol. 2017;26(5):451–4.
23. Yang X, Chen Z, You YP. The comparative study in perioperative temporary balloon occlusion of the distal abdominal aorta and perioperative temporary balloon occlusion of the internal iliac arteries in the therapy of patients with placenta accreta. J Pract Obstet Gynecol. 2016;32(9):684–8.
24. Xie L, Wang Y, Luo FY, Man YC, Zhao XL. Prophylactic use of an infrarenal abdominal aorta balloon catheter in pregnancies complicated by placenta accreta. J Obstet Gynaecol. 2017;37(5):557–61.
25. Ullmark G, Hovelius L, Strindberg L, Wallner A. Reduced bleeding through temporary balloon occlusion in hip and knee revision surgery. J Acta orthopaedica Scandinavica. 2000;1(71):51–4.
26. Ioscovich A, Shatalin D, Butwick AJ, Ginosar Y, Orbach-Zinger S, Weiniger CF. Israeli survey of anesthesia practice related to placenta previa and accreta. Acta Anaesthesiol Scand. 2016;60(4):457–64.
27. Guasch E, Montenegro P, Ochoa C, Schiraldi R, Diez J, Gilsanz F. General anaesthesia and obstetric bleeding in caesarean section. One year's experience in a university hospital. Rev Esp Anestesiol Reanim. 2012;59(8):415–22.
28. Reitman E, Devine PC, Laifer-Narin SL, Flood P. Case scenario: perioperative management of a multigravida at 34-week gestation diagnosed with abnormal placentation. J Anesthesiology. 2011;4(115):852–7.
29. Parekh N, Husaini SW, Russell IF. Caesarean section for placenta praevia: a retrospective study of anaesthetic management. Br J Anaesth. 2000; 84(6):725–30.
30. Turan A, Bajracharya GR, Leung S, Yazici Kara M, Mao G, Botsford T, Ruetzler K, Maheshwari K, Ali Sakr Esa W, Elsharkawy H, Sessler DI. Association of neuraxial anesthesia with postoperative venous thromboembolism after noncardiac surgery: a propensity-matched analysis of ACS-NSQIP database. Anesth Analg. 2019;128(3):494–501.
31. Mauermann WJ, Shilling AM, Zuo Z. A comparison of neuraxial block versus general anesthesia for elective total hip replacement: a meta-analysis. Anesth Analg. 2006;103(4):1018–25.
32. Rollins M, Lucero J. Overview of anesthetic considerations for cesarean delivery. Br Med Bull. 2012;101:105–25.
33. Munoz LA, Mendoza GJ, Gomez M, Reyes LE, Arevalo JJ. Anesthetic management of placenta accreta in a low-resource setting: a case series. Int J Obstet Anesth. 2015;24(4):329–34.

28

Anesthesia management of atrial myxoma resection with multiple cerebral aneurysms

Ran Zhang[1], Zhiyu Tang[1], Qing Qiao[1], Feroze Mahmood[2] and Yi Feng[1*]

Abstract

Background: Embolic stroke is a common complication of atrial myxoma, whereas multiple cerebral aneurysms associated with atrial myxoma is rare. The pathogenesis of the cerebral vascular disease related to an atrial myxoma is still not well known, and there are no guidelines to guide treatment and anesthesia management in such patients.

Case presentation: In this report, we present a 38-year-old woman with occasional dizziness and headache diagnosed as multiple cerebral fusiform aneurysms, in whom transthoracic echocardiography revealed a mass attached to the interatrial septum in the left atrium. Myxoma resection was performed in fast track cardiac surgery pathway without neurological complications, and no intervention was carried out on the cerebral aneurysms. She was discharged home 6 days after the procedure for followed-up. Furthermore, we reviewed and analyzed the literature in the PubMed and Google Scholar databases in order to conclude the optimal treatment in such cases.

Conclusions: Atrial myxoma-related cerebral aneurysms are always multiple and in a fusiform shape in most occasions. Early resection of myxoma and conservative therapy of aneurysm is an optimal treatment. TEE and $PbtO_2$ monitoring play an essential role in anesthesia management. Fast track cardiac anesthesia is safe and effective to early evaluate neurological function. Long term follow-up for "myxomatous aneurysms" is recommended. And outcome of most patients is excellent.

Keywords: Multiple cerebral aneurysms, Atrial myxoma, Anesthesia management

Background

Atrial myxoma is the most common benign cardiac tumor, which represents about 50% of all primary cardiac tumors. Approximately 75% occur in the left atrium [1]. Systemic embolism due to atrial myxoma has been well documented, especially embolic stroke [2]. However, intracranial aneurysms are rarely associated to atrial myxoma [3]. We present the case of a woman with dizziness and headache whose brain computed tomography angiography (CTA) manifested multiple fusiform aneurysms, and transthoracic echocardiography revealed a mass in the left atrium.

The pathogenesis of the cerebral vascular disease related to an atrial myxoma is still not well known, and there are no guidelines to guide treatment and anesthesia management in such patients.

Case presentation

Case report

A 38-year-old woman with no medical history presented 10 days of dizziness and headache without loss of consciousness, dysarthria, weakness, nausea, or vomiting. Neurological examination was normal. The brain CTA manifested two unruptured fusiform aneurysms, which

* Correspondence: doctor_yifeng@sina.com
[1]Department of Anesthesiology, Peking University People's Hospital, No. 11 Xi Zhi Men Nan Da Jie, Xicheng District, Beijing, China

located in left anterior cerebral artery and left posterior cerebral artery, with the size of 9.7 mm × 6.3 mm and 10.2 mm × 7 mm, respectively (Fig. 1). Furthermore, transthoracic echocardiography (TTE) revealed a 4.8 × 2.9 × 2.5 cm^3 mass attached to the interatrial septum in the left atrium, which obstructed the mitral orifice without mitral valve regurgitation (Fig. 2).

According to the recommendation of multidisciplinary team (MDT), myxoma was first considered to be excised, a conservative approach was chosen for cerebral aneurysms, and the fast track cardiac surgery pathway should be performed to evaluate neurological function as soon as possible. The baseline vital signs of this patient were measured before induction of general anesthesia, in order to maintain the fluctuation range of heart rate (HR) and mean arterial pressure (MAP) within 10% throughout the perioperative period. The mass was successfully removed and histological examination confirmed a typical myxoma (Fig. 3). No mitral regurgitation or shunt flow across the atrial septum was revealed by transesophageal echocardiography (TEE) (Fig. 4). Parenchymal brain oxygen ($PbtO_2$) monitoring did not change significantly throughout the procedure. The patient was transported to intensive care unit (ICU) receiving infusion of propofol. After that,

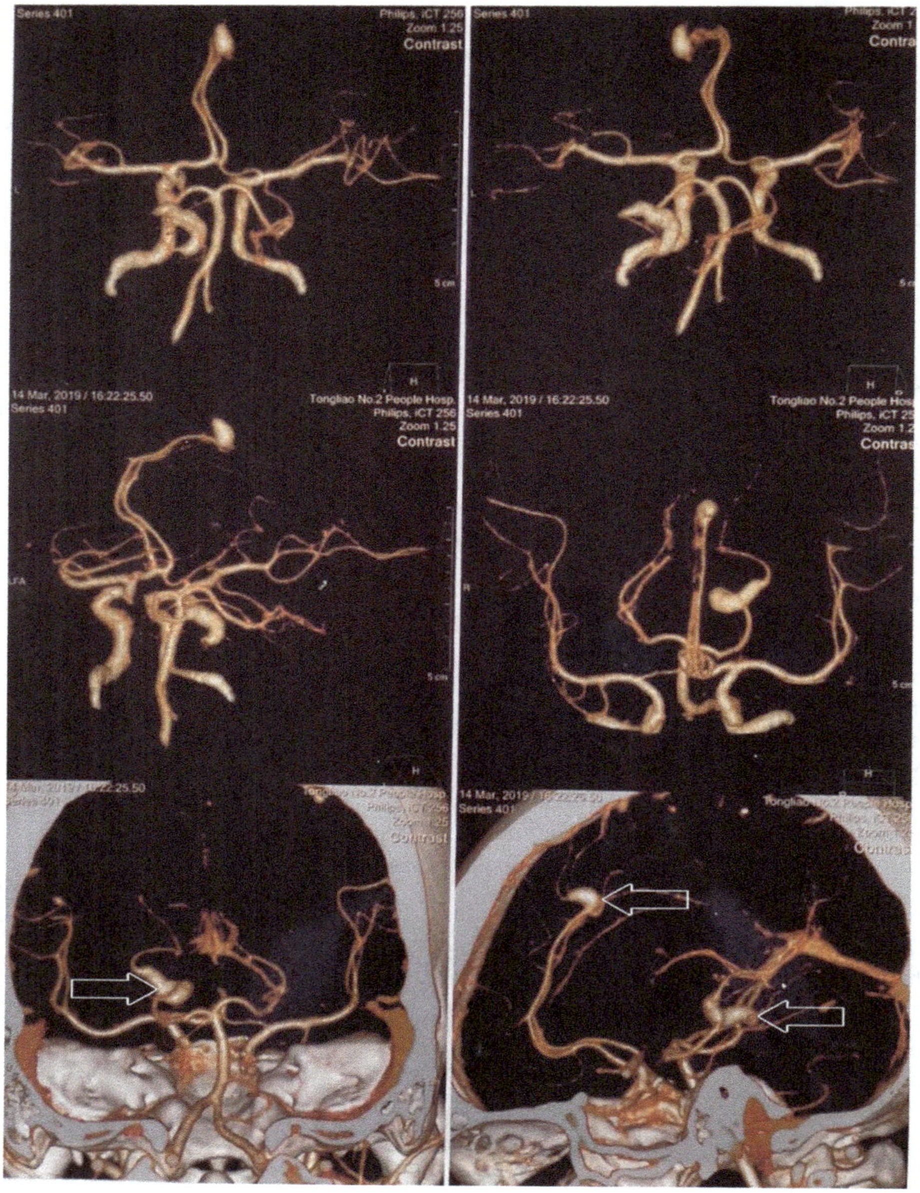

Fig. 1 Two fusiform aneurysms located in left anterior cerebral artery and left posterior cerebral artery, with the size of 9.7 mm × 6.3 mm and 10.2 mm × 7 mm, respectively

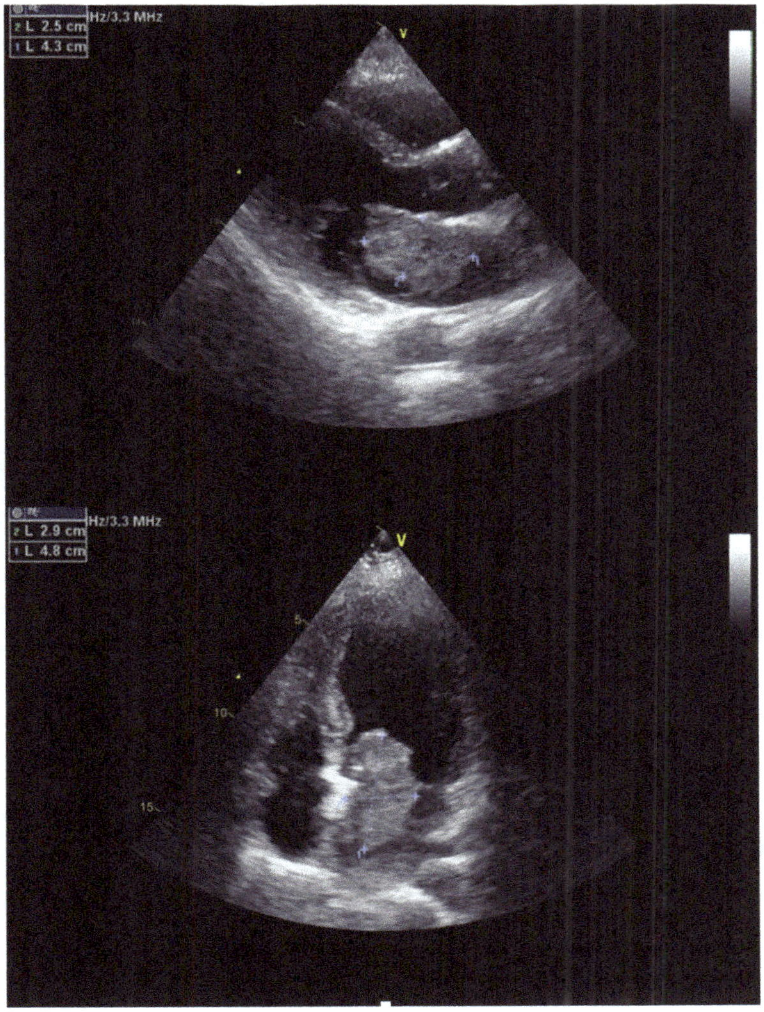

Fig. 2 TTE revealed a $4.8 \times 2.9 \times 2.5$ cm^3 mass attached to the interatrial septum in the left atrium, which obstructed the mitral orifice without mitral valve regurgitation

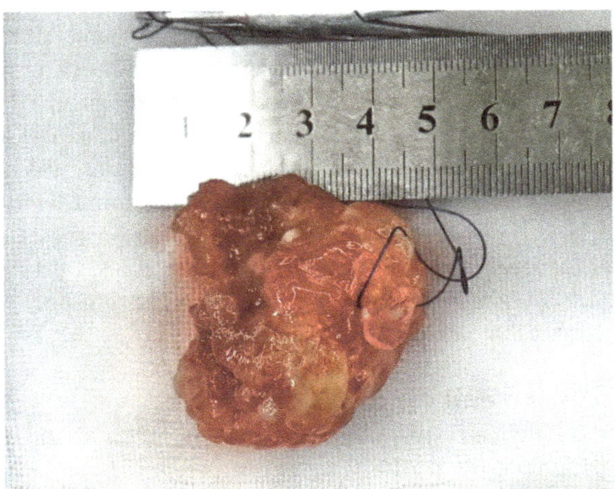

Fig. 3 Polypoid type of atrial myxoma

continuous infusion of fentanyl ($0.3\mu g/kg \times h^{-1}$) was performed to ensure analgesia and attenuate cardiovascular response to tracheal intubation. She was extubated 3 h after surgery without neurological disorder and discharged from ICU on the first day. Intravenous patient-controlled analgesia pump was employed to insure postoperative numeric rating scale (NRS) score lower than 3 (0 = No pain, 10 = worst pain imaginable) [4]. She was fully recovered and discharged home on the sixth day after surgery.

Review and analysis of the literature

The keywords "cerebral aneurysm", "intracranial aneurysm", "myxoma", and "anesthesia" were used for searching in the PubMed and Google Scholar databases. The literature written in English published from January 1966 to April 2019 was reviewed, and articles or abstracts providing the following information were included, for instance, age, gender,

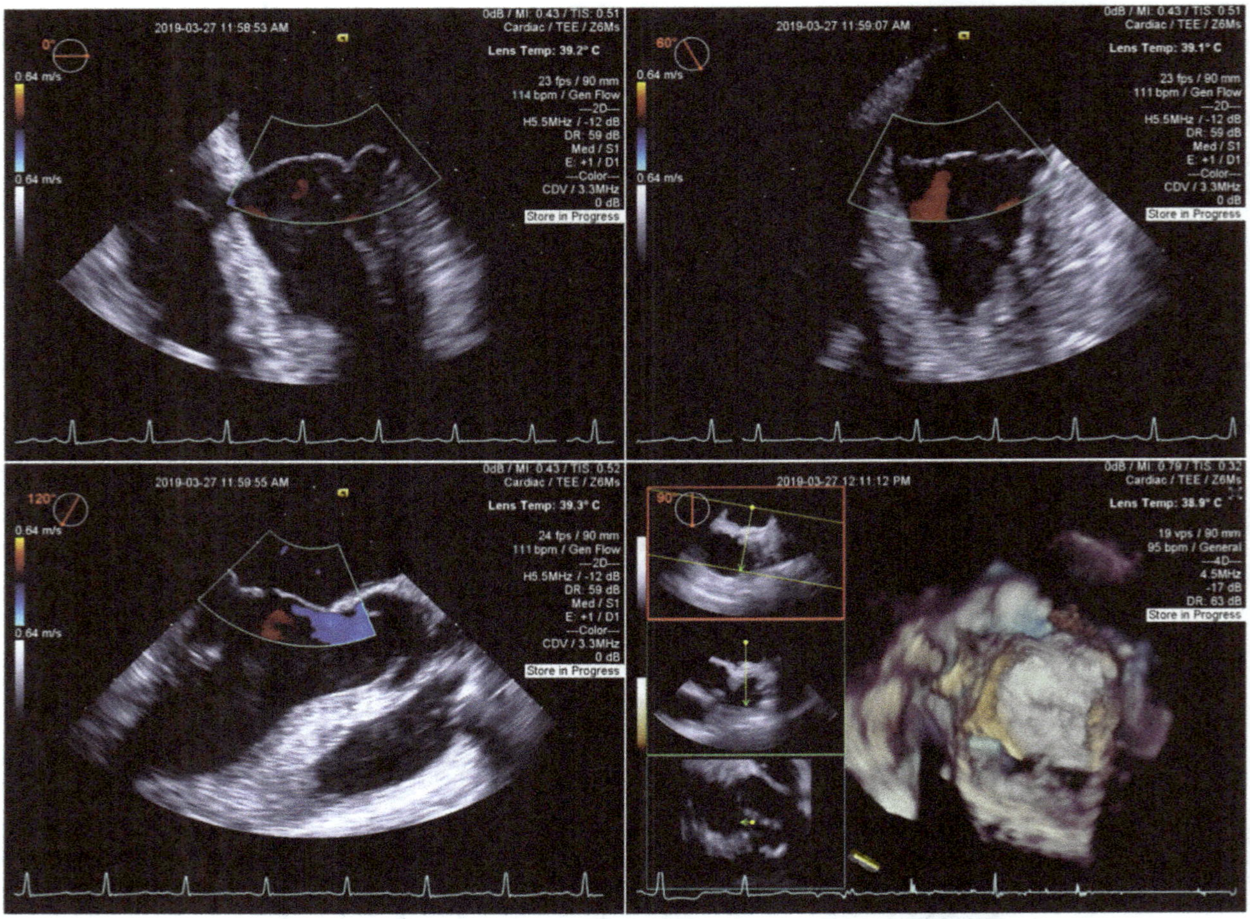

Fig. 4 After resection of myxoma, no mitral regurgitation or shunt flow across the atrial septum was revealed by transesophageal echocardiography

intervention for myxoma and aneurysm, complication, and outcome. Eventually, there were 47 reports of 49 cases and a total of 50 cases analyzed [3, 5–49]. The median age was 38 years (95%CI, 34–42), and female/male ratio was 3.17:1. Resection of atrial myxoma was performed first in 90% (45) cases. Among these, conservative therapy for cerebral aneurysm was performed in 70% (35) cases, including repeated operations of recurrence myxoma in 2 cases [33, 40]. Whereas, craniotomy for aneurysm in 3 cases [8, 11, 19], coiling for 2 cases [15, 34], radiation for 1 case [32], and cytostatic treatment for 1 case was carried out later [12]. Only one case reported craniotomy was performed first and early resection of myxoma was advised [13]. Three patients were dead in the early 1970s due to lack of knowledge and treatment [45, 46, 48]. After resection of myxoma, 13.3% (6/45) patients suffered neurological dysfunction, while acute left hemiparesis appeared during induction of anesthesia and the operation was delayed in one case [5]. Severe neurological complication appeared in one patient with chronic renal failure, who finally died of sepsis [22]. No perioperative subarachnoid hemorrhage (SAH) was reported. Except in one patient, a conservative therapy was attempted, and a myxoma was verified by autopsy with cerebral aneurysms in 1973 [45]. During follow-up period, the rates of stable and regression of aneurysm were 50% (25 cases) and 10% (5 cases) respectively, while enlargement was 10% (5 cases), and new formation was 12% (6 cases). The subgroup of 11 progressive cases was further analyzed, continuous conservative therapy was performed in 4 cases, operation was carried out in 3 cases, and radiotherapy was administered in one case. Further follow-up revealed stable or regression after the treatment. Only one patient suffered SAH [21]. Although anesthesia management was introduced in only one case, it was in craniotomy procedure [13].

Discussion and conclusions

The incidence of primary heart tumors is less than 0.2% in patients. 75% of the tumors are benign, in which approximately 50% are myxomas [1]. Nearly three quarters of myxomas are located in the left atrium, while 15 ~

20% are in the right atrium. Up to 20% of patients can be asymptomatic, whereas in a large case series, mitral valve obstruction, systemic emboli, and constitutional symptoms occurred [50, 51]. Systemic emboli has been well documented, especially embolic stroke [52, 53]. It was reported a villous myxoma might be associated with more chances of metastasis of myxomas, and polypoid type was the only independent predictor of systemic emboli [54]. However, cerebral aneurysms related to atrial myxoma are rare. This patient was asymptomatic with myxoma, and neurological symptoms appeared first, for instance, dizziness and headache. The myxoma was polypoid type in this case.

In 1894, Marchand first reported an interesting phenomenon that cerebral aneurysms were associated with atrial myxoma [55]. Until 2005, Sabolek demonstrated the typical manifestation of aneurysms were multiple with fusiform shape [27]. To date, only around 50 case reports written in English could be found in the literature (Table 1). However, the exact mechanism is still not clear. The hypothesis of "Metastasize and Infiltrate" was considered as an essential mechanism for cerebral aneurysm formation. Myxoma cells may metastasize to the cerebral arteries, infiltrate into the vessel wall through the vasa vasorum or endothelial, interrupt the elastic lamina, and lead to aneurysm formation. Histological examination of the excised cerebral aneurysm verified this hypothesis [29, 36, 48]. Recent reports proposed another hypothesis, which is inflammation reaction arised from myxoma. It is reported that new cerebral aneurysms can form after myxoma resection, without recurrent myxoma or embolism [56]. Some studies found that new aneurysm formed with elevated proinflammation cytokines like interleukin-6 (IL-6) after resection of myxoma [27]. What is more, IL-6 level upregulated by myxoma may contribute to aneurysm formation [57, 58]. Other researches illuminated that IL-6 could promote matrix metalloproteinases expression and activity, which enhance invasion of myxoma cells [23, 59]. Unfortunately, IL-6 level was not tested in our patient.

There are no clinical practice guidelines on such patients. Myxoma was suggested to be resected first to prevent systemic emboli and mitral valve obstruction [1, 10]. In the meantime, fusiform aneurysm is not suitable for clipping or coiling compared to saccular aneurysm, surgical procedure is still an important intervention [60]. Fortunately, the SAH rate of multiple cerebral fusiform aneurysms related to atrial myxoma was low [27]. In addition, it is reported that the cerebral aneurysms regressed after myxoma resection in some cases [3, 5]. Therefore, a conservative treatment approach for cerebral aneurysms was recommended by the preoperative MDT meeting.

Anesthesia management was an enormous challenge. Few piece of evidence was found in the database to guide optimal clinical anesthesia practice. The procedural strategy was to prevent ischemic and hemorrhagic stroke. Intraoperative cerebrovascular monitoring techniques remain controversial [61]. $PbtO_2$ monitoring was recommended to detect brain ischemia and intracranial hypertension in neurocritical care patients [62]. As is known to all, the transmural pressure (TMP) of cerebral aneurysm is equal to cerebral perfusion pressure (CPP), which depends on mean arterial pressure (MAP) and intracranial pressure (ICP).

$$TMP = CPP = MAP - ICP$$

Therefore, an increase in MAP or a decrease in ICP will lead to an increase in CPP, which might increase the risk of rupture of aneurysm. On the contrary, a decrease in MAP or an increase in ICP will increase the risk of cerebral ischemia [63]. Firstly, induction of general anesthesia was an important step. One patient was reported to develop an acute left hemiparesis during induction [5]. Thus, it is crucial to control the TMP diligently. MAP and heart rate (HR) was recommended to close to baseline [64]. Lidocaine is beneficial to such patients, which could not only blunt cerebral hemodynamic response to endotracheal intubation, but also attenuate proinflammatory effects [65, 66]. Besides, esmolol and fentanyl were demonstrated to prevent hemodynamic fluctuation related to intubation in a randomized controlled trial [67]. Secondly, cardiopulmonary bypass (CPB) is a risk factor of stroke, whose pathophysiological mechanisms refer to hemorrhagic, global ischemia, and embolic [68]. TEE plays a vital role in evaluating embolism originated from the heart [69]. On the other hand, it is instrumental to detect the pathogenesis of hypotension, guide fluid replenishment and identify mitral regurgitation and shunt flow [70]. With respect to SAH, perioperative hypertension and anticoagulation are common in the cardiac surgery [68], which may increase the risk of aneurysm rupture. Although a most recent large observational study investigated the risk of postoperative 30-day SAH was 0.29%, not higher than general population [71], it was suggested to decrease CPB time and intensively control the blood pressure [68]. In addition, $PaCO_2$ should be maintained at normal level, and hyperventilation, which will decrease ICP, should be avoided [72]. In this case, the CPB time was 41 min, fluctuation range of MAP was within 10%, and $PaCO_2$ was normal throughout the procedure. Thirdly, the fast track cardiac anesthesia was implemented to evaluate neurological function early after procedure, which aims to extubation within $1 \sim 6$ h postoperation [73]. However, tracheal extubation should be paid more attention, when tachycardia, hypertension and coughing frequently occur [74]. And it would increase the risk of aneurysm rupture. Fentanyl attenuates cough and cardiovascular response effectively, which can be

Table 1 Case reports of multiple aneurysms related to atrial myxoma

	Author	Year	Age	Gender	Procedure (myxoma, aneurysm)	Complication	Outcome
1	This case	2019	38	F	Resection, Conservative	None	Discharge 6 days postoperation and follow-up
2	Coutinho R, et al	2018	46	F	Resection, Conservative	Acute left hemiparesis during induction	Aneurysms completely regressed 18 days later and follow-up
3	Penn DL, et al	2018	12	M	Resection, Conservative	None	1 year follow-up, growth of 2 aneurysms, hybrid procedure, 43 months follow-up, unchanged
4	Flores PL, et al	2018	61	M	Resection, Conservative	None	18 months follow-up, unchanged
5			19	F	Resection, Conservative	None	5 year follow-up, several enlarged, others regressed, asymptomatic, conservative
6	Yoo HJ, et al	2018	20	F	Resection, Craniotomy later	Lost vision in right eye	Not mentioned
7	Quan K, et al	2017	49	F	Resection, Conservative	Not mentioned	Further intracranial lesions resection may be performed
8	Sveinsson O, et al	2015	19	F	Resection, Conservative	None	1 year follow-up, unchanged
9	Zheng J, et al	2015	25	F	Resection first, craniotomy 7 months later	Drowsiness and partial seizure 6 days after craniotomy	Discharge 7 days later, 2 months follow-up, unchanged
10		2015	39	F	Resection 20 years ago, Conservative	None	14 months follow-up, occasional dizziness
11	Vontobel J, et al	2015	41	F	Resection, Cytostatic treatment	None	Follow-up, decreased tracer uptake in PET, stable aneurysm sizes
12	Srivastava S, et al	2014	30	F	None, Craniotomy first	None	Discharge 7 days later, early resection of myxoma was advised
13	Xu Q, et al	2013	46	F	Resection, Conservative	None	Follow-up
14	Al-Said Y, et al	2013	67	F	Resection, Coiling 1 week later	None	1 year follow-up, unchanged
15	Kim H, et al	2012	58	M	Resection, Conservative	None	1 year follow-up, unchanged
16	KJ George, et al	2012	45	F	Resection, Conservative	None	Discharge 2 weeks later, 18 months follow-up, unchanged
17	Lee SJ, et al	2012	55	F	Resection, Conservative	Not mentioned	47 months follow-up, asymptomatic
18	Radoi MP, et al	2012	45	F	Myxoma 1 year ago, Craniotomy twice for 2 lesions	Minor neurological deficits	Discharge 3 weeks later, 12 months follow-up, unchanged
19	Chiang KH, et al	2011	52	F	Resection, Conservative	None	2 years follow-up, unchanged
20	Eddleman CS, et al	2010	18	M	Resection, Conservative	Not mentioned	4 months follow-up, multiple aneurysms formated and hemmorrhage, 3 months later, several aneurysms enlarged and hemmorrhage
21	Koo YH, et al	2009	65	F	Resection, Conservative	None	6 months follow-up, unchanged
22	Shinn SH, et al	2009	48	F	Resection, Conservative	Complex-focal type of status epilepticus	Dead due to sepsis 22 days after surgery
23	Ryou KS, et al	2008	27	F	Resection, Conservative	Intermittent headache	11 years follow-up, unchanged
24	Li Q, et al	2008	27	F	Resection, Conservative	None	2 years follow-up, unchanged
25	Kvitting JP, et al	2008	55	F	Resection, Conservative	None	6 months follow-up, unchanged
26	Sedat J, et al	2007	50	F	Resection, None	None	5 years later aneurysms formated and radiation therapy, 1 year follow-up, one aneurysm regressed
27	Namura O, et al	2007	35	M	Resection, Conservative	Raynaud's phenomenon	10 years follow-up, unchanged

Table 1 Case reports of multiple aneurysms related to atrial myxoma *(Continued)*

	Author	Year	Age	Gender	Procedure (myxoma, aneurysm)	Complication	Outcome
28	Herbst M, et al	2005	31	M	Resection, Conservative	None	2 years follow-up, unchanged
29	Sabolek M, et al	2005	43	F	Resection, Conservative	None	15 months follow-up, one aneurysm regressed
30	Chen Z, et al	2005	19	F	Resection, None	None	2 years later multiple aneurysms formated and conservative therapy, 1 year follow-up, unchanged
31	Josephson SA, et al	2005	33	F	Not mentioned	Not mentioned	8 years follow-up, unchanged
32	Ashalatha R, et al	2005	54	M	Resection, None	None	6 months follow-up, multiple aneurysms formated and Conservative therapy
33	Altundag MB, et al	2005	41	F	Resection, Radiation 1 year later	None	4 years follow-up, unchanged
34	Stock K, et al	2004	22	F	Resection 2 times, conservative	None	11 years follow-up, some aneurysms regressed and some aneurysms smaller, no new aneurysm
35	Yilmaz MB, et al	2003	38	F	Recurrence and resection of myxoma, coil embolization for one giant aneurysm	None	Follow-up, unchanged
36	Furuya K, et al	1995	35	M	Resection, Conservative	None	19 months follow-up, enlarged and craniotomy, another 5 months follow-up, unchanged
37	Mattle HP, et al	1995	49	M	Resection, Conservative	Not mentioned	5 years follow up, aneurysm formated 3 years after surgery, demented 5 years later and continuously progressed
38	Suzuki T, et al	1994	34	M	Resection, Conservative	Not mentioned	Follow-up, aneurysm formated 2 months after surgery, and enlarged 5 months later
39	Chen HJ, et al	1993	68	F	Resection, Conservative	Not mentioned	Craniotomy 1 year later, 2 years follow-up, unchanged
40	Hung PC, et al	1992	10	F	Resection, Conservative	None	8 months follow-up, unchanged
41	Bobo H, et al	1987	15	F	Resection four times for recurrent myxoma, Conservative	None	6 months follow-up, unchanged
42	Reed OM, et al	1986	25	F	Resection, Conservative	Not mentioned	12 years follow-up, clip for a large aneurysm 9 years later
43	Branch CL, et al	1985	53	F	Resection, Conservative	None	18 months follow-up, one aneurysm disappeared
44	Leonhardt ET, et al	1977	31	M	Resection, Conservative	None	2 months follow-up, unchanged
45	Damásio H, et al	1975	43	F	Resection, Conservative	None	1 year follow-up, unchanged
46	Steinmetz EF, et al	1973	48	F	Conservative, Conservative	SAH and hematoma evacuation	Dead 2 months later, autopsy verified myxoma with cerebral aneurysms
47	Burton C, et al	1970	41	F	None, craniotomy first	Not mentioned	Dead in the first day after surgery
48	New PF, et al	1970	41	F	Resection, Conservative	None	8 years follow-up, unchanged
49	Price DL, et al	1970	21	F	Conservative, Conservative	Not mentioned	Dead 11 months later, autopsy verified myxoma with cerebral aneurysms
50	Stoane L, et al	1966	29	M	Resection, Conservative	None	2 months follow-up, slightly larger and conservative therapy

safely used in fast track cardiac anesthesia [75–77]. Fortunately, refined perioperative anesthesia management was performed in this rare case, and the patient recovered uneventfully.

Atrial myxoma-related cerebral aneurysms are always multiple and in a fusiform shape in most occasions. Early resection of myxoma and conservative therapy of aneurysm is an optimal treatment. It is a great challenge to anesthesiologists to prevent stroke perioperatively. TEE and $PbtO_2$ monitoring play an essential role in anesthesia management. Fast track cardiac anesthesia is safe and effective to early evaluate neurological function. Long term follow-up for "myxomatous aneurysms" is recommended. And outcome of most patients is excellent. Further study is needed to reveal the mechanism of atrial myxoma resulting in multiple cerebral aneurysms.

Abbreviations

AMR: Atrial myxoma resection; MCAs: Multiple cerebral aneurysms; CTA: Computed tomography angiography; TTE: Transthoracic echocardiography; MDT: Multidisciplinary team; HR: Heart rate; MAP: Mean arterial pressure; TEE: Transesophageal echocardiography; PbtO2: Parenchymal brain oxygen; ICU: Intensive care unit; NRS: Numeric rating scale; SAH: Subarachnoid hemorrhage; IL-6: Interleukin-6; TMP: Transmural pressure; CPP: Cerebral perfusion pressure; ICP: Intracranial pressure; CPB: Cardiopulmonary bypass

Acknowledgements

We would like to thank Dr. Gang Liu and Dr. ZQ Han from department of cardiac surgery for their understanding, supporting and collaborating in this case. We also thank DL Wang from department of neurosurgery for evaluating the patient and making some pertinent suggestions.

Authors' contributions

RZ implemented perioperative anesthesia management of the patient, analyze the literature and complete the draft manuscript. ZYT helped postoperative follow-up and the collection of clinical data. QQ drew up the anesthesia plan. FM analyzed the data of perioperative transesophageal echocardiography. YF revised the manuscript. All authors read and approved the final manuscript.

Author details

[1]Department of Anesthesiology, Peking University People's Hospital, No. 11 Xi Zhi Men Nan Da Jie, Xicheng District, Beijing, China. [2]Department of Anesthesiology, Beth Israel Deaconess Medical Center, Boston, USA.

References

1. Reynen K. Cardiac myxomas. N Engl J Med. 1995;333(24):1610–7.
2. Lee VH, Connolly HM, Brown RD Jr. Central nervous system manifestations of cardiac myxoma. Arch Neurol. 2007;64(8):1115–20.
3. Sedat J, Chau Y, Dunac A, Gomez N, Suissa L, Mahagne MH. Multiple cerebral aneurysms caused by cardiac myxoma. A case report and present state of knowledge. Interv Neuroradiol. 2007;13(2):179–84.
4. Breivik H, Borchgrevink PC, Allen SM, Rosseland LA, Romundstad L, Hals EK, Kvarstein G, Stubhaug A. Assessment of pain. Br J Anaesth. 2008;101(1):17–24.
5. Renan Coutinho, MAyara Graciani, Livia Afonso, Thiago Teixiera, Beatriz Haynes, Carolina Oliviera, MArco Lima. Brain Aneurysm Associated with Atrial Myxoma Neurology April 10, 2018;90(15 Supplement):6.208.
6. Penn DL, Lanpher AB, Klein JM, Kozakewich HPW, Kahle KT, Smith ER, Orbach DB. Multimodal treatment approach in a patient with multiple intracranial myxomatous aneurysms. J Neurosurg Pediatr. 2018;21(3):315–21.
7. Flores PL, Haglund F, Bhogal P, Yeo Leong Litt L, Sodermann M. The dynamic natural history of cerebral aneurysms from cardiac myxomas: a review of the natural history of myxomatous aneurysms. Interv Neuroradiol. 2018;24(3):277–83.
8. Yoo HJ, Chung J, Ahn JS. Cerebral myxomatous aneurysm treated by M2-M2 bypass: a case report. The Nerve. 2018;4(2):120–2.
9. Quan K, Song J, Zhu W, Chen L, Pan Z, Li P, Mao Y. Repeated multiple intracranial hemorrhages induced by cardiac myxoma mimicking cavernous angiomas: a case report. Chin Neurosurg J. 2017;3(1):3.
10. Sveinsson O, Herrman L. Multiple cerebral aneurysms in a patient with cardiac myxoma: what to do? BMJ Case Rep. 2015;2015.
11. Zheng J, Li S, Cao Y, Wang S, Wang R, Zhao J. Multiple cerebral myxomatous aneurysms: what is the optimal treatment? J Stroke Cerebrovasc Dis. 2015;24(1):232–8.
12. Vontobel J, Huellner M, Stolzmann P. Cerebral 'metastasizing' cardiac myxoma. Eur Heart J. 2016;37(21):1680.
13. Srivastava S, Tewari P. Stroke associated with left atrial mass: association of cerebral aneurysm with left atrial myxoma! Ann Card Anaesth. 2014;17(1):56–8.
14. Xu Q, Zhang X, Wu P, Wang M, Zhou Y, Feng Y. Multiple intracranial aneurysms followed left atrial myxoma: case report and literature review. J Thorac Dis. 2013;5(6):E227–31.
15. Al-Said Y, Al-Rached H, Baeesa S, Kurdi K, Zabani I, Hassan A. Emergency excision of cardiac myxoma and endovascular coiling of intracranial aneurysm after cerebral infarction. Case Rep Neurol Med. 2013;2013:839270.
16. Kim H, Park EA, Lee W, Chung JW, Park JH. Multiple cerebral and coronary aneurysms in a patient with left atrial myxoma. Int J Cardiovasc Imaging. 2012;28(Suppl 2):129–32.
17. George KJ, Rennie A, Saxena A. Multiple cerebral aneurysms secondary to cardiac myxoma. Br J Neurosurg. 2012;26(3):409–11.
18. Lee SJ, Kim JH, Na CY, Oh SS. Eleven years' experience with Korean cardiac myxoma patients: focus on embolic complications. Cerebrovasc Dis. 2012; 33(5):471–9.
19. Radoi MP, Stefanescu F, Arsene D. Brain metastases and multiple cerebral aneurysms from cardiac myxoma: case report and review of the literature. Br J Neurosurg. 2012;26(6):893–5.
20. Chiang K-H, Cheng H-M, Chang B-S, Chiu C-H, Yen P-S. Multiple cerebral aneurysms as manifestations of cardiac myxoma: brain imaging, digital subtraction angiography, and echocardiography. Tzu Chi Med J. 2011;23(2):63–5.
21. Eddleman CS, Gottardi-Littell NR, Bendok BR, Batjer HH, Bernstein RA. Rupture of cerebral myxomatous aneurysm months after resection of the primary cardiac tumor. Neurocrit Care. 2010;13(2):252–5.
22. Shinn SH, Chon SH, Kim HJ. Multiple cerebral aneurysms associated with cardiac myxoma in a patient with chronic renal failure: how can we resolve multiple cerebral aneurysms? Thorac Cardiovasc Surg. 2009;57(1):47–8.
23. Koo YH, Kim TG, Kim OJ, Oh SH. Multiple fusiform cerebral aneurysms and highly elevated serum interleukin-6 in cardiac myxoma. J Korean Neurosurg Soc. 2009;45(6):394–6.
24. Li Q, Shang H, Zhou D, Liu R, He L, Zheng H. Repeated embolism and multiple aneurysms: central nervous system manifestations of cardiac myxoma. Eur J Neurol. 2008;15(12):e112–3.
25. Kvitting JP, Engvall J, Broqvist M, Franzen S, Andersson M, Ohlsson U, Nielsen NE. Recurrence of myxoma in the left ventricle with concurrent cerebral fusiform aneurysms after previous atrial myxoma surgery. J Thorac Cardiovasc Surg. 2008;135(5):1172–3.
26. Namura O, Saitoh M, Moro H, Watanabe H, Sogawa M, Nishikura K, Hayashi J. A case of biatrial multiple myxomas with glandular structure. Ann Thorac Cardiovasc Surg. 2007;13(6):423–7.
27. Sabolek M, Bachus-Banaschak K, Bachus R, Arnold G, Storch A. Multiple cerebral aneurysms as delayed complication of left cardiac myxoma: a case report and review. Acta Neurol Scand. 2005;111(6):345–50.
28. Josephson SA, Johnston SC. Multiple stable fusiform intracranial aneurysms following atrial myxoma. Neurology. 2005;64(3):526.
29. Herbst M, Wattjes MP, Urbach H, Inhetvin-Hutter C, Becker D, Klockgether T, Hartmann A. Cerebral embolism from left atrial myxoma leading to cerebral and retinal aneurysms: a case report. AJNR Am J Neuroradiol. 2005;26(3): 666–9.
30. Chen Z, Wang YL, Ye W, Miao ZR, Song QB, Ling F. Multiple intracranial aneurysms as delayed complication of atrial myxoma. Case report and literature review. Interv Neuroradiol. 2005;11(3):251–4.
31. Ashalatha R, Moosa A, Gupta AK, Krishna Manohar SR, Sandhyamani S. Cerebral aneurysms in atrial myxoma: a delayed, rare manifestation. Neurol India. 2005;53(2):216–8.

32. Altundag MB, Ertas G, Ucer AR, Durmus S, Abanuz H, Calikoglu T, Ozbagi K, Demirkasimoglu A, Kaya B, Bakkal BH, et al. Brain metastasis of cardiac myxoma: case report and review of the literature. J Neuro-Oncol. 2005;75(2):181–4.
33. Stock K. Multiple cerebral aneurysms in a patient with recurrent cardiac myxomas. A case report. Interv Neuroradiol. 2004;10(4):335–40.
34. Yilmaz MB, Akin Y, Guray U, Kisacik HL, Korkmaz S. Late recurrence of left atrial myxoma with multiple intracranial aneurysms. Int J Cardiol. 2003;87(2–3):303–5.
35. Mattle HP, Maurer D, Sturzenegger M, Ozdoba C, Baumgartner RW, Schroth G. Cardiac myxomas: a long term study. J Neurol. 1995;242(10):689–94.
36. Furuya K, Sasaki T, Yoshimoto Y, Okada Y, Fujimaki T, Kirino T, et al. J Neurosurg. 1995;83(1):170–3.
37. Suzuki T, Nagai R, Yamazaki T, Shiojima I, Maemura K, Yamaoki K, Tanaka N, Machida T, Kotsuka Y, Furuse A, et al. Rapid growth of intracranial aneurysms secondary to cardiac myxoma. Neurology. 1994;44(3 Pt 1):570–1.
38. Chen HJ, Liou CW, Chen L. Metastatic atrial myxoma presenting as intracranial aneurysms with hemorrhage: case report. Surg Neurol. 1993;40(1):61–4.
39. Hung PC, Wang HS, Chou ML, Huang SC, Su WJ. Multiple cerebral aneurysms in a child with cardiac myxoma. J Formos Med Assoc. 1992;91(8): 818–21.
40. Bobo H, Evans OB. Intracranial aneurysms in a child with recurrent atrial myxoma. Pediatr Neurol. 1987;3(4):230–2.
41. Reed OM, Mellette JR Jr, Fitzpatrick JE. Cutaneous lentiginosis with atrial myxomas. J Am Acad Dermatol. 1986;15(2 Pt 2):398–402.
42. Branch CL Jr, Laster DW, Kelly DL Jr. Left atrial myxoma with cerebral emboli. Neurosurgery. 1985;16(5):675–80.
43. Leonhardt ET, Kullenberg KP. Bilateral atrial myxomas with multiple arterial aneurysms--a syndrome mimicking polyarteritis nodosa. Am J Med. 1977; 62(5):792–4.
44. Damasio H, Seabra-Gomes R, da Silva JP, Damasio AR, Antunes JL. Multiple cerebral aneurysms and cardiac myxoma. Arch Neurol. 1975;32(4):269–70.
45. Steinmetz EF, Calanchini PR, Aguilar MJ. Left atrial myxoma as a neurological problem: a case report and review. Stroke. 1973;4(3):451–8.
46. Price DL, Harris JL, New PF, Cantu RC. Cardiac myxoma. A clinicopathologic and angiographic study. Arch Neurol. 1970;23(6):558–67.
47. New PF, Price DL, Carter B. Cerebral angiography in cardiac myxoma. Correlation of angiographic and histopathological findings. Radiology. 1970;96(2):335–45.
48. Burton C, Johnston J. Multiple cerebral aneurysms and cardiac myxoma. N Engl J Med. 1970;282(1):35–6.
49. Stoane L, Allen JH Jr, Collins HA. Radiologic observations in cerebral embolization from left heart myxomas. Radiology. 1966;87(2):262–6.
50. Burke A, Jeudy J Jr, Virmani R. Cardiac tumours: an update: cardiac tumours. Heart. 2008;94(1):117–23.
51. Pinede L, Duhaut P, Loire R. Clinical presentation of left atrial cardiac myxoma. A series of 112 consecutive cases. Medicine (Baltimore). 2001;80(3):159–72.
52. Elbardissi AW, Dearani JA, Daly RC, Mullany CJ, Orszulak TA, Puga FJ, Schaff HV. Survival after resection of primary cardiac tumors: a 48-year experience. Circulation. 2008;118(14 Suppl):S7–15.
53. Aggarwal SK, Barik R, Sarma TC, Iyer VR, Sai V, Mishra J, Voleti CD. Clinical presentation and investigation findings in cardiac myxomas: new insights from the developing world. Am Heart J. 2007;154(6):1102–7.
54. Ha JW, Kang WC, Chung N, Chang BC, Rim SJ, Kwon JW, Jang Y, Shim WH, Cho SY, Kim SS, et al. Echocardiographic and morphologic characteristics of left atrial myxoma and their relation to systemic embolism. Am J Cardiol. 1999;83(11):1579–82 A1578.
55. Marchand F. Zur Kenntnis der Embolie und Thrombose der Gerhirnarterien, Zugleich ein Beitrag zur Casuistik der primaren Herztumoren und der gekreuzten Embolie. Klin Wochenschr. 1894;31:1–5.
56. Santillan A, Sigounas D, Fink ME, Gobin YP. Multiple fusiform intracranial aneurysms 14 years after atrial myxoma resection. Arch Neurol. 2012;69(9): 1204–5.
57. Jean WC, Walski-Easton SM, Nussbaum ES. Multiple intracranial aneurysms as delayed complications of an atrial myxoma: case report. Neurosurgery. 2001;49(1):200–2 discussion 202-203.
58. Ezerioha N, Feng W. Intracardiac Myxoma, cerebral aneurysms and elevated Interleukin-6. Case Rep Neurol. 2015;7(2):152–5.
59. Orlandi A, Ciucci A, Ferlosio A, Pellegrino A, Chiariello L, Spagnoli LG. Increased expression and activity of matrix metalloproteinases characterize embolic cardiac myxomas. Am J Pathol. 2005;166(6):1619–28.
60. Barletta EA, Ricci RL, Silva RDG, Gaspar R, Araujo JFM, Neves MWF, de Aquino JLB, Barba Belsuzarri TA. Fusiform aneurysms: a review from its pathogenesis to treatment options. Surg Neurol Int. 2018;9:189.
61. Gruber A, Dorfer C, Standhardt H, Bavinzski G, Knosp E. Prospective comparison of intraoperative vascular monitoring technologies during cerebral aneurysm surgery. Neurosurgery. 2011;68(3):657–73 discussion 673.
62. Oddo M, Bosel J, Participants in the International Multidisciplinary Consensus Conference on Multimodality M. Monitoring of brain and systemic oxygenation in neurocritical care patients. Neurocrit Care. 2014; 21(Suppl 2):S103–20.
63. Cottrell JE, SD. Anesthesia and neurosurgery. 4th ed. St. Louis: Mosby; 2001.
64. Abd-Elsayed AA, Wehby AS, Farag E. Anesthetic management of patients with intracranial aneurysms. Ochsner J. 2014;14(3):418–25.
65. Hamill JF, Bedford RF, Weaver DC, Colohan AR. Lidocaine before endotracheal intubation: intravenous or laryngotracheal? Anesthesiology. 1981;55(5):578–81.
66. Dunn LK, Durieux ME. Perioperative use of intravenous Lidocaine. Anesthesiology. 2017;126(4):729–37.
67. Ugur B, Ogurlu M, Gezer E, Nuri Aydin O, Gursoy F. Effects of esmolol, lidocaine and fentanyl on haemodynamic responses to endotracheal intubation: a comparative study. Clin Drug Investig. 2007;27(4):269–77.
68. Devgun JK, Gul S, Mohananey D, Jones BM, Hussain MS, Jobanputra Y, Kumar A, Svensson LG, Tuzcu EM, Kapadia SR. Cerebrovascular events after cardiovascular procedures: risk factors, recognition, and prevention strategies. J Am Coll Cardiol. 2018;71(17):1910–20.
69. Celeste F, Muratori M, Mapelli M, Pepi M. The evolving role and use of echocardiography in the evaluation of cardiac source of embolism. J Cardiovasc Echogr. 2017;27(2):33–44.
70. Reeves ST, Finley AC, Skubas NJ, Swaminathan M, Whitley WS, Glas KE, Hahn RT, Shanewise JS, Adams MS, Shernan SK, et al. Basic perioperative transesophageal echocardiography examination: a consensus statement of the American Society of Echocardiography and the Society of Cardiovascular Anesthesiologists. J Am Soc Echocardiogr. 2013;26(5):443–56.
71. Nam JS, Jeon SB, Jo JY, Joung KW, Chin JH, Lee EH, Chung CH, Choi IC. Perioperative rupture risk of unruptured intracranial aneurysms in cardiovascular surgery. Brain. 2019;142(5):1408–15.
72. Yao F. Yao and Artusio's anesthesiology. 6th ed. Philadelphia: Lippincott; 2008.
73. Cheng DC. Fast track cardiac surgery pathways: early extubation, process of care, and cost containment. Anesthesiology. 1998;88(6):1429–33.
74. Hartley M, Vaughan RS. Problems associated with tracheal extubation. Br J Anaesth. 1993;71(4):561–8.
75. Tagaito Y, Isono S, Nishino T. Upper airway reflexes during a combination of propofol and fentanyl anesthesia. Anesthesiology. 1998;88(6):1459–66.
76. Nishina K, Mikawa K, Maekawa N, Obara H. Fentanyl attenuates cardiovascular responses to tracheal extubation. Acta Anaesthesiol Scand. 1995;39(1):85–9.
77. Myles PS, Daly DJ, Djaiani G, Lee A, Cheng DC. A systematic review of the safety and effectiveness of fast-track cardiac anesthesia. Anesthesiology. 2003;99(4):982–7.

Effect of opioid-free anaesthesia on post-operative period in cardiac surgery

Pierre-Grégoire Guinot[*], Alexandra Spitz, Vivien Berthoud, Omar Ellouze, Anis Missaoui, Tiberiu Constandache, Sandrine Grosjean, Mohamed Radhouani, Jean-Baptiste Anciaux, Jean-Philippe Parthiot, Jean-Pierre Merle, Nicolas Nowobilski, Maxime Nguyen and Belaid Bouhemad

Abstract

Background: No study has been conducted to demonstrate the feasibility of an opioid-free anesthesia (OFA) protocol in cardiac surgery to improve patient care. The aim of the present study was to evaluate the effect of OFA on post-operative morphine consumption and the post-operative course.

Methods: After retrospectively registering to clinicaltrial.gov (NCT03816592), we performed a retrospective matched cohort study (1:1) on cardiac surgery patients with cardiopulmonary bypass between 2018 and 2019. Patients were divided into two groups: OFA (lidocaine, dexamethasone and ketamine) or opioid anaesthesia (OA) (sufentanil). The main outcome was the total postoperative morphine consumption in the 48 h after surgery. Secondary outcomes were rescue analgesic use, a major adverse event composite endpoint, and ICU and hospital length of stay (LOS).

Results: One hundred ten patients were matched (OFA: $n = 55$; OA: n = 55). On inclusion, demographic and surgical data for the OFA and OA groups were comparable. The total morphine consumption was higher in the OA group than in the OFA group (15 (6–34) vs 5 mg (2–18), $p = 0.001$). The pain score during the first 48 post-operative hours did not differ between the two groups. Creatinine values did not differ on the first post-operative day (80 (IQR: 66–115) vs 77 mmol/l (IQR: 69–95), $p = 0.284$). Incidence of the composite endpoint was lower in the OFA group (25 patients (43%) vs 38 patients (68%), $p = 0.021$). The time to extubation and the ICU stays were shorter in the OFA group (3 (1–5) vs 5 (3–6) hours, p = 0.001 and 2 (1–3) vs 3 (2–5) days, $p = 0.037$).

Conclusion: The use of OFA was associated with lower morphine consumption. OFA might be associated with shorter intubation time and ICU stays. Further randomized studies are needed to confirm these results.

Keywords: Anesthetics, Lidocaine, Intravenous, Propofol, Opioid, Cardiac surgery, Outcomes

Background

Since the 1960s, the systematic administration of opioids has been considered one of the pillars of modern anaesthesia [1]. The use of opioid analgesics has become widespread with the development of new opioid agents. Their use is based on their antinociceptive effects, the control of the autonomic nervous system (ANS) responses to surgical stress, and their induced hypnotic reduction [2]. However, the principle underlying the administration of opioids during anaesthesia has only recently been called into question. Opioids have a number of adverse effects that limit their effectiveness in peri-operative care, the most relevant being respiratory depression, gastrointestinal alterations, hyperalgesia, inflammation modulation, and immunologic modulation [3]. Moreover, the recent opioid epidemic, due in part to persistent use of perioperative opioids, raises questions about the systematic administration of opioids during anaesthesia and the development of new non-opioid strategies.

* Correspondence: guinotpierregregoire@gmail.com
Department of Anaesthesiology and Critical Care Medicine, Dijon University Medical Centre, 21000 Dijon, France

Opioid-free anaesthesia (OFA) is a long-standing concept. It is based on the fact that a sympathetic reaction evidenced by hemodynamic changes in an anesthetised patient does not systematically reflect pain. In addition, a sleeping patient will not recall pain, while hormonal stress and sympathetic and inflammatory reactions can be controlled by therapeutic classes other than opioids [4, 5]. There is an increasing body of literature on OFA, demonstrating its feasibility with a decrease of post-operative morphine consumption and improvement of postoperative well being [6–9]. Several OFA protocols have also been published [10]. The most commonly used nonopioid agents are lidocaine, dexamethasone, and ketamine [10], and all have been studied separately in cardiac surgery. Murphy et al. demonstrated that the administration of dexamethasone decreased morphine consumption and the ICU length of stay [11]. Ketamine was shown to have analgesic effects and opioid-sparing effects [12]. Lidocaine has demonstrated analgesic and opioid-sparing effects in cardiac and non-cardiac surgery [13, 14], and additional studies have found cardioprotective and/or neuroprotective effects [15, 16]. More specifically, the use of lidocaine has been associated with a decrease in arrhythmias and a non-constant improvement in postoperative cognitive functions. All these studies were performed with opioid anaesthesia (OA). In non-cardiac surgery, OFA was demonstrated to be associated with lower post-operative opioid use, and better respiratory outcomes [6, 7, 17]. To our knowledge, no study has evaluated the effect of OFA on morphine consumption and the post-operative course in cardiac surgery patients.

The main objective of the present study was to demonstrate that, compared with OA, OFA lowers postoperative morphine consumption. In addition, we evaluated the effect of OFA on operative hemodynamic stability, postoperative complications assessed by a composite criterion and the length of stay (LOS) in the ICU and in hospital.

Methods

Patients

We performed a retrospective, open-label, matched (1:1), single-centre study in a tertiary university hospital (Dijon, France) between 2018 and 2019. All patients were included within this time frame. The study was recorded on January 25, 2019 to clinicaltrial.gov (NCT03816592). Our team started using an OFA strategy for cardiac surgery in 2017. Consequently, the number of patients receiving OFA has increased steadily since 2017. In practical terms, OFA administration was left to the discretion of the attending anesthetist regardless of a patient's co-morbidities and surgical risk. The study was performed in accordance with the ethical standards outlined in the 1964 Declaration of Helsinki. As the study was observational and used existing, routinely collected data, and in compliance with French law (loi Jardé n° 2012–300) informed consent was not required. We submitted the protocol study to the "Délégation à la Recherche et à l'Innovation (DRCI) », CHU de Dijon, Dijon, France, and followed the MR004 (méthodologie de référence 004) in accordance with the national commission for data protection (CNIL) guidelines. The present report was drafted in line with the STROBE statement [18].

The main inclusion criteria were as follows: age 18 or over, cardiac surgery with the use of cardiopulmonary bypass (CPB) (coronary artery bypass grafting (CABG), the surgical correction of valve disease (aortic, mitral), combined surgery (CABG and valve disease), ascending aortic disease, and left ventricular assist device implantation). The exclusion criteria were: off-pump cardiac surgery, preoperative analgesic use, gabapentin use, antidepressant therapy and preoperative cognitive dysfunction.

Operative management

Maintenance or withdrawal of preoperative medications adhered to international guidelines. Anaesthesia and cardiopulmonary bypass procedures were standardised for all patients. In the OA group, anaesthesia was induced with an intravenous bolus of ketamine (0.3–0.5 mg/kg), propofol (0.4–2 mg/kg) and sufentanil (0.5 ng/ml) until the loss-of-eyelash reflex. Sufentanil was continuously administered using Schneider's target-controlled infusion model. All OA patients had loco-regional analgesia by serratus anterior plane block (thoracotomy, levobupivacaine 0.125 mg/ml, 0.5 ml/kg) or a continuous parasternal infusion of a local anaesthetic (sternotomy, levobupivacaine 0.125 mg/ml continuous infusion 8 ml/h for 48 h). None of the OA patients received intravenous lidocaine. In the OFA group, anaesthesia was induced with an intravenous bolus of dexamethasone (0.1 mg kg^{-1}), intravenous bolus of ketamine (0.3–0.5 mg kg^{-1}), intravenous bolus of lidocaine (1.5 mg kg^{-1} bolus 15 min before the start of propofol) and propofol (0.4–2 mg kg^{-1}) until the loss-of-eyelash reflex. Lidocaine was continuously administered at 1.5 mg/kg/h until the end of surgery.

In both groups, tracheal intubation was facilitated with cisatracurium (0.15 mg kg^{-1}), and neuromuscular blockade was ensured using intermittent bolus of cisatracurium to reach adequate muscle relaxation measured by peripheral nerve stimulation. Sufentanil and lidocaine were discontinued at the end of surgery. In both groups, anaesthesia was maintained by target-controlled infusions of propofol (started at 2–4 ng ml^{-1}). Sedation was titrated using the bispectral index (Covidien, Boulder, CO, USA) to obtain a value between 40 and 60. Arterial hypertension (systolic arterial pressure > 140 mmHg) was treated with esmolol in case of tachycardia (heart rate > 80 bpm) or urapidil/nicardipine if the heart rate dropped below 80 bpm.

Cardiopulmonary bypass was conducted with a heart-lung machine (Stockert Sorin S5 Heart Lung, Milan, Italy) at a target blood flow of 2.4 l min^{-1} m^{-2}. The mean arterial blood pressure (MAP) was maintained at more than 65 mmHg by increasing the pump flow rate or, if required, by administering a bolus of phenylephrine (100 μg) or norepinephrine (5 μg). The CPB circuit was primed with 1500 ml of crystalloids (Plasma-Lyte®; Baxter, Lessines, Belgium) and 5000 ui of heparin. After systemic heparinization (300 ui kg^{-1}) to obtain a hemochron level of 400 s, median sternotomy or thoracotomy was performed and aortic and right auricular cannulations were started. Normoglycemia was maintained using intravenous insulin (intravenous bolus of 5–10 ui) if necessary. Patients with a haemoglobin value below 8 g dl^{-1} received homologous red blood cell transfusions. Heparin was reversed with protamine at a 1:1 ratio.

ICU management

At the end of surgery, all patients were sedated and the lungs were mechanically ventilated until haemodynamic stability and normothermia were obtained and blood loss was considered acceptable (less than 1 ml kg^{-1} h^{-1}). Tracheal extubation was done according to the French guidelines [19]. Patients were managed by a team of physicians trained in postoperative cardiac surgical care which included a cardiologist.

Analgesia was standardised and comprised of intravenous paracetamol (1 g every 6 h) and patient-controlled morphine analgesia. Before extubation, all patients received 1 g of acetaminophen. Immediately after, all patients received titrated intravenous morphine with a bolus of 2 to 3 mg until a score of 3 or less was obtained on the visual analogue pain scale. Patient-controlled analgesia morphine was then started as follows: 1 mg bolus, refractory period of 7 min, maximum dose of 20 mg every 4 h without continuous infusion. The use of complementary analgesics was left to the discretion of the attending physician. According to our institutional protocol, complementary analgesia comprised the use of ketoprofen (50 mg), tramadol (50 mg), and nefopam (20 mg). Pain was assessed every 4 h during the ICU stay with the visual analogue scale. Non-invasive ventilation was left to the discretion of attending physician. Common indications were high-risk patients, atelectasis, hypoxemia, hypercapnia and acute respiratory failure. Patients were discharged from ICU at the discretion of their attending physician. The patients' electrocardiogram, pulse oxygen saturation and central venous blood pressure were continuously monitored. The scheduled blood tests included arterial/venous blood gas measurements on admission to the ICU, and then several times a day on request by the attending physician.

The following variables were continuously recorded in the institutional database: age, gender, body weight, height, personal medical history, ASA score, Euro-SCORE2, Euroscore, type of cardiac surgery, the preoperative left ventricular ejection fraction, the duration of CPB, the duration of aortic clamping, the need for intraoperative blood transfusion, norepinephrine, dobutamine, the use of a antihypertensive agent (nicardipine, urapidil), the use of a short acting beta-blocker (esmolol), troponin values, creatinine value, time to extubation (hours), any occurrence of complications during the stay in the ICU or in the hospital, and the LOS in the ICU.

The primary endpoint was the cumulative dose of postoperative morphine in the first 48 h (in milligrams). The secondary endpoints were: analgesic rescue, a composite endpoint of major adverse events (new onset of atrial fibrillation or flutter, second or third atrio-ventricular blockade, stroke, acute kidney injury, confusion, reintubation, non-invasive ventilation support, and in-hospital death), fluid expansion (ml), total propofol dose (mg), antihypertensive agent use, vasoplegia syndrome, catecholamine use, troponin Ic (ng ml^{-1}), creatinine (mmol l^{-1}), ICU LOS (days), and hospital LOS (days). The secondary composite endpoint was assessed during the hospital stay. All data was extracted from our institutional database and collected by a physician who was not involved in the care of the study patients.

Statistical analysis

The trial was designed to investigate the potential superiority of OFA in terms of postoperative morphine consumption. According to the studies of Berthoud et al., we calculated that 55 patients per group would be sufficient to demonstrate a 10 mg difference in morphine consumption (with a mean consumption of 18 mg) with a power of 0.8 and an alpha risk of 0.05 [20, 21]. Based on known factors associated with postoperative pain and operative course, the database was matched (1:1) on age, body mass index, Euroscore 2, and type of surgery (sternotomy/thoracotomy) [22, 23]. Normal distribution was assessed using the Shapiro-Wilk test. Data are expressed as medians (interquartile range). The Wilcoxon test was used for the comparison of matched continuous variables, and the Cochran-Mantel-Haenszel test with odds ratios (OR) was used or the comparison of categorical variables [21]. The threshold for statistical significance was set at $p < 0.05$. Statistical analyses were performed with SPSS 24 (IBM, France).

Results

Of the 931 patients operated during the study period, 110 were matched and analysed (Fig. 1). The intervention and control groups did not differ significantly in their demographic characteristics and cardiac surgery type (Tables 1 and 2). In the overall study population, the mean age was 69 years (IQR: 63–74, males: $n = 78$), the median EuroSCORE2 was 1.6 (IQR: 0.89–3.01) and the median EuroScore was 6 (IQR: 4.9–8.3).

Analgesia evaluation

The total postoperative morphine dose was significantly different in the OFA and OA groups: 5 (IQR: 2 to 18) vs 15 mg (IQR: 6–34), $p = 0.001$ (Table 3). However, complementary analgesia did not differ significantly: ketoprofen (18% vs 16%, OR = 1.136, $p = 1$ and 150 (IQR: 50–262) vs 125 mg (IQR: 50–263), p = 1)), nefopam (20% vs 13%, OR = 1.714, $p = 0.441$ and 40 (IQR: 20–100) vs 20 mg (20–33), $p = 0.317$), and tramadol (31% vs 31%, OR = 1, p = 1, and 100 (IQR: 50–150) vs 100 mg (IQR: 50–150), p = 1)) were used in equal measures. The pain scores were also similar in the two groups (Table 3).

Secondary endpoints

Operative data differed between groups in terms of vasopressor use, antihypertensive drug use, and total fluid infused (Table 2). More patients in the OFA group were treated with urapidil (50% vs 22%, $p = 0.003$) whereas more patients in the OA group were treated with ephedrine (73% vs 52%, $p = 0.032$). The time to extubation was shorter in the OFA group (3 (IQR: 1–5) vs 5 h (IQR: 3–6), p = 0.001) (Table 3). The composite endpoint was less common in the OFA group (25 (43%) vs 38 patients (68%), OR = 0.373, $p = 0.021$) along with a lower use of non-invasive ventilation (27% vs 49%, OR = 0.389, p = 0.032). Creatinine values did not differ on the first post-operative day (80 (IQR: 66–115) vs 77 mmol/l (IQR: 69–95), $p = 0.284$). The incidence of cardiac and renal outcomes were similar. The OFA group spent less time in the ICU (2 (IQR: 1–3) vs 3 days (IQR: 2–5), $p = 0.037$) though the length of the hospital stay did not differ (8 (IQR: 7–15) vs 10 days (IQR: 8–14), $p = 0.790$).

Discussion

In the present study, we found that OFA was associated with: (1) lower postoperative morphine consumption; (2) higher operative use of antihypertensive agents; (3) a decrease of orotracheal intubation time and the use of non-invasive respiratory support; and (4) shorter ICU stays.

To date, two published case reports and one retrospective study have reported on the use of OFA study in thoracic surgery [7, 24, 25], but no study has focused specifically on the use of OFA in cardiac surgery. In

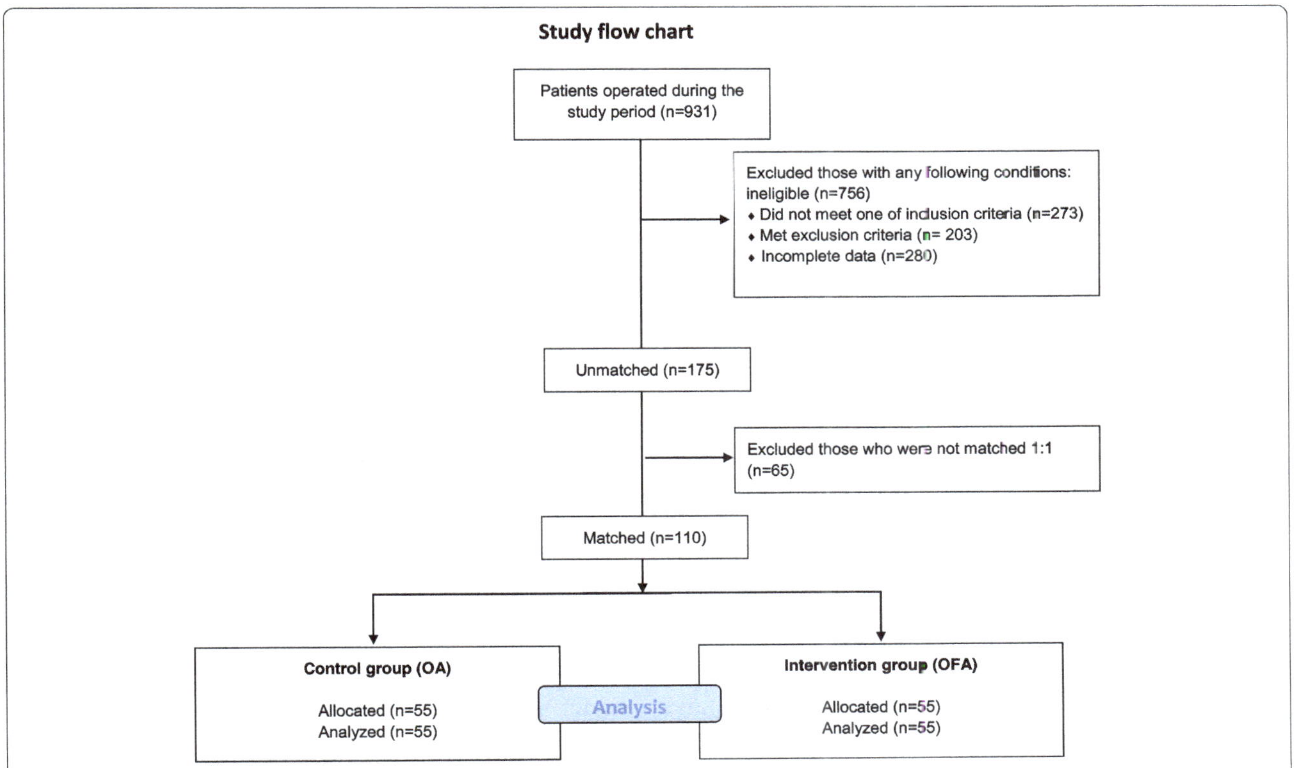

Fig. 1 Flow chart diagram

Table 1 Demographic characteristics of the population. Data are expressed as median (interquartile range), or number (%). The *p*-value always refers to comparison between the OFA group and the OA group

Variables	OFA group (*n* = 55)	OA group (n = 55)	*P*-value
Age, (years)	69 (62–74)	69 (65–74)	0.066
Gender (M), n (%)	43 (78)	35 (64)	0.115
Body mass index (kg m $^{-2}$)	26 (24–30)	26 (23–30)	0.162
ASA, n (%)			
2	3 (5)	7 (12)	
3	41 (75)	38 (69)	
4	11 (20)	10 (19)	
EuroSCORE II (%)	1.51 (0.98–3.1)	1.69 (0.87–3.01)	0.805
Euroscore (%)	6 (5–9)	6 (3–8)	0.238
Medical history, n (%)			
Coronary disease	31 (56)	27 (49)	0.571
Arrhythmia	8 (14)	13 (24)	0.332
Dyslipidaemia	31 (56)	34 (62)	0.556
Smoking history	23 (42)	19 (35)	0.556
High blood pressure	42 (76)	43 (77)	1
Diabetes	15 (27)	15 (27)	1
Chronic renal insufficiency	12 (22)	7 (13)	0.276
Stroke	4 (7)	4 (7)	1
Obstructive sleep apnoea	7 (13)	7 (13)	1
Treatment, n (%)			
Beta blocker	34 (62)	34 (62)	1.00
Calcic channel blocker	9 (16)	6 (11)	0.581
Aspirin	32 (58)	28 (49)	0.596
Clopidogrel	2 (4)	6 (11)	0.261
Angiotensin enzyme converting inhibitor	21 (38)	23 (42)	0.832
Statin	32 (58)	34 (62)	0.832
Diuretics	21 (38)	19 (35)	0.850
Left Ventricular Ejection Fraction (%)	60 (51–65)	60 (50–65)	0.278
Creatinine (mmol l $^{-1}$)	83 (72–96)	84 (70–98)	0.558

non-cardiac surgery with OFA, previous studies have demonstrated decreased postoperative pain scores and opioid consumption [6, 8, 9]. In cardiac surgery, the studies evaluating loco-regional analgesia have demonstrated a decrease in morphine consumption [20]. Despite its retrospective design, the present study confirmed the feasibility of OFA in cardiac surgery. Because OFA is based on the opioid avoidance with a multimodal analgesic treatment, it is associated with lower postoperative morphine consumption and fewer of the adverse effects that result from opioid use. The postoperative pain score did not differ between groups, indicating that OA and OFA provided comparable analgesia.

Yet one important question remains: what is the analgesic/anaesthetic effect of OFA during surgery [26]? OFA is an anaesthesia strategy that replaces opioids (balanced general anesthesia) with non-opioid drugs (multimodal general anesthesia). Opioids are usually administered during anesthesia for their antinociceptive effects, to control the responses of the autonomic nervous system (ANS) to surgical stress, and for their hypnotic effect. Our approach to OFA was based on published literature which demonstrates that each of the effects associated with opioids can be obtained with lidocaine (analgesic, hypnotic, and ANS control), dexamethasone (analgesic) and ketamine (analgesic and hypnotic) [11–13]. The lidocaine dosing regimen was based on the literature published since the 1990s that has demonstrated a safety profile with continuous infusion of lidocaine during cardiac and non-

Table 2 Operative characteristics of the population

Variables	OFA group (n = 55)	OA group (n = 55)	OR ($CI_{95\%}$)	*P*-value
Type of surgery				
Valvular surgery	20 (34)	22 (38)		0.806
Coronary artery bypass graft	11 (22)	9 (19)		0.845
Combined	21 (38)	21 (38)		1
Ascending aorta	1 (2)	1 (2)		1
LVAD	2 (4)	2 (4)		1
Sternotomy/thoracotomy	40/15	39/16		1
Urgent, n (%)	13 (23)	10 (18)		0.641
Anaesthesia time (min)	303 (268–360)	308 (288–360)		0.409
Cardiopulmonary bypass time (min)	118 (102–148)	119 (101–149)		0.505
Aortic cross clamp time (min)	84 (66–119)	94 (72–114)		0.383
Propofol				
mg	1351 (922–1840)	1145 (740–1634)		**0.008**
mg kg^{-1}	17.5 (13.4–22.6)	15.5 (10.9–18.5)		**0.045**
Sufentanil				
Gamma	0	89 (75–120)		**0.0001**
Gamma kg^{-1}	0	1.12 (0.93–1.56)		0.062
Anti hypertensive agents, n (%)				
Urapidil	28 (50)	12 (22)	3.716 (1.620–8.522)	**0.003**
Median dose (mg)	15 (10–20)	10 (5–15)		0.713
Nicardipin	6 (11)	10 (18)	0.551 (0.185–1.639)	0.419
Median dose (mg)	1.5 (1–2)	1 (0.5–2.5)		0.157
Vasopressor, n (%)				
Ephedrine	28 (51)	40 (73)	0.389 (0.176–0.861)	**0.032**
Median dose (mg)	15 (9–28)	26 (15–30)		0.130
Phenylephrine	36 (67)	31 (56)	1.467 (0.679–3.168)	0.588
Median dose (mg)	0.275 (0.15–0.5)	0.35 (0.2–0.55)		0.272
Norepinephrine	40 (73)	30 (55)	2.222 (1.002–4.927)	0.076
Median cumulated dose (mg)	1.24 (0.35–2.4)	1.34 (0.41–2.46)		0.092
Esmolol, n (%)	11 (20)	1 (2)	13.5 (1.677–108.652)	**0.006**
Median dose (mg)	30 (10–46)	73 (73–73)		
Dobutamine, n (%)	7 (13)	8 (15)	0.857 (0.288–2.551)	1
Total fluid administration				
Cumulated in ml	1250 (1000–1500)	1500 (1000–2000)		0.060
Cumulated in ml kg^{-1}	15.2 (10.7–21.4)	21.4 (12.5–27.7)		0.015
Transfusion, n (%)	13 (24)	13 (24)	1 (0.439–2.277)	1

Data are expressed as median (interquartile range), or number (%). The p-value always refers to comparison between the OFA group and the OA group

cardiac surgeries [27, 28]. Lidocaine has effects that depend on the total dose, and detrimental effects can be seen with elevated doses of lidocaine [27]. But lidocaine also has beneficial effects during surgery, providing (a) an anti-inflammatory effect; (b) an increase in the cardioprotective effect of cardioplegia; (c) a decrease in the risk of arrhythmias; and (d) a decrease in the risk of brain inflammation [15, 16, 28, 29].

OFA may be associated with certain adverse effects such as a higher incidence of blood pressure events or adverse effects resulting from toxic plasma levels. We observed a trend towards higher use of norepinephrine and anti-hypertensive agents that may be the result of

Table 3 Post-operative course of primary (total postoperative morphine consumption) and secondary endpoints (complementary analgesia, postoperative complications, ICU and hospital stays)

Variables	OFA group (n = 55)	OA group (n = 55)	OR ($CI_{95\%}$)	*P*-value
Total morphine consumption (mg)	5 (2–18)	15 (6–34)		**0.001**
Additional analgesic (n, %)				
Tramadol	17 (31)	17 (31)	1 (0.445–2.245)	1
Total median dose (mg)	150 (50–262)	125 (50–263)		1
Ketoprofen	10 (18)	9 (16)	1.136 (0.422-3.056)	1
Total median dose (mg)	100 (50–150)	100 (50–150)		1
Nefopam	11 (20)	7 (13)	1.714 (0.611–4.812)	0.441
Total median dose (mg)	40 (20–100)	20 (20–33)		0.317
Visual analog score				
Extubation	0 (0–2)	0 (0–3)		0.324
12 h after ICU admission	0 (0–0)	0 (0–1)		0.777
First postoperative day	0 (0–2)	0 (0–2)		0.665
Second postoperative day	0 (0–2)	0 (0–2)		0.874
Vomiting (n, %)	5 (9)	9 (16)	0.511 (0.160–1.637)	0.393
Creatinine (mmol l^{-1})				
at admission to ICU	83 (72–106)	76 (64–91)		0.105
on first postoperative day	80 (66–115)	77 (69–95)		0.284
Troponin Ic (ng ml^{-1})				
at admission to ICU	6.2 (3.7–10)	7.5 (2.9–20)		0.091
24 h after surgery	4.7 (2.6–8.2)	7 (3.1–16)		0.091
PaO_2				
at admission to ICU	162 (113–195)	155 (114–181)		0.479
24 h after surgery	99 (83–122)	115 (89–138)		0.084
FiO_2				
at admission to ICU	50 (30–60)	50 (50–60)		**0.005**
24 h after surgery	28 (25–32)	32 (30–36)		**0.018**
PaO_2/FiO_2 ratio				
at admission to ICU	357 (275–458)	290 (213-372)		**0.006**
24 h after surgery	355 (261–420)	322 (265–435)		0.919
Time to extubation (hours)	3 (1–5)	5 (3–6)		**0.001**
Catecholamine use, n (%)				
Norepinephrine	26 (32)	31 (38)	0.694 (0.328–1.471)	0.447
Dobutamine	9 (16)	9 (16)	0.766 (0.277–2.115)	0.798
Transfusion, n (%)				
Red blood cell	16 (29)	18 (33)	0.843 (0.375–1.895)	0.837
Endpoint composite score, n (%)	**25 (43)**	**38 (66)**	**0.373 (0.171–0.813)**	**0.021**
Confusion	4 (7)	10 (19)	0.353 (0.103–1.204)	0.151
Stroke	1 (2)	0		1
Seizure	1 (2)	0		1
Atrial fibrillation,	15 (27)	22 (40)	0.563 (0.252–1.254)	0.228
Ventricular tachycardia or fibrillation	1 (2)	3 (5)	0.315 (0.032–3.125)	0.599
Atrio-ventricular block requiring pacemaker implantation	2 (4)	1 (2)	2.038 (0.179–23.151)	1
Acute renal failure	12 (22)	14 (26)	0.817 (0.338–1.974)	0.823

Table 3 Post-operative course of primary (total postoperative morphine consumption) and secondary endpoints (complementary analgesia, postoperative complications, ICU and hospital stays) *(Continued)*

Variables	OFA group (n = 55)	OA group (n = 55)	OR ($CI_{95\%}$)	*P*-value
Reintubation	1 (2)	3 (6)	0.321 (0.032–3.186)	0.612
Non-invasive ventilation	15 (27)	27 (49)	0.389 (0.176–0.861)	**0.032**
Mortality	1 (2)	1 (2)	1 (0.061—16.401)	1
ICU stays (days)	2 (1–3)	3 (2–5)		**0.037**
Hospital stays (days)	8 (7–15)	10 (8–14)		0.790

Data are expressed as median (25th to 75th percentiles), or number (%). The p-value always refers to comparison between the OFA group and the OA group

several factors: the increasing use of propofol, the half-life of urapidil/nicardipine (mostly used before CPB), and the vasoactive effect of lidocaine. Several studies have already underlined the growing incidence of hypertensive episodes and the higher use of anti-hypertensive agents [6, 7]. Bakan et al. also found that a higher total dose of propofol was needed to maintain OFA [6]. According to the literature, the dosage regimen used in the present study may be associated with low to moderate plasma values of lidocaine, which are associated with vasoconstriction [27]. Because blood pressure may be high, physicians frequently use anti-hypertensive agents. On the contrary, because the hypnotic effect of lidocaine may be less marked than that of opioids, physicians increase propofol doses which can potentially cause arterial hypotension. Finally, the combination of high-dose propofol and the increasing use of anti-hypertensive agents may increase the need for vasopressors during CPB. Accordingly, we did not demonstrate a higher incidence of postoperative vasoplegic syndrome. To date, we do not have observed clinical signs of local anaesthetic toxicity (arrhythmia, atrial-ventricular block, seizure) with our protocol, which confirms the existing data on lidocaine plasma levels [27–29].

Though we did not use dexmedetomidine in our protocol because it is not available in our department, the uses of an alpha$_2$ agent may have several advantages. First, the combination of dexmedetomidine and lidocaine was shown to provide better postoperative pain relief than the use of each agent individually [14]. Also, in cardiac surgery, a recent meta-analysis confirmed that dexmedetomidine provided good hemodynamic stability during surgery with less tachycardia and arterial hypertension [30]. Moreover, studies suggest a positive effect on confusion and atrial fibrillation, with a shorter time to extubation and a shorter ICU length of stay [31, 32]. According to the literature, the combination of lidocaine and dexmedetomidine should improve hemodynamic stability and decrease the need for antihypertensive agents.

We demonstrated that OFA resulted in lower intubation time and use of non-invasive ventilation. The respiratory effects may be explained by the avoidance of opioids and better pain relief. In our experience, patients anesthetized with OFA have a shorter period of respiratory inhibition during surgery than patients anesthetized with opioids. Spontaneous breathing returns sooner following OFA and patients seem to become alert more quickly after orotracheal extubation. In our results, oxygen requirements and non-invasive ventilation was lower in the OFA group. These effects may be associated with the respiratory depression and cognitive dysfunction that are well-known effects of opioid sedation [8, 33].

The present study had several limitations. Our study was a single retrospective study, which implies a certain number of design-related limitations. Despite protocol management for sedation and analgesia, bias may have been introduced by the attending physician and nursing staff. In addition, some patients received analgesia in addition to patient-controlled morphine analgesia, suggesting postoperative multimodal analgesia. Nevertheless, the protocol for postoperative intravenous analgesic use was similar in the two groups. Similar limitations should be mentioned for non-invasive ventilation and ICU stays, which were left to the discretion of the attending physician. Only controlled prospective randomized studies can confirm the present results. Moreover, further studies are needed to determine the optimal associations, dosages, and infusion protocols during cardiac surgery. We have included two types of surgery (sternotomy and thoracotomy) than could be not equivalent in term of pain. Because the matching was based on this aspect, the two groups did not differ in term of type of surgery. The relatively small number of patients in our population might also limit our study's external validity. Nevertheless, we calculated a sample size based on morphine consumption, which has been demonstrated to be associated with OFA, and we included a mixed cardiac surgery population. We believe our results demonstrate the feasibility of OFA in several cardiac surgery subtypes. Our team currently uses OFA in cardiac surgery on a daily basis without any restrictions other than contraindications to lidocaine use.

Conclusion

The present study demonstrated that OFA was associated with a decrease in postoperative morphine consumption. OFA might have beneficial effects of on the post-operative course of patients undergoing cardiac surgery with CBP. Further randomized studies are needed to confirm these results.

Abbreviations

CPB: Cardiopulmonary bypass; ICU: Intensive care unit; LOS: Length of stay; MAP: Mean arterial pressure; OA: Opioid anesthesia; OFA: Opioid-free anesthesia

Acknowledgements

Thank you to Suzanne Rankin for proofreading and reviewing the English manuscript.

Authors' contributions

Study design: PGG. Data acquisition: AS. Data analysis: PGG, MN. Data interpretation: PGG, OE, VB, MR, TC, AM, JBA, JPP, JPM, SG. Manuscript preparation: PGG, MN, BB, NN. Manuscript revision: all authors. Final approval: all authors.
All authors read and approved the manuscript.

References

1. Scholz J, Steinfath M, Schulz M. Clinical pharmacokinetics of alfentanil, fentanyl and sufentanil. An update. Clin Pharmacokinet. 1996;31:275–92.
2. Fawcett WJ, Jones CN. Bespoke intra-operative anaesthesia - the end of the formulaic approach? Anaesthesia. 2018;73:1062–6.
3. Khademi H, Kamangar F, Brennan P, Malekzadeh R. Opioid therapy and its side effects: a review. Arch Iran Med. 2016;19:870–6.
4. Lavand'homme P, Estebe J-P. Opioid-free anesthesia: a different regard to anesthesia practice. Curr Opin Anaesthesiol. 2018;31:556–61.
5. Veyckemans F. Opioid-free anaesthesia: still a debate? Eur J Anaesthesiol. 2019;36:245–6.
6. Bakan M, Umutoglu T, Topuz U, Uysal H, Bayram M, Kadioglu H, et al. Opioid-free total intravenous anesthesia with propofol, dexmedetomidine and lidocaine infusions for laparoscopic cholecystectomy: a prospective, randomized, double-blinded study. Braz J Anesthesiol. 2015;65:191–9.
7. Bello M, Oger S, Bedon-Carte S, Vielstadte C, Leo F, Zaouter C, et al. Effect of opioid-free anaesthesia on postoperative epidural ropivacaine requirement after thoracic surgery: a retrospective unmatched case-control study. Anaesth Crit Care Pain Med. 2019.
8. Frauenknecht J, Kirkham KR, Jacot-Guillarmod A, Albrecht E. Analgesic impact of intra-operative opioids vs. opioid-free anaesthesia: a systematic review and meta-analysis. Anaesthesia. 2019.
9. Hontoir S, Saxena S, Gatto P, Khalife M, Ben Aziz AM, Paesmans M, et al. Opioid-free anesthesia: what about patient comfort? A prospective, randomized, controlled trial. Acta Anaesthesiol Belg. 2016;67:183–90.
10. Mauermann E, Ruppen W, Bandschapp O. Different protocols used today to achieve total opioid-free general anesthesia without locoregional blocks. Best Pract Res Clin Anaesthesiol. 2017;31:533–45.
11. Murphy GS, Sherwani SS, Szokol JW, Avram MJ, Greenberg SB, Patel KM, et al. Small-dose dexamethasone improves quality of recovery scores after elective cardiac surgery: a randomized, double-blind, placebo-controlled study. J Cardiothorac Vasc Anesth. 2011;25:950–60.
12. Peltoniemi MA, Hagelberg NM, Olkkola KT, Saari TI. Ketamine: a review of clinical pharmacokinetics and pharmacodynamics in anesthesia and pain therapy. Clin Pharmacokinet. 2016;55:1059–77.
13. Koppert W, Weigand M, Neumann F, Sittl R, Schuettler J, Schmelz M, et al. Perioperative intravenous lidocaine has preventive effects on postoperative pain and morphine consumption after major abdominal surgery. Anesth Analg. 2004;98:1050–5 table of contents.
14. Xu S-Q, Li Y-H, Wang S-B, Hu S-H, Ju X, Xiao J-B. Effects of intravenous lidocaine, dexmedetomidine and their combination on postoperative pain and bowel function recovery after abdominal hysterectomy. Minerva Anestesiol. 2017;83:685–94.
15. Fiore AC, Naunheim KS, Taub J, Braun P, McBride LR, Pennington DG, et al. Myocardial preservation using lidocaine blood cardioplegia. Ann Thorac Surg. 1990;50:771–5.
16. Klinger RY, Cooter M, Berger M, Podgoreanu MV, Stafford-Smith M, Ortel TL, et al. Effect of intravenous lidocaine on the transcerebral inflammatory response during cardiac surgery: a randomized-controlled trial. Can J Anaesth J Can Anesth. 2016;63:1223–32.
17. Aronsohn J, Orner G, Palleschi G, Gerasimov M. Opioid-free total intravenous anesthesia with ketamine as part of an enhanced recovery protocol for bariatric surgery patients with sleep disordered breathing. J Clin Anesth. 2019;52:65–6.
18. von Elm E, Altman DG, Egger M, Pocock SJ, Gøtzsche PC, Vandenbroucke JP, et al. The strengthening the reporting of observational studies in epidemiology (STROBE) statement: guidelines for reporting observational studies. Int J Surg Lond Engl. 2014;12:1495–9.
19. Quintard H, l'Her E, Pottecher J, Adnet F, Constantin J-M, De Jong A, et al. Experts' guidelines of intubation and extubation of the ICU patient of French Society of Anaesthesia and Intensive Care Medicine (SFAR) and French-speaking Intensive Care Society (SRLF) : In collaboration with the pediatric Association of French-speaking Anaesthetists and Intensivists (ADARPEF), French-speaking Group of Intensive Care and Paediatric emergencies (GFRUP) and Intensive Care physiotherapy society (SKR). Ann Intensive Care. 2019;9:13.
20. Berthoud V, Ellouze O, Nguyen M, Konstantinou M, Aho S, Malapert G, et al. Serratus anterior plane block for minimal invasive heart surgery. BMC Anesthesiol. 2018;18:144.
21. Niven DJ, Berthiaume LR, Fick GH, Laupland KB. Matched case-control studies: a review of reported statistical methodology. Clin Epidemiol. 2012;4:99–110.
22. Ip HYV, Abrishami A, Peng PWH, Wong J, Chung F. Predictors of postoperative pain and analgesic consumption: a qualitative systematic review. Anesthesiology. 2009;111:657–77.
23. Kara KA, Caner T. Comparison of pain in the early post-operative period using VAS score in patients after cardiac surgery who had minimally invasive incisions vs. full median sternotomy. Ann Ital Chir. 2019;90:3–9.
24. Chanowski EJP, Horn J-L, Boyd JH, Tsui BCH, Brodt JL. Opioid-free ultra-fast-track on-pump coronary artery bypass grafting using erector spinae plane catheters. J Cardiothorac Vasc Anesth. 2019;33:1988–1990.
25. Landry E, Burns S, Pelletier MP, Muehlschlegel JD. A successful opioid-free anesthetic in a patient undergoing cardiac surgery. J Cardiothorac Vasc Anesth. 2018;18:S1053–0770.
26. Cividjian A, Petitjeans F, Liu N, Ghignone M, de Kock M, Quintin L. Do we feel pain during anesthesia? A critical review on surgery-evoked circulatory changes and pain perception. Best Pract Res Clin Anaesthesiol. 2017;31: 445–67.
27. Hsu Y-W, Somma J, Newman MF, Mathew JP. Population pharmacokinetics of lidocaine administered during and after cardiac surgery. J Cardiothorac Vasc Anesth. 2011;25:931–6.
28. Gholipour Baradari A, Habibi MR, Habibi V, Nouraei SM. Administration of lidocaine to prevent cognitive deficit in patients undergoing coronary artery bypass grafting and valve plasty: a systematic review and meta-analysis. Expert Rev Clin Pharmacol. 2017;10:179–85.
29. Baraka A, Kawkabani N, Dabbous A, Nawfal M. Lidocaine for prevention of reperfusion ventricular fibrillation after release of aortic cross-clamping. J Cardiothorac Vasc Anesth. 2000;14:531–3.
30. Duncan D, Sankar A, Beattie WS, Wijeysundera DN. Alpha-2 adrenergic agonists for the prevention of cardiac complications among adults undergoing surgery. Cochrane Database Syst Rev. 2018;3:CD004126.
31. Nguyen J, Nacpil N. Effectiveness of dexmedetomidine versus propofol on extubation times, length of stay and mortality rates in adult cardiac surgery patients: a systematic review and meta-analysis. JBI Database Syst Rev Implement Rep. 2018;16:1220–39.
32. Wang G, Niu J, Li Z, Lv H, Cai H. The efficacy and safety of dexmedetomidine in cardiac surgery patients: a systematic review and meta-analysis. PLoS One. 2018;13:e0202620.
33. Hudetz JA, Iqbal Z, Gandhi SD, Patterson KM, Byrne AJ, Hudetz AG, et al. Ketamine attenuates post-operative cognitive dysfunction after cardiac surgery. Acta Anaesthesiol Scand. 2009;53:864–72.

Permissions

All chapters in this book were first published by BioMed Central; hereby published with permission under the Creative Commons Attribution License or equivalent. Every chapter published in this book has been scrutinized by our experts. Their significance has been extensively debated. The topics covered herein carry significant findings which will fuel the growth of the discipline. They may even be implemented as practical applications or may be referred to as a beginning point for another development.

The contributors of this book come from diverse backgrounds, making this book a truly international effort. This book will bring forth new frontiers with its revolutionizing research information and detailed analysis of the nascent developments around the world.

We would like to thank all the contributing authors for lending their expertise to make the book truly unique. They have played a crucial role in the development of this book. Without their invaluable contributions this book wouldn't have been possible. They have made vital efforts to compile up to date information on the varied aspects of this subject to make this book a valuable addition to the collection of many professionals and students.

This book was conceptualized with the vision of imparting up-to-date information and advanced data in this field. To ensure the same, a matchless editorial board was set up. Every individual on the board went through rigorous rounds of assessment to prove their worth. After which they invested a large part of their time researching and compiling the most relevant data for our readers.

The editorial board has been involved in producing this book since its inception. They have spent rigorous hours researching and exploring the diverse topics which have resulted in the successful publishing of this book. They have passed on their knowledge of decades through this book. To expedite this challenging task, the publisher supported the team at every step. A small team of assistant editors was also appointed to further simplify the editing procedure and attain best results for the readers.

Apart from the editorial board, the designing team has also invested a significant amount of their time in understanding the subject and creating the most relevant covers. They scrutinized every image to scout for the most suitable representation of the subject and create an appropriate cover for the book.

The publishing team has been an ardent support to the editorial, designing and production team. Their endless efforts to recruit the best for this project, has resulted in the accomplishment of this book. They are a veteran in the field of academics and their pool of knowledge is as vast as their experience in printing. Their expertise and guidance has proved useful at every step. Their uncompromising quality standards have made this book an exceptional effort. Their encouragement from time to time has been an inspiration for everyone.

The publisher and the editorial board hope that this book will prove to be a valuable piece of knowledge for researchers, students, practitioners and scholars across the globe.

List of Contributors

Arthur Neuschwander and Julien Josserand
Anesthesiology and Intensive Care Department, European Hospital Georges-Pompidou, Assistance Publique - Hôpitaux de Paris (AP-HP), 20 rue Leblanc, 75015 Paris, France

Benoit Champigneulle
Anesthesiology and Intensive Care Department, European Hospital Georges-Pompidou, Assistance Publique - Hôpitaux de Paris (AP-HP), 20 rue Leblanc, 75015 Paris, France
West francilian network for organ and tissue procurement, Paris, France

Régis Bronchard and Olivier Bastien
Agence de la Biomédecine, Direction Prélèvement Greffe Organes-Tissus, Saint-Denis La Plaine, France

Gersende Favé
Anesthesiology and Intensive Care Department, European Hospital Georges-Pompidou, Assistance Publique - Hôpitaux de Paris (AP-HP), 20 rue Leblanc, 75015 Paris, France
Paris Descartes University, Sorbonne Paris Cité, Paris, France

Benjamin Lebas
Anesthesiology and Intensive Care Department, Hautepierre Hospital, Strasbourg, France

Romain Pirracchio
Anesthesiology and Intensive Care Department, European Hospital Georges-Pompidou, Assistance Publique - Hôpitaux de Paris (AP-HP), 20 rue Leblanc, 75015 Paris, France
Paris Descartes University, Sorbonne Paris Cité, Paris, France
Département de biostatistiques et d'informatique médicale, INSERM U-1153, Équipe ECSTRA, Université Paris Diderot; Hôpital Saint-Louis, AP-HP, Paris, France

Stefan Felix Ehrentraut, Barbara Schroll, Stefan Lenkeit, Heidi Ehrentraut, Christian Bode, Stefan Kreyer, Florian Kögl, Felix Lehmann, Thomas Muders, Martin Scholz, Claudia Strater, Folkert Steinhagen, Nils Ulrich Theuerkauf, Carsten Weißbrich, Christian Putensen and Jens-Christian Schewe
Department of Anaesthesiology and Intensive Care Medicine, University Hospital Bonn, Sigmund-Freud-Str. 25, 53105 Bonn, Germany

Yuqing Zeng
The First Clinical Medical College, Guangzhou University of Chinese Medicine, 16 Jichang Road, Baiyun District, Guangzhou 510405, Guangdong Province, People's Republic of China
Department of Orthopaedics, Tongde Hospital of Zhejiang Province, Hangzhou, Zhejiang Province, People's Republic of China

Junming Wan, Haiyong Ren, Jianwei Lu and Fuhua Zhong
Department of Orthopaedics, Tongde Hospital of Zhejiang Province, Hangzhou, Zhejiang Province, People's Republic of China

Shu Deng
Department of Hematology, The First Affliated Hospital of Zhejiang Chinese Medical University, 54 Youdian Road, Hangzhou, Zhejiang Province, People's Republic of China

Nishma Hindocha
Department of Ear, Nose, Throat and Maxillofacial Surgery, Zealand University Hospital, Koege, Denmark

Filip Manhem
Public Dental Service Östergötland, Linköping, Region Östergötland, and Department of Biomedical and Clinical Sciences, Linköping University, Linköping, Sweden

Emmanuel Bäckryd
Pain and Rehabilitation Center, and Department of Medical and Health Sciences, Linköping University, Linköping, Sweden

Mats Bågesund
Centre for Orthodontics and Paediatric Dentistry, Norrköping, Public Dental Service Östergötland, Region Östergötland, and Department of Biomedical and Clinical Sciences, Linköping University, Linköping, Sweden

Ivar N. Omenås
Division of Emergencies and Critical Care, Oslo University Hospital, Oslo, Norway

Christian Tronstad
Department of Clinical and Biomedical Engineering, Oslo University Hospital, Oslo, Norway

Leiv Arne Rosseland
Division of Emergencies and Critical Care, Oslo University Hospital, Oslo, Norway
Institute of Clinical Medicine, University of Oslo, Oslo, Norway

Silvia Loggi, Nicoletta Mininno, Elisa Damiani, Benedetto Marini, Erica Adrario, Claudia Scorcella, Roberta Domizi, Andrea Carsetti, Simona Pantanetti and Abele Donati
Anaesthesia and Intensive Care Unit, Department of Biomedical Sciences and Public Health, Università Politecnica delle Marche, via Tronto 10/a, 60126 Torrette di Ancona, Italy

Gabriele Pagliariccio and Luciano Carbonari
Unit of Vascular Surgery, Azienda Ospedaliera Universitaria "Ospedali Riuniti Umberto I – Lancisi – Salesi" of Ancona, Ancona, Italy

Shihoko Iwata, Sumire Yokokawa, Mihoshi Sato and Makoto Ozaki
Department of Anesthesiology, Tokyo Women's Medical University Hospital, 8-1 Kawada-cho, Shinjuku-ku, Tokyo 162-8666, Japan

Asuka Kitajima, Yuji Otsuka and Masamitsu Sanui
Department of Anesthesiology and Critical Care Medicine, Jichi Medical University Saitama Medical Center, 1-847 Amanumacho, Omiyaku, Saitama 330-8503, Japan

Alan Kawarai Lefor
Department of Surgery, Jichi Medical University, 1-3311 Yakusiji, Shimono, Tochigi, Saitama 329-0498, Japan

L. Kaufner, P. Niggemann, T. Baum, C. D. Spies and A. Henkelmann
Department of Anaesthesiology and Operative Intensive Care Medicine (CCM, CVK), Charité-Universitätsmedizin Berlin, Corporate Member of Freie Universität Berlin, Humboldt-Universität zu Berlin, and Berlin Institute of Health, Campus Virchow-Klinikum, Augustenburger Platz 1, 13353 Berlin, Germany

S. Casu and C. von Heymann
Department of Anaesthesia, Intensive Care Medicine, Emergency Medicine and Pain Therapy, Vivantes Klinikum im Friedrichshain, Berlin, Germany

J. Sehouli
Department of Gynaecology, Charité-Universitätsmedizin Berlin, Berlin, Germany

A. Bietenbeck
Institut für Klinische Chemie und Pathobiochemie, Klinikum rechts der Isar der Technischen Universität München, Munich, Germany

M. Boschmann
Experimental & Clinical Research Center, ECRC, Charité-Universitätsmedizin Berlin CCB, Berlin, Germany

Won Jung Hwang, Min A. Joo and Jin Joo
Department of Anesthesiology and Pain Medicine, Seoul St. Mary's Hospital, College of Medicine, The Catholic University of Korea, 222 Banpodaero, Seocho-gu, Seoul 06591, South Korea

Khaled El-Radaideh, Rawand A. Alzoubi and Mohammad I. Abu-Shehab
Department of Anesthesia and Recovery, Faculty of Medicine, Jordan University of Science and Technology, Irbid, Jordan

Adel M. Bataineh
Department of Anesthesia and Recovery, Faculty of Medicine, Jordan University of Science and Technology, Irbid, Jordan
Department of Anaesthesia and Recovery, King AbduLLAH-I University Hospital, Irbid, Jordan

Ibraheem Y. Qudaisat
Department of Anesthesia and Intensive Care, School of Medicine, University of Jordan, Amman, Jordan

Lin Li, Yi Pang, Yongchao Wang, Qi Li and Xiangchao Meng
Department of Thyroid, Breast, Hernia Surgery, Tianjin the third Central Hospital, NO.83, Jintang Road, Tianjin 300170, China

Dan Tan
Editorial Office, Journal of New Medicine, Zhongnan Hospital of Wuhan University, No.169 Donghu Road, Wuchang District, Wuhan 430071, Hubei Province, China

Haifa Xia, Shujun Sun and Fuquan Wang
Department of Anesthesiology, Institute of Anesthesia and Critical Care, Union Hospital, Tongji Medical College, Huazhong University of Science and Technology, Wuhan, China

Hiroshi Hanamoto, Hiroharu Maegawa, Mika Inoue, Aiko Oyamaguchi, Chiho Kudo and Hitoshi Niwa
Department of Dental Anesthesiology, Osaka University Graduate School of Dentistry, 1-8 Yamada-Oka, Suita, Osaka 565-0871, Japan

Ohseong Kwon
Department of Urology, Hallym University Kangnam Sacred Heart Hospital, Seoul, South Korea

Jung-Man Lee
Department of Anesthesiology and Pain Medicine, SMG-SNU Boramae Medical Center, Seoul, South Korea

Juhyun Park, Min Chul Cho, Hwancheol Son and Hyeon Jeong
Department of Urology, SMG-SNU Boramae Medical Center, Seoul, South Korea

Seung Hoon Ryang and Sung Yong Cho
Department of Urology, Seoul National University Hospital, 101, Daehak-ro Jongno-gu, 03080 Seoul, Republic of Korea

Alexis R. Tovar and Allison L. Thoeny
University of Arizona, 1501 N Campbell Ave, Room 4401, Tucson, AZ 85724, USA

Kavya N. Reddy
Saint Louis University, St. Louis, USA

Shabaaz M. Baig, Meenu Batra, Anna Korban and Shridevi Pandya Shah
Department of Anesthesiology, Rutgers New Jersey Medical School, 185 South Orange Ave, MSB-E 577, Newark, NJ 07103, USA

Kevin Colodner
University of Maryland, College Park, USA

Uchenna Madubuko
New York Medical College, Valhalla, USA

Sirirat Tribuddharat, Thepakorn Sathitkarnmanee, Naruemon Vattanasiriporn, Maneerat Thananun, Duangthida Nonlhaopol and Wilawan Somdee
Department of Anesthesiology, Faculty of Medicine, Khon Kaen University, 123 Mitrapap road, Ampur Muang, Khon Kaen 40002, Thailand

X. Q. Cao, L. L. Gui and W. Mei
Department of Anesthesiology and Pain Medicine, Tongji Hospital, Tongji Medical College, Huazhong University of Science and Technology, 1095 Jiefang Road, Wuhan 430030, People's Republic of China

K. Joypaul
Department of Anesthesiology, Flacq Hospital, Hospital Road, Centre-de-Flacq, Mauritius

F. Cao
Department of Psychiatry, University of Missouri-Kansas City, 5100 Rockhill Road, Kansas City 64110, MO, USA

J. T. Hu
Department of Anesthesiology, Wuhan No.4 Hospital, 473 Hanzheng Road, Wuhan 430033, People's Republic of China

Hyongmin Oh, Hansol Kim, Hyun-Kyu Yoon, Hyung-Chul Lee and Hee-Pyoung Park
Department of Anesthesiology and Pain Medicine, Seoul National University Hospital, Seoul National University College of Medicine, 101, Daehak-ro, Jongno-gu, Seoul 03080, South Korea

Yuval Baar and Idit Matot
Division of Anesthesia, Intensive Care, and Pain Management, Tel-Aviv Medical Center, 6 Weizmann St., 6423906 Tel-Aviv, Israel

Barak Cohen
Division of Anesthesia, Intensive Care, and Pain Management, Tel-Aviv Medical Center, 6 Weizmann St., 6423906 Tel-Aviv, Israel
Outcomes Research Consortium, Cleveland Clinic, Cleveland, OH, USA

Shai Fein
Division of Anesthesia, Operating Rooms, Pain, and Critical Care, Samson Assuta Ashdod University Hospital, Ben-Gurion University of the Negev, Ashdod, Israel

Robert W. Arnold and Aleah N. Bond
Alaska Children's EYE & Strabismus, 3500 Latouche St #280, Anchorage, Alaska 99508, USA

Melissa McCall and Leif Lunoe
Providence Anesthesia Group, Anchorage, Alaska, USA

Ana M. Araújo and Humberto S. Machado
Serviço de Anestesiologia, Centro Hospitalar Universitário do Porto, Largo Prof. Abel Salazar, 4099-001 Porto, Portugal

Amílcar C. Falcão
Laboratory of Pharmacology, Faculty of Pharmacy, University of Coimbra, Pólo das Ciências da Saúde, Azinhaga de Santa Comba, 3000-548 Coimbra, Portugal

Patrício Soares-da-Silva
Department of Biomedicine, Unit of Pharmacology and Therapeutics, Faculty of Medicine, University of Porto, Alameda Prof. Hernâni Monteiro, 4200-319 Porto, Portugal

Frank Fideler and Christian Grasshoff
Departmnt of Anesthesiology and Intensive Care Medicine, University Hospital Tuebingen, Tübingen, Germany

Michael Walker
Clinic for Anesthesiology, Intensive, Emergency- and Pain-Therapy, Ludwigsburg, Germany

David W. Tscholl, Lucas Handschin, Julian Rössler, Donat R. Spahn and Christoph B. Nöthiger
Institute of Anesthesiology, University and University Hospital Zurich, Raemistrasse 100, 8091 Zurich, Switzerland

Mona Weiss
Department of Management, School of Business and Economics, Free University of Berlin, Garystrasse 21, 14195 Berlin, Germany

Zhuqing Yang and Qinye Shi
Department of Anesthesiology, the Fourth Affiliated Hospital of Zhejiang University School of Medicine, N1 Shangcheng Road, Yiwu, Zhejiang Province, China

Fangping Bao
Department of Anesthesiology, the Fourth Affiliated Hospital of Zhejiang University School of Medicine, N1 Shangcheng Road, Yiwu, Zhejiang Province, China
Department of Anethesiology, the First Affiliated Hospital of Zhejiang University School of Medicine, 79 Qingchun Road, Hangzhou, Zhejiang Province, China

Peng Li, Xiangkui Li and Xinchuan Wei
Department of anesthesiology, Sichuan Academy of Medical Sciences & Sichuan Provincial People's Hospital, Chengdu, Sichuan, China

Xia Liu
North Sichuan Medical College, Nanchong, Sichuan, China

Juan Liao
Department of Stomatology, Sichuan Academy of Medical Sciences & Sichuan Provincial People's Hospital, Chengdu, Sichuan, China

Ran Zhang, Zhiyu Tang, Qing Qiao and Yi Feng
Department of Anesthesiology, Peking University People's Hospital, No. 11 Xi Zhi Men Nan Da Jie, Xicheng District, Beijing, China

Feroze Mahmood
Department of Anesthesiology, Beth Israel Deaconess Medical Center, Boston, USA

Pierre-Grégoire Guinot, Alexandra Spitz, Vivien Berthoud, Omar Ellouze, Anis Missaoui, Tiberiu Constandache, Sandrine Grosjean, Mohamed Radhouani, Jean-Baptiste Anciaux, Jean-Philippe Parthiot, Jean-Pierre Merle, Nicolas Nowobilski, Maxime Nguyen and Belaid Bouhemad
Department of Anaesthesiology and Critical Care Medicine, Dijon University Medical Centre, 21000 Dijon, France

Index

www.ingramcontent.com/pod-product-compliance
Lightning Source LLC
LaVergne TN
LVHW060512210926
848485LV00005B/1066